See What Others Have to Say About *The Complete Idiot's Guide to T'ai Chi and QiGong,* Acclaimed Primer and Reference Used by Top T'ai Chi, QiGong, and Health Professionals

"I highly recommend this book to all seeking to enhance their physical, mental, and spiritual potential. Quantum Physics and leading-edge cell biology emphasize the primal role of energy in our lives. In a user-friendly and meaningful style, Bill Douglas offers a compelling and easy-to-understand description of ancient Asian energy exercises that effectively reduce stress and improve health."

—Bruce H. Lipton, Ph.D., Cellular Biologist and best-selling author of *The Biology of Belief: Unleashing the Power of Consciousness, Matter & Miracles*

"Visionary! If you only buy one book on T'ai Chi, *then this is the book.* This book is all you ever needed to know to change your life. I have taught T'ai Chi for several decades myself, yet I have now read Bill's book from cover to cover *seven times,* and *still* get something new from it each time."

—Dr. Michael Steward Sr., D.MA, Ph.D., MA, Senior Coach for Team USA, Inductee of the World Sports Medicine and World Martial Arts Hall of Fame

"[I was] living an extremely unhealthy lifestyle … taking numerous medications for arthritis, depression, and pain. … ['T']hen one day while browsing in the library I discovered a book … *The Complete Idiot's Guide to T'ai Chi and QiGong.* I was so impressed that I ordered Bill's videos. … Now that I am practicing T'ai Chi and QiGong daily, I am off most of my medications. People keep telling me I look 'different' and that I look happy. Well, I am happy and I feel great! … Thank you! Thank you! Thank you!"

—Dave Long, Washington

"I had the privilege of studying T'ai Chi with this book's author, Bill Douglas. As a practicing physician, there are certainly times when stress can seem to be the norm. I found T'ai Chi to be profoundly beneficial in reducing stress, increasing mental clarity, and improving my emotional as well as physical health. Where else can you find such a highly effective tool to achieve these worthwhile goals without fancy equipment or complicated formulas? If T'ai Chi can help with stress in an ER room where lives often hang in the balance, imagine what it can do for everyone else!"

—John D. Hernandez, M.D., Integrative Medicine

"Sometimes Chinese culture can be difficult to explain. Sifu Bill Douglas successfully uses American culture to explain the art of T'ai Chi Chuan. He simplifies difficult concepts, making them easier to understand. This book takes the best parts of T'ai Chi and makes them understandable [to Westerners] without requiring a grounding in Chinese culture and history."

—Sifu Yijiao Hong, USA All-Tai Chi Grand Champion and USA Team member; Certified International Coach and Judge, International Wushu Federation

"Douglas has achieved for QiGong what Apple did for the computer. He's brought it to the people … great place to start for beginners. … Teachers may also find this an excellent manual 'on how to explain these concepts to the general public ….'"

—R. Poccia, stress management instructor, Beyond Anonymous, San Francisco

"It has been a year since I began practicing T'ai Chi under the teaching of the author of this book, Bill Douglas, and his associate instructor, Erik Feagans. This span of time certainly allows me to evaluate the result of this gentle 'martial art,' not only as stress management therapy, but, more impressively, with regard to its effect on my physical health.

"Suffering for years from chronic neck pain consequent to a whiplash injury, and also suffering from a limited motion of the right shoulder, I approached the T'ai Chi course with some skepticism. The course was initiated after unsuccessful sessions of physical therapy, including mobilization, ultrasounds, heat application, etc. After two months of T'ai Chi, the pain in the cervical region disappeared while the range of motion of my right shoulder returned completely to normal. This achievement remained unchanged during the past winter up until now.

"I would not hesitate to recommend T'ai Chi to individuals suffering from the same ailments, as well as to mature persons who are seeking to maintain or improve their health and to remain free of chronic pain due to the aging process."

—Loredana Brizio-Molteni, M.D., F.A.C.S.

"After leaving my very first T'ai Chi class with the author of this book, I remember driving home, and it was as if someone had opened up every one of my senses. It was an overwhelming sense of happiness that swept over me. It was at that very moment I knew T'ai Chi is something I want in my life forever."

—Lisa Shikles, Shawnee, Kansas

"Because of my practice of T'ai Chi and QiGong, my barometer for detecting 'dis-ease' within myself earlier allows me to prevent serious infection and speed up healing. I feel T'ai Chi is a wonderful part of a revolution in health care, whereby each of us takes much more responsibility for our own health and healing."

—Susan Norman, C.I.M.T.

"I found you by accident while looking for an alternative to back surgery … with three ruptured discs in my lower back. … I read your book from cover to cover. … I am also now over halfway through your second tape, and my range of motion is better than it has been in years. I have also managed to lose a few pounds. … Recently, I went to my regular medical doctor. … [H]e told me he was very pleased with my range of motion and my attitude. … He was so intrigued by my description of your program that he has borrowed my book and the tapes I have finished."

—Mark Herndon, Georgia

"Since beginning Bill Douglas's T'ai Chi program, I have taught the exercises I learned for the past five years in our Pain Management multidisciplinary program at Research Medical Center. My clients have found improved breathing, larger mobility, better posture, improved balance and coordination, flexibility, increased endurance and strength, and relaxation."

—Berni Wheeler, occupational therapist

"I have found so many health benefits since beginning Bill Douglas's T'ai Chi program, which I began during a nervous breakdown with panic, chest pains, fatigue, and chronic migraines. I saw Bill's T'ai Chi and QiGong program information, and I gave it a try. I felt sudden and immediate benefits. My chest pains started to go away, my heavy fatigue went away, my nervousness calmed. My migraines are now nonexistent, as is the severe hay fever I'd had since childhood. And if that isn't enough, I have also lost my craving for fatty foods I once used to soothe my stress, and am now losing weight."

—Tina Webb, Shawnee, Kansas

"As a physical therapist assistant, I believe that these techniques that are taught by Bill through his book and tapes will become one of the essential tools to be utilized in medical facilities as an adjunct to standard therapy.

"Not a day goes by when I am not able to help an individual find pain control using Bill's QiGong techniques, and many find increased balance and coordination, even after a small taste of Tai Chi, seeing an automatic difference. Personally, tests show me with a 90 percent improvement in overall balance and in one test a 105 percent improvement in balance since beginning Tai Chi."

—Joyce Rupp, physical therapist assistant, Hays, Kansas

"From the perspective of a health psychologist serving patients who are coping with chronic illness and stressful life events, I see the gentle mindfulness exercises of T'ai Chi and QiGong relaxation therapy as potentially useful for a broad spectrum of people. The author of this book, Bill Douglas, explains the complexities of T'ai Chi and QiGong in the form of an invitation, easing his students into a greater understanding of the usefulness and purpose of this ancient form of meditative movement."

—Kristy Straits-Troster, Ph.D., clinical psychologist, Primary Care Medicine

"Dizziness is one of the more common reasons for a doctor visit, particularly in patients over the age of 50. Because the causes of dizziness can range from benign self-limiting conditions to potentially life-threatening ones, a thorough medical evaluation is essential before embarking on any form of therapy. Persistent dizziness certainly has a distinct impact on the quality of life and emotional well-being of the patient. Falls, hip fractures, and lack of confidence in public often create a feeling of helplessness.

"In over 20 years of experience as a clinical neurologist, I find that extensive and expensive medical evaluation, including CAT scans, MRI scans, and vascular imaging studies, as well as prescription medications, adds little to alleviating the problem. I have found vestibular rehabilitation exercises in the form of T'ai Chi classes to be a cost-effective mode of therapy. Many of my patients have opted for this nonmedication approach to treatment and have developed a sense of self-confidence through this form of exercise. In short, as a traditional medical practitioner, I frequently recommend T'ai Chi for my patients with dizziness and disequilibrium."

—Charles D. Donohoe, M.D., neurologist

"Since beginning Bill's T'ai Chi program, my resting heart rate has gone from 81 to 61. It's amazing!"

—Anne Bauman, Kansas

"I found the Energy Work (Sitting QiGong) and breath work learned in Bill's T'ai Chi program to be calming and to have that effect on those around me as well, including a returning patient who was hallucinating and having panic attacks. By walking with him and breathing deeply, the patient eventually calmed and lay down breathing evenly to await the doctor."

—Psychotherapist, Kansas City area

"Rx: Continue T'ai Chi. — Dx: Hypertension."

—An actual physician's prescription for a patient to continue in Bill Douglas's hospital T'ai Chi and QiGong classes

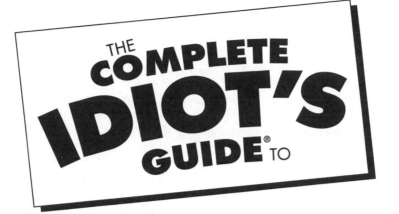

T'ai Chi and QiGong

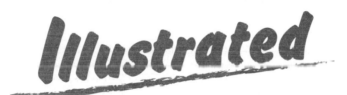

Third Edition

by Bill Douglas

ALPHA

A member of Penguin Group (USA) Inc.

In loving memory of my father, William Edward Douglas Sr., a man who endured the horror of war and hardship like few others … yet from that experience hungered for a world of justice and peace for all peoples of the world. Your Herculean efforts to heal your life serve as an example, enabling me to open to the profound healing T'ai Chi and QiGong offer me and the world. I hope you are up there enjoying the sight of Germans and Americans, Jews and Arabs, all playing T'ai Chi together every year. I dedicate World T'ai Chi and QiGong Day to your memory.

ALPHA BOOKS

Published by the Penguin Group

Penguin Group (USA) Inc., 375 Hudson Street, New York, New York 10014, U.S.A.

Penguin Group (Canada), 10 Alcorn Avenue, Toronto, Ontario, Canada M4V 3B2 (a division of Pearson Penguin Canada Inc.)

Penguin Books Ltd, 80 Strand, London WC2R 0RL, England

Penguin Ireland, 25 St Stephen's Green, Dublin 2, Ireland (a division of Penguin Books Ltd)

Penguin Group (Australia), 250 Camberwell Road, Camberwell, Victoria 3124, Australia (a division of Pearson Australia Group Pty Ltd)

Penguin Books India Pvt Ltd, 11 Community Centre, Panchsheel Park, New Delhi—110 017, India

Penguin Group (NZ), cnr Airborne and Rosedale Roads, Albany, Auckland 1310, New Zealand (a division of Pearson New Zealand Ltd)

Penguin Books (South Africa) (Pty) Ltd, 24 Sturdee Avenue, Rosebank, Johannesburg 2196, South Africa

Penguin Books Ltd, Registered Offices: 80 Strand, London WC2R 0RL, England

International Standard Book Number: 1-59257-420-3
Library of Congress Catalog Card Number: 2005930983

08   07   06   05   8   7   6   5   4   3   2   1

Interpretation of the printing code: The rightmost number of the first series of numbers is the year of the book's printing; the rightmost number of the second series of numbers is the number of the book's printing. For example, a printing code of 05-1 shows that the first printing occurred in 2005.

Printed in the United States of America

Note: This publication contains the opinions and ideas of its author. It is intended to provide helpful and informative material on the subject matter covered. It is sold with the understanding that the author and publisher are not engaged in rendering professional services in the book. If the reader requires personal assistance or advice, a competent professional should be consulted.

The author and publisher specifically disclaim any responsibility for any liability, loss, or risk, personal or otherwise, which is incurred as a consequence, directly or indirectly, of the use and application of any of the contents of this book.

Most Alpha books are available at special quantity discounts for bulk purchases for sales promotions, premiums, fund-raising, or educational use. Special books, or book excerpts, can also be created to fit specific needs.

For details, write: Special Markets, Alpha Books, 375 Hudson Street, New York, NY 10014.

Publisher: *Marie Butler-Knight*
Editorial Director/Acquiring Editor: *Mike Sanders*
Senior Managing Editor: *Jennifer Bowles*
Development Editor: *Christy Wagner*
Senior Production Editor: *Billy Fields*
Copy Editor: *Krista Hansing*

Cartoonist: *Shannon Wheeler*
Cover/Book Designer: *Trina Wurst*
Indexer: *Aamir Burki*
Layout: *Becky Harmon*
Proofreading: *John Etchison*

Contents at a Glance

Appendixes

Contents

Foreword

As Bill explains in this book, although T'ai Chi and QiGong are exercises, they are integral parts of Traditional Chinese Medicine (TCM). As alternative medicine and therapies sweep the Western world, doctors now prescribe QiGong and T'ai Chi for treating stress problems, illnesses, and injuries, while many people use it as a tonic to extend their peak performance into old age. Robert Parish, one of the great NBA players, claimed T'ai Chi extended his career, making him one of the oldest *dominant* starting players in NBA history. Just as T'ai Chi protected Mr. Parish's body from the intense stress of professional basketball, it can help each of us protect ourselves from the relentless stress of a rapidly changing world.

In my 48 years of experience in Traditional Chinese Medicine, here and in the Orient, I have never heard anyone explain the premise of T'ai Chi and QiGong as succinctly as Bill does. He has the most unusual ability to explain concepts he's spent a lifetime learning in a way that is tangible and applicable to the novice student the very first day of class. You will happily realize that this book offers you, the reader, a humorous and enjoyable journey deep into the world of T'ai Chi and QiGong. After providing an extensive understanding of T'ai Chi and QiGong's profound potential, the book proceeds to very practically explain how you can dive into T'ai Chi and QiGong by clarifying such basic concepts as what to wear to class and what to call your teacher.

This book provides ways T'ai Chi can be integrated into your life on many levels through your work, social recreation, and health care, just as it has been in China for many years. Bill shares and eloquently articulates my vision that Traditional Chinese Medicine is leading a transformation in Western health care that will financially save you, the patient, untold dollars and much needless pain and suffering. This book will facilitate that transformation by making the everyday person comfortable with the commonsense approach health tools like T'ai Chi and QiGong make, and we will all be better for it.

This book, with humor and gentleness, guides you through T'ai Chi and QiGong to help you boost your immune system, sleep better, and improve everything about you effortlessly. This book is for everybody living with stress, but a must for every corporate wellness director, health-care worker, and activities director. Here you can learn why T'ai Chi is the fastest-growing exercise and healing balm for modern life!

—Richard Yennie, D.C., Dipl. Ac. (NCCA), Deputy Director, China Medical Association, Research Committee, Taipei, Taiwan; President, QiGong Society of America; U.S. Representative, World Academic Society of Medical QiGong; President, Acupuncture Society of America, Inc.; Faculty Member, Waseda Acupuncture College, Tokyo, Japan; Visiting Professor at Beijing University of Chinese Medicine, Beijing, China

Introduction

Before I began T'ai Chi and QiGong classes, my stress was unbearable, and depression and anxiety were almost a way of life. I actually thought at the time that that's just the way life was. It's funny what we'll settle for, when all the while there are powerful and exciting opportunities to change—just waiting for us to reach out and grab them. Back then, I returned home every night from a job I didn't like and used greasy food, overspending, too much TV, or whatever else could help me handle the stress of a life I didn't really feel too good about. I really didn't see much hope for finding any "real joy" in my life.

Then a friend suggested a T'ai Chi class. From that day, my life began to change, to loosen, to expand and open, becoming more than I ever dreamed possible. Today I travel the world, sharing the most exciting life possibilities with fascinating people all seeking to expand their lives into more than they ever imagined.

T'ai Chi enabled me to let go of my tight, rigid grip on what I thought was possible in life. As it taught me to breathe deeply and allow my body's rigid muscles to let go and relax, my mind and heart began to do so as well. An open mind and open heart expanded outward into an open world. When we begin to live for what we love, the world begins to love us for it. T'ai Chi and QiGong help us loosen up so the love within us can expand outward into all aspects of our lives. This is how we become "lovely" in the truest sense of the word. There is such beautiful potential awaiting all of us, and I am so proud and so grateful that this book has been a part of so many people's expansion—just as T'ai Chi and QiGong have been a part of mine. Enjoy!

How to Use This Book

Although some chapters of this book use particular T'ai Chi styles to give readers an experience of T'ai Chi and QiGong, the majority of this book and the DVD are profoundly useful to anyone interested in any style of T'ai Chi or QiGong and are used by teachers worldwide, from many different styles, as a primer and textbook for their students. Its easygoing, accessible style has helped T'ai Chi and QiGong teachers find fresh, user-friendly explanations to help students "get T'ai Chi or QiGong" more quickly and easily by relaxing into it.

This book is divided into six parts, plus the supporting DVD. Each part's information will prepare you for the next, opening your mind and imagination to concepts that will unlock your ability to expand your awareness of T'ai Chi and QiGong even more. The 1½-hour DVD supports many sections of the book's chapters with carefully selected visual information that text and illustrations simply cannot convey.

Here's what you get:

The DVD, *Visual Support for This Book's Instruction,* is a powerful new addition, with 1½ hours of exhibitional inserts to support the text and illustrated instruction and general information throughout this book. The DVD is created from excerpts of two of my acclaimed fully instructional DVD programs that total well over 5 hours in content. Obviously, it was impossible to include the entire contents of these programs in this book's highly useful 1½-hour DVD; therefore, carefully selected excerpts were chosen to powerfully augment the information and instructions provided within the book. As you read through the book's six parts, you'll be directed at appropriate points to view the DVD provided with this book to expand your understanding of the book's instructions and information. As various sections of the book refer you to the same video excerpts, you'll discover a multidimensional quality to the DVD, encouraging you to see T'ai Chi and QiGong's many subtle aspects and qualities. (See Appendix C for more details on my multi-hour fully instructional DVD programs.)

Part 1, "T'ai Chi: Relax into It," explains how T'ai Chi and QiGong can change every part of your life for the better, with visual support from the DVD. Part 1 concludes by explaining how T'ai Chi and QiGong work by introducing you to Traditional Chinese Medicine (TCM) and explaining how modern Western science is now beginning to understand how this ancient wisdom works.

Part 2, "Suiting Up and Setting Out," prepares you to dive into T'ai Chi and QiGong "big time" or "little time," depending on how much of T'ai Chi's magic you want to experience. In this part, you learn the nuts and bolts of how classes are taught (with DVD visuals), along with T'ai Chi etiquette, terms, wardrobe, and all the things that will enable you to choose the best class for you. You also discover the underlying tenets of T'ai Chi and QiGong, which will dramatically enhance the benefit you get from class or video instruction beyond this book's voluminous resources.

Part 3, "Starting Down the QiGong Path to T'ai Chi," explains how QiGong works and then leads you into an experience that is exquisite beyond words. Part 3 ends with an introduction to Moving QiGong exercises including the warm-ups that prepare your mind and body to dive into an ocean of T'ai Chi experience (with references to the DVD). *T'ai Chi* literally means "the supreme ultimate," so hold on for an incredible ride!

Part 4, "Kuang Ping T'ai Chi: Walk on Life's Lighter Side," illuminates the history of T'ai Chi and how the Kuang Ping Yang Style was brought to the West by Master Kuo Lien Ying. Then you are led through the entire 64 postures of this powerful ancient form (with visual support for some select postures' instructions and an entire *Exhibition of the T'ai Chi Long Form* on the DVD) and instructed on a few of the benefits of each movement. Yet remember, the benefits are endless, and because this book is about 350 pages long, to discover them you must experience them yourself as they unfold beautifully within you every day for the rest of your life.

Part 5, "T'ai Chi's Buffet of Short, Sword, and Fan Styles," exposes you to the many incredibly beautiful forms of T'ai Chi (with visual exhibitions on the DVD) available to you today. Remember that only about 30 years ago, these arts were secrets of China, so we are very lucky to have these exquisite art forms available to us now in our lifetimes. Part 5 gives you a small yet delicious taste of what is available. If you seek, ye shall find.

Part 6, "Life Applications," shows that T'ai Chi is much more than just a "physical exercise." T'ai Chi can help heal every aspect of our lives, our relationships, and our world (the DVD's visual images complement these points). To that end, Part 6 explains how T'ai Chi and/or QiGong can be used to help treat almost any illness or physical malady. It also explains to what extent T'ai Chi can be a powerful adjunct therapy for many mental or emotional problems, as well as a powerful tool that helps you increase your productivity and creativity in your professional life. But even beyond healing, you will see how T'ai Chi can help the world realize a much more expansive vision of possibility for our ever-evolving future.

T'ai Chi Pearls

Throughout this book, I've included five types of extra information for your enlightenment:

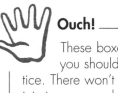

Ouch!

These boxes alert you to any caution you should observe in T'ai Chi practice. There won't be many of these; T'ai Chi injuries are nearly nonexistent when done correctly.

Know Your Chinese

These boxes give you definitions for Chinese medical and philosophical terms related to T'ai Chi and QiGong, including pronunciation aids.

A T'ai Chi Punch Line

These boxes are full of fun anecdotes and trivia about the fascinating world of T'ai Chi and QiGong, modern and old.

T'ai Sci

These boxes provide you modern scientific terms and insights into the world of T'ai Chi's ancient discoveries.

Sage Sifu Says

These boxes offer you tips on living the principles of T'ai Chi and maximizing your understanding of T'ai Chi's subtle layers to help you get the most out of it. Sifu (pronounced *see-foo*) means "one who has mastered an art"—but not only martial arts; a master chef or artist might be a sifu.

Acknowledgments

A great thanks to the many dedicated Chinese creators of T'ai Chi who've spent lifetimes developing this wonderful art and health science the world now has access to. T'ai Chi and QiGong are great gifts the Chinese culture has provided for the world, and I offer the creators a deep and heartfelt thank you. Their efforts leave me convinced that every culture on this planet has treasures to offer the rest, and I hope we all can open our hearts and minds to truth and value, no matter where it comes from.

A profound thanks to my teacher, Master Jennifer Booth; her teacher, Gil Messenger; their teacher, Russell Schofield; and our grand master, Kuo Lien Ying, who made the daunting journey from China to San Francisco, as did many other courageous masters of other styles of T'ai Chi and forms of QiGong. Their courage in migrating to strange lands made it possible for millions of people in many nations to have access to the beauty and power of Kuang Ping Yang T'ai Chi Ch'uan and the other wonderful forms, including Chen, Yang, Wu, Sun, Mulan, and others. I would further like to thank my teacher, Ms. Booth, for focusing intensely on the *healing* aspects of T'ai Chi and QiGong and for imparting that importance to me.

I would like to thank my brilliant sister Diane Douglas, her associates Jay and Sandra, my brother Ed, and my sisters Barbara and Peggy, without whose insights and support, none of this would have been possible. My wife, Angela, and her mother, Shun Oi Wong, were an integral part of my T'ai Chi journey, and my father-in-law, Bonwyn Wong, embodied the humility and infinite wisdom Chinese people are famous for. My children, Isaac, Andrea, and Michael, led me to the doorway of change through their innocent examples of wisdom, and my parents, Evelyn and William Douglas, showed me that even the harshest tests can produce pearls in us beautiful creatures known as human beings.

Thanks to Mulan Quan instructors Angela Wong-Douglas and Andrea Mei-Wah Douglas for their wonderful exhibitions and insights into the elegant art form of Mulan Quan Basic, Fan, and Sword Style. Thanks always to Mike Sanders, Christy Wagner, Krista Hansing, and Billy Fields for their patience and profound editing expertise, to Susan Norman for her sage advice on holistic living; and to Betty Wyckoff for her research work.

With the modern stress plague ravaging the world, I want to thank the visionary educators beginning to incorporate T'ai Chi and QiGong into education systems worldwide. When every graduating senior is a T'ai Chi master, how much less drug and alcohol abuse, and how much less violence and fewer children in prisons will there be? Thank you all for your courage, vision, and open-heartedness, to see the profound value of these tools even though they come from another culture. Thanks to all the innovative T'ai Chi teachers who are discovering new ways to teach these ancient arts, to make them fun and contemporary so modern children (and adults) in all societies can learn to love them. All the T'ai Chi and QiGong teachers working to educate the world on the last Saturday of April each year on World T'ai Chi and QiGong Day (and all year) are pioneers whose health education work will benefit the world in ways we cannot yet even imagine.

Last, but not least, I'd like to thank illustrator Jenny Hahn Neely (shikuns@mindspring.com) for her work on the more than 200 instructional sketches and her dedication to this project. Ms. Neely is an extraordinary artist with an ability to capture complex and *even internal* T'ai Chi concepts in her illustrations. Her work has set a new standard for T'ai Chi book instruction. Also, thanks to Jessica Kincaid for her computer graphics (www.filigree.com) and to master photographer David Larson for his brilliant photos. Thanks to Andrea Mei-Wah Douglas for her wonderful cover photo, and to Dominic Orr for providing his spectacular home as that photo's location.

Special Thanks to the Technical Reviewer

The Complete Idiot's Guide to T'ai Chi and QiGong was reviewed by an expert who double-checked the accuracy of what you'll learn here, to help us ensure that this book gives you everything you need to know about T'ai Chi and QiGong. Special thanks are extended to Master Jennifer Booth.

Trademarks

All terms mentioned in this book that are known to be or are suspected of being trademarks or service marks have been appropriately capitalized. Alpha Books and Penguin Group (USA) Inc. cannot attest to the accuracy of this information. Use of a term in this book should not be regarded as affecting the validity of any trademark or service mark.

In This Part

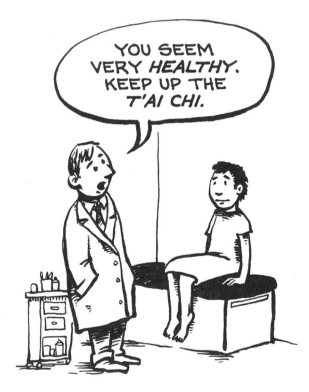

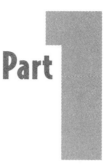

Part 1

T'ai Chi: Relax into It

Part 1 explains why a simple, easy-to-do, 2,000-year-old Chinese martial art is the most popular exercise in the world today and is practiced in corporations, hospitals, living rooms, and backyards just like yours around the world.

If you want to find a calm center in the middle of life's storm of change while also toning your muscles and healing your mind and body, T'ai Chi and QiGong are just what the doctor ordered—literally. *Ask your doctor!* Whether you seek a simple, easy-to-do exercise; a stress-management tool; or a profoundly healthy philosophy of life, T'ai Chi may just be what you've been looking for.

This edition's new exhibitional DVD, containing excerpts from my fully instructional multi-hour DVD (see Appendix C), provides powerful support for this book's descriptions and instructions. Throughout all the parts of the book, you are directed at various points to view video support for text explanations.

In This Chapter

- ◆ The reasons behind T'ai Chi's exploding popularity

- ◆ The root of T'ai Chi

- ◆ A brief history of T'ai Chi

- ◆ Powerful benefits from *all* styles of T'ai Chi

- ◆ On the DVD: visualize T'ai Chi's soothing, unhurried flow

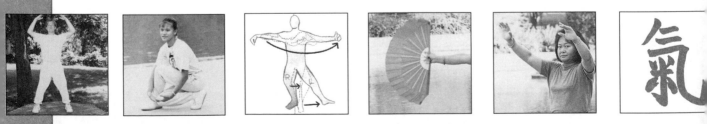

Chapter 1

Why Practice T'ai Chi?

T'ai Chi comes in several excellent styles. While some chapters in this book relate to particular T'ai Chi styles, you'll find this book to be a valuable resource to anyone exploring any form of T'ai Chi or QiGong, which is why it is used as a primer and textbook by teachers of many styles, and in several languages, worldwide.

About 20 percent of the world's population practices T'ai Chi or QiGong, and it's fast becoming the most popular exercise in the world today. Its rapid expansion is largely due to one important fact—*it feels really good.* T'ai Chi is increasingly offered in businesses, hospitals, and schools everywhere. T'ai Chi is not only a valuable tool for improving health—it is a powerful business tool as well. Companies see that T'ai Chi improves productivity by helping employees be happy, relaxed, and creative. Hospitals see T'ai Chi as a potent yet cost-effective therapy for nearly any condition. T'ai Chi classes can be found almost anywhere nowadays. In this chapter, I give you a whirlwind tour of the reasons behind T'ai Chi's growing popularity and what T'ai Chi can do for you.

Exploring the Reasons Behind T'ai Chi's Popularity

Do you ever feel like life is getting more stressful? *It is.* The increasing stress in today's world is one reason for T'ai Chi's growing worldwide popularity. T'ai Chi was designed to help people go through change with less damage by improving the way we handle stress. Studies show change is stressful, and *even though change is often good*, if the stress that change causes isn't managed, it can damage your health and outlook on life. About 90 percent of the discoveries made in the history of the human race have been made in our lifetime, so it's safe to say we are all going through some serious change—*and stress.* T'ai Chi's ability to help practitioners "let go" of this stress more easily is just what the doctor ordered—*literally.*

Imagine that life is a carousel upon which we ride. When life gets spinning really fast, T'ai Chi seems to slow things down, like a hand pulling us away from the edge back to the center of life's carousel. Here, in the center, we can let life spin even faster and not feel like throwing up (well, hardly ever, anyway). In fact, by practicing T'ai Chi as you ride life's carousel, you might even catch yourself going *"Wheeee!"* a lot more often.

Whether you are stressed out, continually exhausted, treating a health problem, or just wanting to get in shape and feel young again, T'ai Chi is just what you need. T'ai Chi goes right to the heart of everything we do by healing and cleansing the central nervous system. T'ai Chi helps us let go of all the nervous tension that bogs down our mental computer system (like getting a general tune-up every day). This makes everything inside us work better, which often makes the world around us seem better, too. So T'ai Chi is really a self-improvement tool that will make you a better "anything-you-want-to-be." Unless, of course, you want to be stressed out, exhausted, and uninspired, and feel old and out of shape. In that case, T'ai Chi won't help.

People everywhere in the world are rapidly embracing T'ai Chi as "their" exercise. Although T'ai Chi originates in China, it is now seen so commonly in the West that soon it will be thought of as an American thing, a British thing, a Canadian thing, or whatever. If you ask American kids what their favorite American food is, many will reply, "Pizza!" (which is originally Italian). And someday, when asked what their favorite American pastime is, Americans will say, "T'ai Chi!"

T'ai Chi Relaxes the Mind, the Body, and Our Lives

Just as we flow through the changes of life (or not), our life energy, or *Qi*, flows through us (or not, if we are stressed out). Qi is the energy of life and flows through all living things. Qi animates, heals, and nurtures life. When the stress of change makes us tense, we squeeze off the flow of life energy. Physically, this feels like tension. T'ai Chi and QiGong are easy, simple, yet sophisticated relaxation exercises that encourage the muscles to let go of tension, the mind to let go of worry, and the heart to let go of angst. Tension, worry, and angst all block our Qi flow.

Know Your Chinese

The Chinese call life energy **Qi** (pronounced *chee*). The character for Qi is also the character for air or breath. QiGong (pronounced *chee kung* and often spelled Chi-Gong) means "breath work" or "energy exercise." There are about 7,000 QiGong exercises in the Chinese Medica (the bible of Chinese Medicine). T'ai Chi is a moving form of QiGong. There are sitting and lying forms of QiGong, but all T'ai Chi is done standing and moving.

Tension, worry, and angst are usually the result of our mind, heart, or body being unable to "let go" of something. The goal of T'ai Chi is to move through a series of choreographed movements like a slow martial arts routine, but *very* slowly and in a state of absolute relaxation. To do this, we have to let go of our mental/physical tensions, grudges, prejudices, and anything that keeps us tied to the past. This enables us to flow more easily into the future by clearing our mind and body of old stress so we constantly get a "fresh" perspective on life.

T'ai Chi is simple and easy to do, yet it benefits us on many deep and complex levels. T'ai Chi's slow, relaxed movements incorporate breathing and relaxation techniques that cleanse our mind, body, and emotions each time we go through the gentle movements. T'ai Chi is designed to uncover and release every single place we hold tension or blocked energy. When our mind or heart holds on to issues (fears, obsessions, angers, and so on), our body literally squeezes itself with tension. Going slowly through the movements is like doing an internal scan of our entire body to clear and release any place it is gripping tension. No exercise on Earth can help you go through this wild ride toward the future quite like T'ai Chi can—which is why T'ai Chi is truly the exercise of the future.

Ouch!

Nearly one third of the adult U.S. population has chronic high blood pressure. Because some medications have side effects, physicians need to be made aware that T'ai Chi can sometimes lower high blood pressure as effectively as medication. Ask your doctor to look into T'ai Chi. However, never adjust medication levels on your own without consulting your physician.

T'ai Chi Promotes Internal Strength for Young and Old

T'ai Chi looks very much like slow-motion kung fu. David Carradine performed a form related to T'ai Chi as Kwai Chang Caine on the television series *Kung Fu*. And although T'ai Chi shares some similarities with kung fu, don't let that scare you away. T'ai Chi can be practiced by anyone at any age and in any condition.

In martial arts circles, T'ai Chi is known as an internal martial art. T'ai Chi promotes internal strength physically, mentally, and emotionally, which is why it can be a powerful training tool for martial artists. But you don't have to be a martial artist to benefit from T'ai Chi because it can also be practiced, with great results, even by those in wheelchairs.

Unlike karate, T'ai Chi has no belt or ranking system because the benefits of T'ai Chi can be only *felt*, not seen. You practice T'ai Chi to live better—more calmly, clearly, healthfully, and productively. T'ai Chi is a tonic for life. You will gauge your progress by how you feel, how spry you look in the mirror, how much you love life, and how healthy you are. Isn't that much better than owning a black belt? However, if you do karate, T'ai Chi can help you get that black belt by improving your internal function and grace.

Also, T'ai Chi differs from most martial arts in that people of all ages can practice it. Many people with disabilities and ailments practice T'ai Chi as therapy. No one is restricted from practicing T'ai Chi, and T'ai Chi can benefit the fittest athletes just as much as it benefits elderly arthritis sufferers. T'ai Chi clubs are sprouting up all over the world, with people from all walks of life.

T'ai Chi: Finally an Exercise That *Feels Good!*

T'ai Chi is popular because it is easy to do and provides a gentle workout that doesn't leave you drained, but *energized!* T'ai Chi's "effortless" nature is a big stretch for most of us, however, because we associate exercise with *force, pain,* and *tension.* In fact, some exercise actually contributes to stress. When I played junior high football in west Texas many years ago, the coaches determined that we were finished running when one of us started throwing up. That's right, upchucking. It was the only time in my life I ever hoped to see someone throw up.

T'ai Chi is helping the world get a healthful, enjoyable view of exercise. As a nation, we have adopted a mutant notion of exercise, exemplified by the mantra "No pain, no gain." This has traumatized many Americans, including myself, leaving an indelible mark on how we view exercise. In T'ai Chi, we have a mantra, too: "If your exercise causes pain, you'll get so sick of the thought of it that you'll never want to do it again." Do T'ai Chi because it feels good, and you will look forward to it. Each morning you will find yourself grateful that you're alive and able to practice this cool exercise called T'ai Chi.

You Are Perfect—and Perfect for T'ai Chi

T'ai Chi doesn't begin with the premise that there is "something wrong" that needs to be fixed, sculpted, lost, or burned off. It is a very accepting exercise, and it helps us remember we are already *perfect* … but our ability to get better is *limitless*. Everyone is qualified to do T'ai Chi. You don't have to look good in tights or Spandex to do T'ai Chi (although if you do T'ai Chi enough, you'll look pretty good in whatever you like to wear).

Ouch!

Beginning T'ai Chi is a *big step* for many of us, and it is easy to psych yourself out of taking it up—just like the first day we went to kindergarten and thought of all the "big, bad" stuff that would probably happen. But for most of us, none of that materialized, and in fact, we actually had a lot of fun. Take a chance. Dive into life by entering the waters of T'ai Chi and QiGong.

T'ai Chi and QiGong are for anybody who is dealing with stress—in other words, *everybody*. Anybody can do T'ai Chi. If you've picked up a book on T'ai Chi, you've probably experienced the *acute stress* of imagining yourself in some of those incredible (seemingly impossible) positions. Relax. Those people are often T'ai Chi athletes. Most people do T'ai Chi just the way you will do it—easily and effortlessly. Although T'ai Chi was one of the original

martial arts, it is now practiced all over the world as a relaxation technique by people of all ages in the same shape you are in—and sometimes in even worse shape!

When you begin an exercise class, you may have the illusion that everybody other than you "belongs" there and that they are all "good" at it. You will find that everybody goes through the same trials and tribulations. As you lighten up on yourself, you'll see struggling, growing, and healing everywhere around you. Breathe and enjoy; you are among friends.

When you first begin practicing T'ai Chi out in the backyard or in your local park, people may stare. Before long, though, your unique practice of T'ai Chi becomes part of the rich texture of the neighborhood, and if you move away, they will miss you. Just as T'ai Chi adds to your personal internal charm, your practice adds to the charm of your community.

T'ai Chi Goes to the Root of Problems

Life is very complicated, and T'ai Chi cannot solve all your problems. However, T'ai Chi can help you simplify your life in a big and relaxing way.

Imagine you're a tree. While your mind and body are the trunk of that tree, all your "life stuff" is like the tree's many leaves. Your job, relationships, hobbies, hopes, and problems are all dangling out there on the tips of your life. When your health is bad or you can't sleep well, that affects the whole tree. You may have problems with your job that may strain your relationships, which, in turn, will drain the energy you need to pursue your hobbies, making you too tired to have hopeful dreams, *and causing your problems to get seemingly bigger and bigger.* When you're already beat, trying to figure out how to heal all these sick, shriveled leaves is too much to even think about.

The Least You Need to Know

◆ T'ai Chi reduces stress and slows the aging process.

◆ Everybody can do T'ai Chi. *Everybody.*

◆ T'ai Chi restores the power of youthful exuberance.

◆ T'ai Chi is an efficient therapy that can improve all aspects of your life.

◆ By clearing the mind, T'ai Chi reminds you that life is a miracle.

In This Chapter

- ◆ A tune-up for the whole you
- ◆ The benefits of innercise versus outercise
- ◆ The ultimate performance booster
- ◆ The difference and similarities between T'ai Chi and yoga
- ◆ On the DVD: *innercise, dan tien, vertical axis*, and the low-impact aspect of T'ai Chi

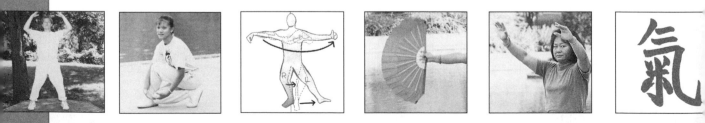

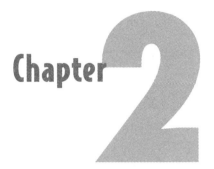

Let's Get Physical

T'ai Chi is perhaps the best physical exercise in the world. Unlike higher-impact exercises, T'ai Chi does not harm the body. In fact, its gentle movements help the body strengthen bone mass and connective tissue, and it is lower impact than even brisk walking. T'ai Chi also works on a cellular level to physically cleanse and tone the body in deep ways that you never see, and can help beautify the external physical body.

Depending on the type of T'ai Chi, you may not even break a sweat doing T'ai Chi. Therefore, T'ai Chi is a great workout you can do during a 15-minute coffee break at work, in your regular work clothes, or in your pajamas when you get up. It won't leave you out of breath and fatigued, but it will leave you feeling clear, peaceful, and at one with the universe.

According to research, T'ai Chi burns nearly as many calories as downhill skiing and provides many of the same health benefits as low-impact aerobic exercises. T'ai Chi provides balance and coordination improvements that are nearly twice as effective as the best balance-training exercises in the world.

For athletes, T'ai Chi could be the best training you can do to improve your game. Golfers sometimes add a hundred yards to their drives after "playing" T'ai Chi for just a few months, while weight lifters often see results immediately. Yet even if your main physical activity is mowing the lawn and carrying groceries, the same things T'ai Chi does to benefit athletic performance will increase your physical power and dramatically reduce the likelihood of injury when you're working around the house. (See Chapter 20 on T'ai Chi and sports performance.)

There is no single exercise that can do what T'ai Chi does for you physically. This is why T'ai Chi is becoming the most popular exercise in the world today. This chapter tells you what you can expect from a T'ai Chi workout.

T'ai Chi Acupuncture Tune-Up

T'ai Chi is a very slow exercise, performed as if you were swimming through water—or the air, in T'ai Chi's case. This has many benefits. You cannot injure yourself when doing T'ai Chi correctly because the slowness allows you time to hear your body's pain signals and stop any movement that doesn't feel right. You simply adjust the T'ai Chi movements to fit your own range of mobility.

> **T'ai Sci**
>
> Acupuncture stimulates points on the body that affect the flow of Qi, or life energy. *Acupressure* is acupuncture without the needles. By massaging acupuncture points, you are performing acupressure and getting much the same benefit.

T'ai Chi's slow, standing movements also thoroughly massage the bottoms of the feet. Acupuncture points on the feet affect every part of the body, including every major organ. Therefore, the slow, gentle massaging your feet get from a 20-minute T'ai Chi routine treats your entire body. By the end of your T'ai Chi play time, every cell of your body will be relaxed and opened to a smoother flow of life energy. You will feel clear, bright, and renewed. (The science of acupuncture is explained in greater detail in Chapter 3.)

Innercise vs. Outercise

T'ai Chi is a mind/body exercise, or an *innercise*. That is, T'ai Chi aids the mind and body simultaneously to powerfully center us physically and emotionally (see Chapter 4). T'ai Chi's an innercise because it uniquely focuses the mind on the *internal condition* of the body rather than on an external performance. Therefore, whereas practicing baseball makes you better at baseball and playing ping-pong makes you a better ping-pong player, T'ai Chi practice makes you better at everything you do!

Advantages of Innercise

T'ai Chi improves our overall performance on a physical level because it provides us with a daily picture of how we operate. Through its slow, deliberate movements, we can, with a kind of inner sight, see inside ourselves to observe our breath, posture, and tension levels, correcting problems before they become illnesses or injuries. (For an example of what's meant by innercise, check out the DVD's *Moving QiGong Warm Ups Excerpt*.)

Some athletes use medication to cover existing pain. T'ai Chi is the opposite of a painkiller. T'ai Chi helps us become aware of problems *before* they become acute. We do not want to hide pain, because pain is the body's way of telling us that some part of us needs healing attention. However, as T'ai Chi and QiGong help the body get gentle healing attention, they also help relieve chronic pain conditions. They help heal injuries or illnesses that pain alerts us to, and they also help us deal with the pain as those conditions are allowed to heal. Painkillers, on the other hand, separate our mind from our body and neither heal nor grant us the awareness needed to avoid further injuries.

This is not an either/or situation. Use medication as needed, and use T'ai Chi and QiGong as needed. The two can work in concert to help you recover. As always, discuss this with your doctor.

Ouch! _____

> With pain medication, there are no absolutes. When pain medication is needed, it is a wonderful thing to have and should be used. No one should force him- or herself to be in agony needlessly. However, if QiGong and T'ai Chi can help reduce the need for pain medication, or help prevent injury that might result in that need, it is a very healthful option.

T'ai Chi tones the muscles, increases breathing capacity, lowers stress levels, improves organ function, and corrects poor posture. All these things help the body maximize its self-healing potential, which is discussed in Chapter 3.

Problems with Outercise

We in the West suffer from the delusion that we can get our bodies fit, or even get our lives in order, without our minds being involved. For example, if you go to the health club, it will most likely have televisions above the stationary bikes or stair-climbing machines. The idea is that we can get healthy, lose stress, and get "buns of steel" while having our minds bombarded with CNN visions of world problems or the top 10 songs blasting in our ears. Of course, we can get buns of steel, but we can't get *truly* healthy that way. We've erroneously equated a hard body with health.

An overemphasis on the development of muscles, built up to look good to the outer world and not necessarily for health reasons, can interfere with our energy flow and natural health processes. The slow, mindful exercises of T'ai Chi give us a healthy muscle tone and also seem to support our immune system function so we get sick less often.

To see the effortless, soothing qualities of T'ai Chi, watch the DVD's *Exhibition of the T'ai Chi Long Form* and *Mulan Style Basic Short Form* (excerpts from the instructional videos listed in Appendix C).

Sage Sifu Says _____

> The Taoist philosopher Lao Tzu recognized that overconditioning just to look good to the outside world would not produce the desired result of health.
>
> > Stretch a bow out all the way,
> > And you'll regret that you didn't stop in time.
> > Sharpen a sword to its finest edge,
> > And the edge will break very quickly.
> > Rest when you've achieved your goal,
> > This is the way of heaven.
>
> In other words, if you drive yourself to pump up your muscles, you'll likely not stick with an exercise program because its goal is in excess of your health needs. It's easier and wiser to do an exercise to make you healthy rather than just to *look good*. This is what T'ai Chi is all about.

Overemphasizing our outer appearance is a *yang* obsession and can discount our internal, or *yin*, needs. T'ai Chi's goal is balance, and regular practice can help achieve this balance as T'ai Chi healthfully tones muscles while attending

The Health Benefits of T'ai Chi

We live in a stressful world; only recently has Western medical research come to recognize that stress is at the root of most health problems. Therefore, the health crisis that stress is causing in the West has actually created a great opportunity for us because it is opening us up to the wonders of TCM and tools like T'ai Chi and QiGong. In fact, the following list of T'ai Chi's measurable health benefits indicates how this opening to T'ai Chi may save us from our health-care crisis. T'ai Chi can ...

- ◆ Boost the immune system.
- ◆ Slow the aging process.
- ◆ Reduce anxiety, depression, and overall mood disturbance.
- ◆ Lower high blood pressure.
- ◆ Alleviate stress responses.
- ◆ Enhance the body's natural healing powers, such as recovering from injury.
- ◆ Increase breathing capacity.
- ◆ Reduce asthma and allergy reactions.
- ◆ Improve balance and coordination *twice* as well as the best balance-conditioning exercises in the world.
- ◆ Help ensure full-range mobility far into old age.
- ◆ Provide the lowest-impact weight-bearing exercise known.

However, before adding T'ai Chi to your physical therapy program, consult your physician to see if T'ai Chi might affect your medication levels. For example, many with high blood pressure find that their blood pressure lowers after playing T'ai Chi for a while. Your physician should know if T'ai Chi can alter your current therapy for such conditions and then

can lower your medication safely. (See Chapter 20 for other conditions T'ai Chi or QiGong may benefit—and show it to your doctor.)

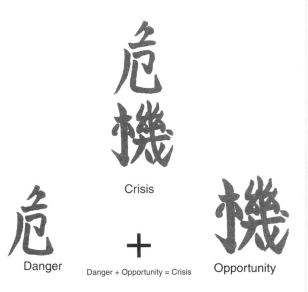

The Chinese character for "crisis" is a combination of two other characters—one for "danger" and the other for "opportunity."

Mind over Matter

The Chinese realized that our mind or consciousness is the root of who we are. Our health and our lives are merely reflections of our state of mind. T'ai Chi's mindful quality incorporates the mind and body into a powerful healing force.

Interestingly, Western science now sees that TCM's ancient insights were right on the money. A new science called *psychoneuroimmunology* has found that our mind constantly communicates to every cell of our body.

Emotional chemicals, known as neuropeptides, flow throughout our bodies, communicating every feeling to the entire body. So when hitting every red light on the street aggravates us or we become anxious in every line we stand in, we walk around in a state of perpetual panic (or as Bruce Springsteen sang, "Yer life is one long emergency"). This negatively affects our heart, brain, and entire circulatory system. In fact, those effects, in turn, affect other organs, which can cause a breakdown of the entire system over time, causing, for example, kidney failure, heart enlargement, and hardening of the arteries.

T'ai Sci

Psychoneuroimmunology is a modern science studying how the mind's attitudes and beliefs affect our physical health. *Psycho* means "mind," *neuro* means "nervous system," and *immunology* means "system of health defenses."

T'ai Chi helps us do just the opposite. We can decide to let issues slide right off us, literally breathing fears out with every sigh and yawn. As we sit in QiGong meditation or move in T'ai Chi's soothing postures, we let a nourishing healing flow of Qi, or life energy, fill every cell of our body.

Don't try too hard to memorize any of these details on TCM or Western medicine. Rather, let the concepts wash over your relaxed mind. The important stuff will stick, and you can always go back and look up details later.

To fully appreciate T'ai Chi's medical benefits, it may be helpful to understand how TCM views the body. TCM has known for centuries what Western science is only now discovering—that the mind and body are two inseparable things. There's a joke in TCM that "the only place the mind, body, emotions, and spirit are separate is in textbooks." In real life and T'ai Chi, it just isn't so. T'ai Chi's slow, mindful movements are the epitome of this union of mind and body. Now Western medicine is becoming increasingly conscious of it as well.

Comedian George Carlin joked, "After hundreds of years of medical research, we have finally discovered the head *is* connected to the body."

So when your body's muscles are rigid, your thinking will likely be more rigid, too. Likewise, if your thinking is harsh and rigid, in time, this will be reflected in stiffness in your muscular frame. This stiffness impedes the flow of Qi, which diminishes your health. Therefore, your mind and your thoughts have as much, or maybe more, to do with your health than the food you eat or the exercise you get.

Energy meridians, or *jing luo*, link all the organs and the entire physical body to the mind and emotional systems. This explains how T'ai Chi and QiGong's mind/body exercises integrate all aspects of the self into a powerful self-healing system.

T'ai Sci

Traditional Chinese Medicine (TCM) differs from the Western approach to medicine in that its focus is holistic. *Holistic* means it views the body as an integrated whole. A TCM doctor does not treat only symptoms, but rather tries to discover the root of health problems.

For example, if we have allergy problems, Western pharmaceuticals might send chemical missiles in to dry out the sinuses. This does stop the runny nose, but some medications may result in irritating the surrounding tissue by drying it out or causing other undesirable side effects. Acupuncture, on the other hand, or T'ai Chi, in the long run, will enable the body's natural balancing to occur, reducing the incidence of sinus problems in a way that nurtures the tissue. This is done by reestablishing the blocked flow of Qi that is at the root of the problem.

Know Your Chinese

The body's energy meridians, or **jing luo**, are a network of channels that move Qi through the body. *Jing* literally means "to move through," and *luo* means "a net."

What are these energy meridians that T'ai Chi helps unblock? By now you know that Qi flows through and powers every cell in your body, the way electricity powers your house. Without Qi, the cell would be dead, for Qi is the life force. Qi gets to the cells through the meridians. You can't see these meridians; you can only detect the energy that moves through them, just as you cannot see an ocean current in the water, but you can detect its motion.

Ancient maps of these meridians, made thousands of years ago by Traditional Chinese doctors, show 14 main energy meridians that carry Qi throughout the body internally and externally. The names follow, listed first by the modern acupuncture abbreviation, then by the English name, and a few followed by the Chinese name in italics:

- ◆ CV = Conception Vessel, or *Ren Mai*
- ◆ CX = Pericardium Channel
- ◆ GB = Gallbladder Channel
- ◆ GV = Governing Vessel, or *Du Mai*
- ◆ HE = Heart Channel
- ◆ KI = Kidney Channel
- ◆ LI = Large Intestine Channel
- ◆ LU = Lung Channel
- ◆ LV = Liver Channel
- ◆ SI = Small Intestine Channel
- ◆ SP = Spleen-Pancreas Channel
- ◆ ST = Stomach Channel
- ◆ TW = Triple Warmer, or *San Jiao* Channel
- ◆ UB = Urinary Bladder Channel

Acupuncture and T'ai Chi

Three aspects make up TCM: acupuncture, herbal medicine, and T'ai Chi/QiGong. All three share a common premise that Qi pours through the body and our health is diminished when the energy flow gets blocked.

So whether an acupuncturist is treating you with needles, an herbalist is prescribing herbs, or you are practicing T'ai Chi, you are trying to balance the imbalances, or unblock the energy that flows throughout your body. Millions of Americans now use alternative therapies like acupuncture and herbs. If you practice T'ai Chi daily, your relaxed state will help herbs or acupuncture work even more effectively.

The energy meridians, which flow throughout the interior of the body, have 361 points that surface at the skin. These are the most common treatment points acupuncturists use. But the whole body and even the mind can be treated with acupuncture because the meridians that surface at the skin also flow inside the body, through the brain and other organs.

T'ai Sci

Modern acupuncturists often call the Qi meridians *bioenergetic circuits*.

T'ai Chi and QiGong affect the same energy flow that acupuncture does, although acupuncture can be better for acute problems, whereas T'ai Chi is a daily tune-up. Acupuncturists may recommend T'ai Chi to their patients, and T'ai Chi teachers may recommend acupuncture to their students with chronic or acute conditions as a supplement to the students' standard medical treatments. T'ai Chi and acupuncture are very complementary.

Say "OOOOHHHHHMMMMMM"— OHMMeter, That Is

It is mind-boggling when you consider that many modern acupuncturists find acupuncture points with electronic equipment, not unlike an Ohmmeter, a device used to measure electrical resistance. What's more amazing is that acupuncture maps were made long before electronics was developed.

How did they know where those points were back then? They might have felt them. As you practice T'ai Chi and QiGong, you will eventually begin to feel the Qi flowing from your hands or in your body.

Get an Acupuncture Tune-Up

Acupuncture sees the body holistically, meaning that each small part of the body contains connections to the whole body. Therefore, an acupuncturist can treat any problem in the whole body through, for example, the ears. Likewise, any part of the body, or even the mind, can be treated through the hands or the feet.

One of the powerful health benefits T'ai Chi provides is a daily acupuncture tune-up. Because T'ai Chi is so slow and the weight shifts so deliberate, with the body very relaxed, the feet are massaged by the earth during a T'ai Chi exercise. The bottoms of the feet have acupuncture points that affect the entire body as well as the mind. The acupressure foot massage you get during a 20-minute T'ai Chi session stimulates all the acupuncture points on the foot, treating the whole body. This type of slow, relaxed motion makes T'ai Chi unique in providing you an acupuncture tune-up each time you do your daily exercise.

View the noninstructional *Exhibition of the T'ai Chi Long Form* and *Mulan Style Basic Short Form* on the DVD to visually understand the flow and effortless slowness of the forms that

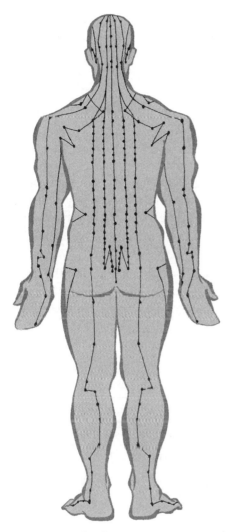

Here is an example of an acupuncture meridian map. This map also comes in a three-dimensional model.

A T'ai Chi Punch Line

There are also acupuncture maps for animals. In fact, some racing horses have their own personal acupuncturists. Many veterinarians are beginning to use acupuncture as part of their practice.

result in stimulating the acupressure points on the feet and throughout the entire body. *No other exercise provides this.*

Don't Be Zang Fu-lish

Another profound benefit T'ai Chi provides is a gentle massaging of the internal organs. Because T'ai Chi moves the body in about 95 percent of the possible motions it can go through, it not only clears the joints of calcium deposits, but it also gently massages the internal organs.

In TCM, this is a powerful therapy for optimum health. TCM recognizes that the body is an integrated whole whereby all the parts are connected by the flow of Qi. In fact, the Chinese system of medicine is built upon a *Zang*

Fu graph, which shows how organs interact with and depend on one another for good, healthy function.

Know Your Chinese

Literally translated, **Zang Fu** means "solid-hollow." Organs within the body considered to be hollow, like the stomach or large intestines, are Fu organs, while the solid organs, such as liver and lungs, are Zang organs.

Because T'ai Chi massages all the organs through its gentle full rotations, it helps balance all the integrating activities of the Zang Fu systems.

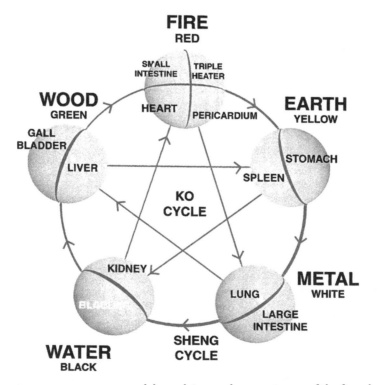

The Zang Fu system uses a memory model, applying each organ to one of the five elements of the earth. The Chinese see the world as made of Earth, Metal, Water, Wood, and Fire. The energy flow affects different organs through the Sheng Cycle and the Ko Cycle. This figure shows how organs are interactive and interdependent on one another for healthful function.

Be Kind to Your Emotions

Acupuncture, herbal medicine, and T'ai Chi/QiGong use the Zang Fu system to understand how the body, mind, and emotions integrate. A problem with a particular organ may have emotional symptoms. Likewise, a chronic emotional state may have a physical impact on the organs. The following list explains the Zang Fu connection between organs and emotions commonly related to imbalances with those organs or their energy channels:

◆ Liver = depression, anger
◆ Heart = excess joy (such as manic behavior), excess mental function
◆ Spleen = obsession
◆ Lung = anguish, grief, melancholy
◆ Kidney = fear, fright

Sage Sifu Says

If you go to a Traditional Chinese physician, he or she may likely ask you about your emotions as well as your physical symptoms because emotional states may help lead him or her to understand which organ's energy is deficient or in excess.

T'ai Chi benefits the mental and emotional states, not only by encouraging us to let go of the day's problems by focusing on breath and movement, but in other ways as well. T'ai Chi stimulates the organs with gentle massage, while stimulating the acupressure points on the feet and throughout the body with its gentle, relaxed postures. The breathing in T'ai Chi is full yet effortless, encouraging internal releases of mental and emotional blocks that also help the internal Zang Fu systems become less restricted, more free-flowing, and more healthful on mental, emotional, and physical levels. (Chapter 4 explains how T'ai Chi and QiGong can provide mental and emotional healing.)

Increase Flexibility

T'ai Chi increases flexibility not only by regularly stretching the muscles very gently, but through the Zang Fu system as well. As we age—especially but not exclusively men—we often find a depletion in our kidney energy. The kidney energy is responsible for the function of the liquid systems of the body. Therefore, the decrease in kidney energy that accompanies aging causes our connective tissue, such as tendons, to become brittle. We are then much more likely to tear or otherwise injure our bones or joints when we stumble or fall.

The tremendous balance improvements T'ai Chi offers are only part of why T'ai Chi practitioners are much less likely than other people to suffer falling injuries. The improved performance of all organ functions enhances the entire physical body's health. In fact, in this way, Sitting QiGong may also increase flexibility, even though it is a nonphysical exercise.

Western Medicine's Research on T'ai Chi and QiGong

After reading this section, you should be satisfied beyond a doubt that *T'ai Chi works*. When you get to the QiGong and T'ai Chi exercises in Parts 3, 4, and 5, you won't have to think about their benefits. The mind is the greatest healer; if you believe in the value of your therapy, it will be much more effective for you.

Stress Is the Symptom

By now you know that stress is the chief cause of illness in the modern world. As Western medicine discovers that T'ai Chi and QiGong are effective stress-reducing exercises, these powerful mind/body health tools are being used in more and more hospitals and prescribed by more and more doctors.

Studies show that reaction to stress can damage the entire body. It causes chronic hypertension (high blood pressure), which can cause the arteries to harden, and causes kidney damage and enlargement of the heart. Stress also has been shown to impair our ability to think and actually shrinks the hypothalamus and the hippocampus parts of the brain. Yikes!

A T'ai Chi Punch Line

TCM sees the body and mind intertwined. A rigid body can cause us to think rigidly as well. Or perhaps more accurately, a rigid mind can cause us to have a rigid body.

Who Ya Gonna Call?

T'ai Chi is a stress buster. An article in *Occupational Therapy Week* explains that T'ai Chi's emphasis on posture (see *Sinking into the Horse Stance* and *Locating your Dan Tien and Vertical Axis* sections on the DVD for proper posture examples) and diaphragmatic breathing (breathing from your diaphragm) accounts for a practitioner's reduction in muscular tension and the stress it causes. Patients using T'ai Chi report a greater ability to cope with fear and anxiety, as that physical relaxation is reflected in their mental attitude.

Bellevue Psychiatric Hospital in New York City provided T'ai Chi to both staff and patients. Its activity therapy supervisor said, "T'ai Chi is a natural and safe vehicle to *neutralize* rather than resist the stress in our personal lives, an ability which we greatly need to nurture in our modern, fast-paced society." View the noninstructional *Exhibition of the T'ai Chi Long Form* and *Exhibition of the Mulan Basic Short Form* sections on the DVD to see the *resistance-free* model of motion and the *slowing down* of mind and body T'ai Chi promotes. *You will likely find yourself feeling calmer from just watching the forms being performed!*

T'ai Chi Is Your Heart's Best Friend

Harvard Medical School's *Women's Health Watch Journal* reported that "T'ai Chi has *salubrious* effects" and that "practicing T'ai Chi regularly may delay the decline of cardiopulmonary function in older adults … T'ai Chi was found to be as effective as meditation in reducing stress hormones."

A Duke University study recently announced that managing stress controls heart disease even more effectively than exercise. Because T'ai Chi provides both powerful stress management and gentle exercise, T'ai Chi is your heart's very best friend. Now, go out and play nice with your new friend.

T'ai Chi Reduces Mental Stress

A study cited in the *Journal of Psychosomatic Research* claimed T'ai Chi study subjects reported less tension, depression, anger, fatigue, confusion, and anxiety. They felt more vigorous and, in general, had less total mood disturbance.

The *Journal of Black Psychology* states that many African Americans suffer from chronic high blood pressure. The article explains that hypertension is a physical result of psychological stress and proposes T'ai Chi as a holistic way of treating psychosomatic illnesses, or those illnesses caused by stress.

T'ai Chi may also help us think better. Research has shown that stress can limit the development of the hippocampus, the part of the brain that deals with learning and memory. T'ai Chi's ability to reduce stress responses may actually enhance our ability to learn and remember.

Sage Sifu Says

With all these T'ai Chi and QiGong facts swimming through your mind, now is a good time to practice QiGong's mind-clearing tools. Take a deep breath from your abdomen to your chest, and on the sighing exhale, let your shoulders relax away from your neck as they sink toward the floor. Repeat this several times, and as you release the breath, imagine that every cell in your body is relaxing as you release each breath.

Ironically, you will find that the more your mind lets go of trying to hold on to facts, the more easily it can absorb information.

T'ai Chi Lowers Body Stress

In an article on T'ai Chi, *Working Woman* magazine noted that "increasingly mind/body workouts are replacing high-impact aerobics, and other body punishing exercises of the 1980s. These mind/body workouts are kinder to the joints and muscles and can reduce the tension that often contributes to the development of disease, which makes them especially appropriate for high-powered, stressed-out baby boomers."

A Boost to Your Immune System

Prevention magazine reported a study on T'ai Chi's effects on the immune system. It found that regular T'ai Chi practice may increase the body's production of T-cells. These T-cells are T-lymphocytes. "Lympho-whats?" you might ask. It doesn't matter. What matters is that these little T-cells help the immune system destroy bacteria and possibly even tumor cells. If T'ai Chi can make more of these little buggers, what are we waiting for? Let's T'ai Chi one on!

Know Your Chinese

T'ai Chi and QiGong have long been known to boost the immune system. Ancient Chinese medicine understood the concept of the immune system, which the Chinese called *bu qi, bu xue,* meaning "tonify the Qi and blood." When Qi and blood are strengthened, we are better able to fight off infection and disease.

In China, QiGong is commonly prescribed as an adjunct to chemotherapy and radiation. Studies indicate that when QiGong is combined with standard cancer treatments, favorable results are obtained, treating virtually all forms and stages of cancer. Part of the reason for this success is that QiGong helps patients feel less helpless. Studies show that feelings of self-empowerment can have powerful healing benefits on the course of almost any disease, including cancer.

A T'ai Chi Punch Line

I was once studying T'ai Chi and QiGong in Hong Kong. Because of the time difference, I was waking up at 3 A.M. With nothing else to do, I became a particularly diligent student and practiced Gathering Qi or Standing Post for nearly an hour and a half each morning. After about a week of this, I began to visually see the Qi flowing around people, especially their heads. I noticed that those who seemed to be enjoying the day had large pluming expanses of energy around them, while those appearing driven and stressed had tiny, restricted energy emanating from them.

How Does T'ai Chi Fight for the Immune System?

American QiGong master Kenneth S. Cohen has dubbed a hormone called DHEA the Health Hormone. In his *brilliant* book, *The Way of Qigong: The Art and Science of Chinese Energy Healing*, Mr. Cohen explains that this hormone is believed to be linked to Qi.

DHEA is short for dehydroepiandrosterone. Yeah, I know, *forget about it.* But don't forget that DHEA is related to youthfulness, less disease, and a more functional immune system. According to Cohen, low DHEA levels have been directly linked to cancer, diabetes, obesity, hypertension, allergies, heart disease, and most autoimmune diseases.

When we are under a lot of stress, our body exhausts itself of this important hormone. Therefore, by practicing T'ai Chi, we can increase DHEA levels, thereby increasing our immune system's ability to fight whatever steps in the ring with it. Let's rumble!

T'ai Chi does two wonderful things to help us age healthfully: it maximizes the body's full potential to regenerate healthy cells, which actually slows the aging process. And it promotes a deep self-acceptance and self-awareness so that as our body goes through the challenges of aging, we are much better able to handle and adjust to those changes, both physically and emotionally.

DHEA and T'ai Chi, Back Together Again

DHEA is also involved in the aging process. Levels of DHEA tend to decline with age, but the decline is much worse when you're under chronic stress. Add natural aging and chronic stress, and you have an express train to an old body. Once again our old friend T'ai Chi comes to the rescue. T'ai Chi's gentle movements and breathing techniques promote the serenity that can keep DHEA from being depleted.

Know Your Chinese

Fan lao huan tong means "reverse old age and return to youthfulness." This is what the Chinese believe T'ai Chi and QiGong offer, and, of course, Western scientific methods are beginning to tell us how and why that happens. East meets West.

Of course, the increased circulation of blood and Qi also fully oxygenates the skin, which provides nourishment to your outer beauty. The Zang Fu system's being balanced by T'ai Chi's stimulation of acupressure points and massage of the internal organs also moves the liquids and oils of the body to the tissue that needs them, further adding to your external beauty and internal health.

Aging's Radical, Dude! (Free Radicals, That Is)

There's a pesky little *free radical* atom in your body called *superoxide* that causes the body to age. Not only does it cause wrinkles and age spots, but it can also weaken cartilage and joints. In fact, this superoxide may even induce cancer or other immune system disorders. *Obnoxious little thing, isn't it?*

T'ai Sci

Free radicals are atoms with an extra electron that bounce around wreaking havoc throughout the body. We see this with our eyes as aging. The calming effects of T'ai Chi and QiGong not only affect the mind, but can also reduce the damage done by free radicals, thereby slowing the aging process.

However, regular T'ai Chi and QiGong practice can protect your body from these pesky free radicals by activating an enzyme called *superoxide dismutase* (or *SOD*). SOD is our cellular superman and defends our cells from the ornery superoxides that break down our health systems.

A study of those who practiced QiGong for a half-hour a day for 1 year showed that their levels of SOD increased dramatically compared to people not doing QiGong. Another study showed a large increase in SOD after only 2 months of QiGong practice.

Make No Bones About It, T'ai Chi Does Your Body Good

The National Institute of Mental Health (NIMH) released a study showing that women under chronic stress with depression had weaker bones than those in normal emotional states. In fact, the stressed/depressed women had the bones of 70 year old women, even though they were only 40 years old.

T'ai Chi lessens the incidence of depression and the body's stress responses and is a gentle, weight-bearing exercise. These qualities might make T'ai Chi the best thing you can do to keep your bones healthy, even into old age.

T'ai Chi Does an Incredible Balancing Act!

For aging Americans, the simple act of stumbling and falling can often be fatal. The sixth-largest cause of death for older Americans is complications from falling injuries. This costs our country about $10 billion a year and causes tremendous suffering for older people as well as their families. We are all paying for our nation's poor balance in human suffering and in higher health-care and health insurance costs.

T'ai Chi was part of a balance study by Harvard, Yale, the Centers for Disease Control and Prevention, Washington University School of Medicine, and Emory University. T'ai Chi practitioners fell and injured themselves only half as much as those practicing other balance training. This is an amazing finding that can change the lives of older Americans.

Although many of us are not in the age group likely to suffer serious injury from falling, we can all benefit greatly by having better balance. Better balance puts much less stress on the body throughout the workday, and as T'ai Chi practice improves your balance, you will find that you have much more energy.

T'ai Chi Is Dirt Cheap—and Can Be Done on Grass!

Compared to the best balance training in the world, T'ai Chi is about twice as effective. Some of the other balance exercises studied in an Ivy League study on balance were very expensive computer models that required participants to go into a lab and practice. The simple exercises of T'ai Chi are not only much more effective than the other exercises, but they are very cheap!

T'ai Chi Is Gentle for Arthritis and Your Joints

T'ai Chi is an exercise few doctors will ever tell patients to *stop* practicing. It provides perhaps the lowest-impact weight-bearing exercise there is. We all need weight-bearing exercise to help build bone mass and connective tissue, but for those with rheumatoid arthritis or some other conditions, weight-bearing exercise is a problem. For these people, weight-bearing exercise can aggravate joints, causing tenderness or swelling.

However, a study cited in the *American Journal of Physical Medicine and Rehabilitation* wanted to see if T'ai Chi would harm rheumatoid arthritis patients. To the researchers' pleasant surprise, T'ai Chi did no damage whatsoever and provided the study participants with the safe weight-bearing exercise they seriously needed. The forms were modified for these patients, and everyone with arthritis or knee problems should be sure they do only forms that feel good to them, but this T'ai Chi discovery is good news for all of us because it gives us all a weight-bearing exercise that is safe even into old age.

T'ai Chi Is the Health Care of the Future

Most Chinese hospitals have long integrated Western crisis medicine with TCM. This is now rapidly happening in the United States as well. The American Medical Association recently recognized acupuncture as a valid treatment, which is causing Western doctors to look at T'ai Chi and QiGong even more intently.

Growing numbers of neurologists, cardiologists, general practitioners, physical therapists, hypertension specialists, and psychologists are already prescribing T'ai Chi and/or QiGong as treatment or supplemental treatment for many conditions. (See Part 6 for examples of T'ai Chi prescribed for specific conditions.)

As more Western scientific research is completed on the benefits of T'ai Chi and QiGong, this trend will expand. The result will be lower health-care costs for all of us.

T'ai Chi and QiGong's Healing Powers

When you first hear of the benefits of T'ai Chi and QiGong, effective for helping treat *all things* on *all levels*, it may sound like snake oil. "How can it do that?" you might ask. It's simple: it does this by connecting us to the most powerful healing tool there is—the healing power of the mind. The power of the mind is at the heart of our healing.

It is estimated that placebos can positively treat about 60 percent of our health problems. Placebos are sugar pills (or fake treatments) doctors sometimes give to fool patients into curing themselves. This gets the mind/body to trigger its own internal healing processes, by the mind simply telling itself it's okay for the body to heal. This indicates that the body has a tremendous potential to *self*-heal, *if we believe in the cure*.

T'ai Chi and QiGong are not placebos. They are powerful health tools that can give us access to the tremendous natural healing power of the body, the power *behind* the placebo. Many of these healing benefits are documented, and new research is emerging all the time. It's important for you to understand just how powerful these tools are so your mind will allow them to do their magic.

氣 A T'ai Chi Punch Line

Studies have shown that if patients "believe" something can cure them, the possibility that it actually will is much higher. Cynicism is found to be one of the single most hazardous behaviors for our health. If I have a choice between being smart enough to realize I'm incurable, or stupid enough to fool myself into curing myself—I'll be the fool any day.

The Least You Need to Know

◆ T'ai Chi facilitates the flow of Qi and health to your cells.

◆ Narrow thinking squeezes off life energy.

◆ T'ai Chi integrates the mind, body, and emotions.

◆ By toning our Qi, we tone all our healing systems.

◆ Only T'ai Chi provides an acupressure treatment and organ massage while promoting circulation and centeredness.

◆ You don't have to memorize how T'ai Chi and QiGong work. Just relax and do it!

becoming more efficient. If this sounds impossible, read on.

Frantic Action vs. Efficiency

T'ai Chi's ability to calm, energize, heal, strengthen, and tone the mind and body in a short, half-hour workout is unequaled. However, if you try to do T'ai Chi efficiently, it doesn't work as well. It's when you relax and don't try that T'ai Chi works its magic.

The idea that we can get something very worthwhile done without having high anxiety to hurry up and do it is a new concept for most of us. When you're viewing T'ai Chi exhibitions on this book's DVD, notice how *unhurried* and how powerful the movements look.

T'ai Chi Is Smelling the Roses

Our heart and mind seem to be in a constant state of turmoil. With the tidal wave of data the Information Age has swept into our lives, it's easy to always feel two steps behind the pack. We struggle to understand the latest technology, knowing full well that a newer version will be out before we learn the one that just came out. We forget to breathe and enjoy the *learning* in life, which, when you get down to it, is pretty much all there is to life. We are not and never will be done learning. So we might as well smell the roses on the way.

Learning to "love the learning" of T'ai Chi is one of the most important lessons T'ai Chi offers our frantic lives. Students sometimes come to T'ai Chi classes gung-ho to learn one set of forms and then move on. The concept that T'ai Chi is a lifelong process comes as a big shock. Students think they can hurry in, get fixed, get calmed, get healthy, and then get going. They want to hurry up and *finish* so they can hurry up to finish the next thing they want to hurry up and do. But by living this way, our lives just become a lot of hurrying. There is no finish in T'ai Chi or in life.

Ouch!

Many Western students feel hopeless upon learning that T'ai Chi is a lifelong process. We in the West are conditioned to expect immediate, short-term results. Don't be discouraged. T'ai Chi is a lifelong process that gives immediate results. Even if you just took one T'ai Chi class and practiced what you learned, you would get great benefit. It just gets better and better for the rest of your life.

T'ai Chi's calming effects can be felt immediately the very first day of practice, but not if you hurry up to feel them. You have to let go of the outcome and let the nice feelings be a pleasant surprise rather than an urgent demand.

T'ai Chi's movements flow one into the other, just as life's events do. By learning how to breathe and relax the body while moving through these events, we become an island of soothing calm even when we're in the center of the rat race. Our habit of letting go of the frantic demands of the day that fill our minds becomes easier and easier as we practice T'ai Chi.

Remember to Breathe (Everything Else Takes Care of Itself)

As a student in a T'ai Chi class (or at home), the very first thing you should do is close your eyes and breathe. Take deep breaths all the way into the bottom of your lungs and then let go of your breath, your muscles, and your day. Let go of everything you've done before getting here and everything you plan to do later. Just be here and now, breathing.

As your mind fills with remembering to breathe through your T'ai Chi movements and gravity forces you to focus on your balance, you must let go of the worries of the day. You cannot do T'ai Chi without letting go of thoughts about what to defrost for dinner or the laundry that needs to be done.

T'ai Chi does not advocate starvation or wearing dirty clothes. It does, however, advocate being 100 percent in the moment, whether you're doing T'ai Chi or washing clothes. This is what is called *mindfulness*, or being here and now. You'll find that the more you can let go of the dinner and the laundry to feel your breath, your muscles releasing, and the silken flow of your T'ai Chi movements, the more you'll enjoy doing the laundry or cooking dinner when you do get to it. The T'ai Chi practice of being here and now will seep into your daily life by reminding you to breathe as you move. While making dinner, you'll relax and breathe, enabling you to truly smell the fragrance of dinner.

We don't have to race if we are always where we like being. Then we never have to fear looking in the mirror and seeing a racing rat.

Sage Sifu Says

As T'ai Chi helps us "feel good" on a regular basis, we want more of that feeling. You might spend more time with people who nurture you and less time with those who put you down. This is a powerfully healthful, transformative part of doing T'ai Chi. As the movements in T'ai Chi teach you to ease around areas of discomfort in the body so as to expand mobility without injury, this echoes out into our lives. You begin to find nurturing ways to move and live socially.

The Power of Effortlessness

In our fast-paced, dog-eat-dog world, it's hard to believe that we can be more powerful when we are not straining. However, that is exactly when we are most powerful, not only mentally and emotionally, *but also physically*. Because we are so conditioned to be mentally and emotionally straining all the time, many students feel "guilty" for taking quiet, still time to heal their minds and emotions from the strains of the day. Those students need a real physical example of how we function more effectively when relaxed.

The Unbendable Arm

The Unbendable Arm exercise is a terrific physical example of the concept of "effortless action" and how powerful that kind of action is. In the West, we tend to think of big, straining muscles and huge forehead veins whenever we think of power.

T'ai Chi can rescue us from that sweaty, head-pounding delusion. In T'ai Chi, our goal is to move and stand with as little effort as possible. Ancient *Taoist* poets tried to explain in words the seemingly limitless power found in living lives of effortlessness with calm minds and quiet hearts. However, the concept of effortless power is so strange to Westerners that the following demonstration of the Unbendable Arm is worth a thousand words. (*Note:* If you have any arm or shoulder injuries, you may not want to do the Unbendable Arm exercise. Also, if you have difficulty performing this exercise, you may want to practice the Sitting QiGong exercise in Part 3 and then try again.)

T'ai Sci

Many Western psychotherapists use Taoist philosophy as they encourage patients to let go of obsessing on the outcome and rather enjoy the "process" of life. In fact, T'ai Chi exercises are recommended as an active model to achieve these healing ends.

The Unbendable Arm is a powerful physical example of the principle of effortless power. In my class demonstrations, I ask the largest, most powerful-looking student to try to bend my arm. Resisting with all my muscular strength, they nevertheless eventually bend my arm. However, when I completely relax my mind and body, thinking of an empty flow, or of airy relaxation pouring through my head, shoulder, arm, and on out my fingers through the walls of the building, they can't bend it. The students strain to bend my relaxed arm, yet they cannot.

Know Your Chinese

The focus of the ancient Chinese **Taoist** (pronounced *dowist*) philosophy is the invisible force of nature's laws. Its premise is that life flows through all living things the way ocean currents flow through the ocean. The Tao nurtures life and cannot be defined because it applies to all things. When we are calm and still in our hearts, minds, and bodies, we can "feel" or "sense" the subtle direction of Tao. Living the Tao is the most effortless, meaningful way to live, flowing with the Tao, the way a surfer rides the waves, while adding our own flair and best intentions to its currents. In the West, we may call the sense of the Tao a hunch or an intuition, or what feels right. Renowned physicist Brian Greene refers to a "sense of elegance" when choosing a direction in research. I think that aptly describes sensing the Tao.

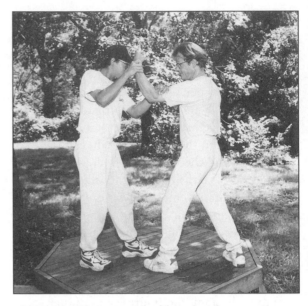

Notice that the person is able to bend my arm even as I use all my muscular strength to resist.

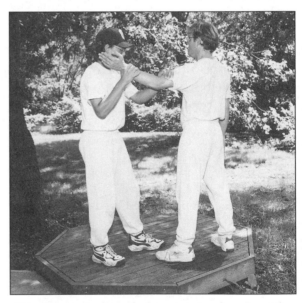

However, notice here that my arm is relaxed, yet the other person cannot bend it.

Our Flexibility Is Our Strength

This Taoist principle of effortless power is even more meaningful in our mental and emotional lives.

I use the Unbendable Arm not to demonstrate the physical power of effortless motion (although it does demonstrate that), but to dispel the myth that our straining is equivalent to productivity. When we breathe and relax while typing at the keyboard or answering the phone, we are so much more effective and real. We have time for the people in our lives instead of always rushing past them to get to the next urgent task.

Patterns vs. Chaos

T'ai Chi helps our bodies be more effective by relaxing our muscles. This allows a more ordered pattern of muscle use so our muscles aren't fighting other muscles. T'ai Chi also has the same effect on the mind. By quieting the mind of all the daily "noise," our mind can open to more orderly patterns of thought. The DVD's T'ai Chi exhibitions show the exhibitioners' awareness seems to be "inside themselves" on the process of effortless motion, not elsewhere, wrapped up in life's problems.

Coaching the Mind Team

Similar to the way the body fights itself physically with muscle tension, the mind also keeps itself in needless chaos with noisy thoughts spinning around in it. T'ai Chi and QiGong can end this internal battle and enhance the power of the mind and imagination. The slow, deliberate motions of T'ai Chi that calm the body and get the muscles to work together more powerfully (as demonstrated by the Unbendable Arm) organizes the mind, too.

Imagine life is like a football game and we keep getting batted around by really big linemen we call problems. The noise in our heads is deafening, as every time we get up from being knocked down, another big problem bangs into us. It's hard to even think about solutions when big problems bang into us one after another.

A T'ai Chi Punch Line

When studying T'ai Chi in Hong Kong as a young man, I was intrigued by the construction workers there. At the time I was in great shape, being a karate enthusiast who trained very hard. However, I was humbled by the much smaller, thinner Chinese construction workers who hauled enormously heavy bags of cement up bamboo scaffolds on their thin shoulders. They showed barely any exertion. Whether the workers practiced T'ai Chi or not, they had obviously absorbed some of its principles.

Now, imagine we could somehow be lifted up above the chaos to look down on what's happening from a higher, clearer angle, like a coach in the upper deck of the stadium. We would see patterns, or plays, forming. We would see how waves of linemen or problems flow. We could make adjustments before problems are right in our face, enabling us to choose the path of least resistance, not only making it easier, but getting much more yardage, or success, with each play. T'ai Chi practice continually lifts our mind to that higher, clearer perception.

Sage Sifu Says

The Taoist philosophers took a holistic approach to the world, meaning that they saw each little thing as kind of a model for bigger structures. For example, each cell in our body makes up the whole body; as individuals, we make up our family; our family makes the neighborhood, which makes the city, state, and society. Therefore, the most powerful contribution we can make to the world is to be the healthiest we can be, physically, mentally, and emotionally. If our health heals the world around us, then a healthier world around us also heals us. This is the kind of cycle that needs to spin out of control.

Innercise Integrates Outer Relationships

Phil Jackson, former head coach of the World Champion Chicago Bulls, is a Zen practitioner, and he introduced the entire Chicago Bulls basketball team to Zen exercises. T'ai Chi and QiGong exercises are from the same roots as Zen exercises and are often indistinguishable from them.

A T'ai Chi Punch Line

The Chinese character for Qi, or life energy, and the Latin root *spir*, as in *spirit*, mean "the air we breathe." Both ancient cultures obviously saw how our breath connects us to the life force. When considering that each of us has breathed an atom of oxygen that was breathed by Jesus, Buddha, and Mohammed, the Taoist claim that we are all connected becomes a very real concept.

The year the Bulls were introduced to Zen practices was the year they became the winningest team in the history of the NBA. This is no coincidence. The choreography the Bulls displayed that year was mind-boggling; the team often resembled one living entity rather than five separate players. As Zen exercise allows the mind to clear itself of its daily chatter or rubble, it also clarifies the communication between people. So just as the Bulls players began to quiet and clarify their own internal function by relaxing muscles and quieting thoughts they didn't need, they simultaneously clarified their player-to-player communication. This clarity is what we saw in the incredible plays the Bulls made that year.

This same clarity we cultivate through our daily T'ai Chi or QiGong exercises can help us clarify our relationships with others at work or home. Most social breakdowns are rooted in a lack of clarity, for if we aren't clear on what we want and need, we can never expect others to support our efforts. Whether it's our love life, our family, our work, or our social relationships, T'ai Chi's soothing way of moving through life will make relationships more healing and effortless.

People around us become easier to deal with when we are easier to deal with. T'ai Chi shows us how much of the external world reflects what goes on in our own heart and mind. *Dressage*, the national magazine for the Olympic horseback riding style, promotes T'ai Chi as perhaps the most effective exercise a rider can perform to enhance riding skills. What's fascinating is why: the article said that a horse picks up on the rider's mental and emotional stress levels. Therefore, if the rider does T'ai Chi before mounting his horse, the horse gives a smoother and quicker ride.

Imagine how much your unconscious mental and emotional turmoil affects those around you at home or work. Then think of how much your life would change if you did T'ai Chi before riding it.

Sage Sifu Says

The life force is clarity and simplicity and holds no need to compete. By letting go of desires, utmost calm is realized, and all the world arrives at effortless peace.

T'ai Chi-*Hut-Hut-BREAK* from Old Patterns

This is what T'ai Chi and QiGong can do. T'ai Chi's physical model of moving with the muscles relaxing off the bones is a model for letting go of mental and emotional obsessions. T'ai Chi allows us to let go of the chaos of life and lets our mind lift and observe, unattached to outcomes, grudges, or obsessive desires. It allows us to see more clearly the patterns that cause us to bump our head into the same old walls again and again.

Letting go of attachments or stepping out of the game from time to time gives us a fresh perspective. Fresh perspective is what allows us to exercise our "imagination muscle." It's the most effortless thing you can do. However, it's not always easy because it requires you to let go of all your thoughts, plans, and regrets. Creating space or breathing room in our busy days with T'ai Chi and QiGong helps our mind let go of old patterns. This allows our mind to open to the pure inspiration that wants to bubble up inside it.

T'ai Chi Dispels the Idea of Wrongness

The most mentally and emotionally healing concept T'ai Chi has to offer our hypercritical world may be that T'ai Chi dispels the idea of "wrongness." When you practice T'ai Chi, you never, ever do it "wrong." You just do it. Each time you do it, you relax a little more, you breathe a little easier, and your T'ai Chi gets a little better. On the DVD's T'ai Chi exhibitions, you may notice the practitioner's reveling in the simple pleasure of relaxed motion.

Ouch! _____

If the T'ai Chi instructor you study with is hypercritical, you may want to find another one who has more fun with T'ai Chi. However, be aware that if you are hypercritical of yourself by nature, you may unconsciously project that onto the instructor. Relax and enjoy yourself when in T'ai Chi class and when practicing at home. This will help your instructor relax, too.

T'ai Chi Is a Model for Life

The effortless sustenance T'ai Chi offers our lives is the understanding that we are always "perfect," that our lives are ever-evolving perfection. When we learn things about T'ai Chi that we can improve, it is much easier to adopt the new ways if the old ways don't have to be "wrong." This is one of the ways T'ai Chi makes a terrific model for life in general.

Our culture's concepts of wrongness constipate the ability to let go of old ways and move into new ways more easily. If something must be wrong before it can be discarded, we judge ourselves as wrong for having done it that way. If we see things in an ever-evolving state of improvement, then nothing is wrong and there are always better ways. Then we can see that we were right for having done it the old way, but can be even "righter" for doing it a new way.

The only wrong thing you can do in T'ai Chi is to tell yourself you're wrong.

T'ai Chi Breaks Limits

T'ai Chi's way of seeing exercise (and life) as a process leaves us always content with where we are, while always taking us past our old limits. When we obsess over getting things "right," whether we know it or not, we limit ourselves by thinking we are "done" when we get it "right." By giving up that myth, we begin to feel a limitlessness to life. T'ai Chi helps us feel bigger, dream bigger, and love bigger.

Each time you do T'ai Chi, you relax a little more deeply and become a little more self-aware, enabling you to continually improve your T'ai Chi.

When we stick with T'ai Chi long enough, we realize that our T'ai Chi improves each time we do it. More important, it helps us see that we never did T'ai Chi "wrong," for T'ai Chi is not a destination where a fixed level of perfection exists. Like our lives, T'ai Chi is an unfolding rose of improvement that blooms endlessly, more perfectly, and more beautifully each new day we practice it. An 80-year-old T'ai Chi teacher was being interviewed about his 60 years of T'ai Chi practice. The interviewer asked him, "At what point did you feel you mastered T'ai Chi?" The old teacher replied, "I'll let you know as soon as I do."

Sage Sifu Says

When problems arise, use your energy to fix the problem rather than wasting energy fixing the blame. Fix the problem, not the blame. This concept goes right to the heart of what T'ai Chi offers our harried lives.

T'ai Chi Enhances Life

Does T'ai Chi make life perfect? No, not more perfect than it already is. And it is always perfect, although sometimes it may seem perfectly miserable. T'ai Chi encourages you to let go of outcomes and simply pour your energy into whatever nourishes life—your life and all life. The flow of Qi through the body is like water through the roots of a plant. It doesn't fix anything in particular; it just enhances life. As the Taoist philosopher Lao Tzu put it, "The best people are like water. Water nurtures all things and never is in competition with them."

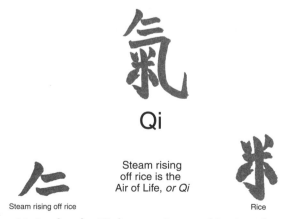

Qi

Steam rising off rice is the Air of Life, *or Qi*

Steam rising off rice

Rice

Notice that the Qi character is a combination of steam or air (the top half) and rice (the lower half). The character for Qi (pronounced *chee*) represents steam rising from rice, meaning "the air of life," a symbol for effortless sustenance.

T'ai Chi and QiGong Strengthen the Imagination Muscle

Sitting QiGong is a motionless exercise. So if the slowness of T'ai Chi makes it seem ineffective to many Westerners, the stillness of QiGong may seem like a colossal waste of time. However, this could not be further from the truth.

These slow, mindful exercises bring the brain into a very calm state known by scientists as the *alpha state*. This is a highly creative state of mind. In fact, three of the great discoverers of our time had their greatest insights while in alpha states. Albert Einstein, Thomas Edison, and Nikolai Tesla all claimed to get their greatest discoveries while in a state of mind that Einstein called "wakeful rest."

Know Your Chinese

The **alpha state** is a frequency of brain waves that occurs during a state of relaxed concentration. It is one of four brain wave frequencies: delta is the slowest, prevalent during infancy or in adults during sleep; theta is present in drowsy, barely conscious states; alpha is during QiGong relaxation exercises; and beta is common when the mind is busy or restless.

Why is the alpha state such a creative state of mind? For one thing, when our mind is filled with normal daily worries, plans, and television/radio noise, there's no room left for creative thought. Also, there may be a deeper knowledge within our minds that we can't access when our minds are busy with daily problem-solving. Psychologist Carl Jung said there is a "collective unconscious" that holds great knowledge, and that we all have access to of our awareness. Our thoughts and emotions, and lastly our physical bodies, are results or reflections of an even deeper part of us. That deeper part is the unmanifest part of ourselves. QiGong and T'ai Chi's ability to connect us to that deeper, unmanifest part of ourselves is a potent self-improvement tool.

Imagine that our lives are like a big, clear glass of 7Up. If you stand up and look down into it, you see only the bubbles bursting up into the air from the surface. This represents the manifest, or obvious, part of life. From this angle, you don't see the deep liquid below that formed these bubbles.

As we experience events in our lives, we are seeing only the bubbles popping up from the surface, not what formed them. These emerging bubbles may take the form of successes or recurring problems. Perhaps we go from one bad relationship to another or constantly fight with our kids.

However, T'ai Chi meditation, and especially QiGong meditation, lets us sit down and look at the "7Up glass of life" from the side, allowing us to see the source of the bubbles. From that angle, we can see that those bubbles, or events of our lives, actually form way down below the surface. This is the unmanifest, or unconscious, part of life.

So our quiet meditations place us sitting on the side, observing the true depth of life. Here we see that experiences are really end results rather than big surprises. Events in our lives are actually results of patterns or habits we have below the level of what we usually see and feel. We set ourselves up for success or failure by how we think of ourselves every day. If we think of ourselves as valuable human beings capable of success, then we're much more likely to form bubbles that pop on the surface of our lives in the form of success stories.

Likewise, if we continually think of ourselves as bad or worthless, we will probably create bubbles to reflect that worthlessness in the form of relationship problems. If we believe that we are worthless, we will attract people into our lives who will reinforce that reality. *Pop, pop, pop.* Seeing only the pops makes us feel like victims of life. (See Chapter 11's Sitting QiGong exercise for a personal experience of this deeper awareness. See Appendix C for information on my audio CD program that includes this and three other sitting exercises to further expand your internal journey.)

Masters Are No Longer Victims

Being a T'ai Chi or QiGong master means we are no longer content to remain ignorant of the unmanifest part of life. However, it's not enough just to know that our responses and actions in life have deeper roots. We have to find ways to change the patterns that form those bubbles way down below the surface of our lives. T'ai Chi and QiGong can help us do this. By quieting our minds and bodies, they can enable us to feel inside where we hurt or hate. By feeling the source inside, we can begin to let it go. For example, if we have a grudge or unresolved hatred in our hearts, we may walk around with a chip on our shoulders. The world will quickly give us confirmation of that grudge or hatred because people we meet will seem cold to us as we greet everyone with the chip on our shoulders, which makes us seem cold to them.

Another example: sometimes I get angry with my kids, but what I'm actually responding to are things I hold inside. When I realize this, my responses change. I find that practicing my quiet T'ai Chi or QiGong meditation when I get home allows me to be clearer with my kids. I clear out stuff inside so that if I do have a problem with their blasting stereo or whatever, I am responding to that and not to something I brought home from the office (or from my childhood).

By being more aware of the dynamics of our lives, we feel less like victims. We can begin to affect our world more clearly.

As our lives become less cluttered with bubbles of discord, there is more room for a limitless flow of life energy or Qi to course through us. We become a geyser, watering and nurturing everyone and everything lucky enough to be around us.

T'ai Chi and QiGong's daily pattern of reminding us that we can *change* with ease, and feel safe in the world without constant muscle-tensing apprehension, is a powerful tool. Sometimes it seems as though the body literally squeezes past burdens within each and every cell. T'ai Chi's ability to allow the body to release those burdens held from the past so each cell can fill with and be nurtured by life energy is a powerful way to affirm that we are worthy of success and love. On levels deeper than we can ever understand, T'ai Chi's easy and pleasant tools help create bubbles in the deepest part of our hearts and minds that burst outward and upward in lives that reflect our very best potential. Cheers, Master! Yeah, that's you.

Ouch!

Modern psychology says we are bombarded on many levels by information and stress that we never consciously perceive. Therefore, trying to attach mental reasons to feelings of being out of control, frightened, or stressed is often a futile exercise. T'ai Chi helps us let go of stress on deep levels that we will never even notice.

Master Your Own Self

As discussed earlier, the six leading causes of death are stress related. Because stress is something we *can* control by practicing T'ai Chi and QiGong, using these tools means we can powerfully affect our future in a positive way.

Luck of the Draw

We all are born with natural tendencies to height or weight, or for some, diabetes or heart disease. Our genes give us those tendencies. However, we can play a big role in how those genes play out. If we drink or smoke heavily and ignore a healthful diet, we can help increase the possibility of the onset of diabetes and heart disease, while likely stunting our growth and expanding our waistline.

On the other hand, we have been lucky enough to live in an age when T'ai Chi is as available as Coca-Cola. We have the ability to put an eternal ace up our sleeve, which heavily stacks the odds in our favor to live long, healthful, productive lives.

Gut Feelings: Tuning Your T'ai Chi Antennae

My T'ai Chi classes for children always began with one simple question: "Can you feel the inside of your bodies?" With little hands pressing into tiny rib cages, their puzzled faces usually answered no. My next question was, "Have you ever felt a stomachache or a headache?" Obviously, they all had.

T'ai Chi and QiGong are about moving the body, but they are also about feeling the body from the inside. We can feel pain inside, so we can also feel pleasure. Awareness of these feelings enables us to detect normal or abnormal function at a very early stage. By becoming attuned to our internal function, by quieting down, moving slowly, and listening to the signals inside our body, we tune our T'ai Chi antennae. We become conscious of our heartbeat and our respiration rate. The T'ai Chi players in the T'ai Chi exhibitions on the DVD are obviously

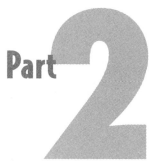

Part 2

Suiting Up and Setting Out

Part 2 prepares you for your first T'ai Chi class, fashionwise and otherwise. However, for those with T'ai Chi experience, it may also provide valuable insights on how to make your ongoing T'ai Chi experience even more meaningful, both internally and externally.

Knowing when and where to do T'ai Chi can enrich your T'ai Chi experience and can even help treat certain health conditions. You will also learn the ins and outs of T'ai Chi etiquette and how to get the most out of T'ai Chi by becoming aware of the different ways it is taught.

Even advanced T'ai Chi students can benefit from Part 2's explanation of some of the mental and emotional challenges T'ai Chi practitioners encounter. If you're an advanced student, this part will validate your experiences. If you're a beginner, these insights will prepare you for those same challenges so you can ride them out and hang in there for the long, beautiful haul with T'ai Chi. If you're a teacher, this part will help you and your student through those rough spots.

In This Chapter

◆ Finding a place to learn

◆ Choosing a T'ai Chi or QiGong class

◆ Choosing an instructor and style of T'ai Chi or QiGong that's right for you

◆ On the DVD: the basic tenets of T'ai Chi *posture*, *speed of motion*, plus *Fan and Sword form samples*

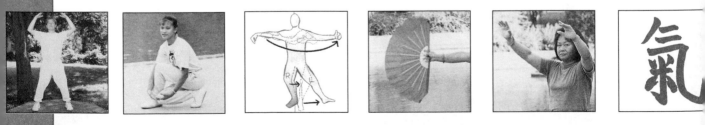

Chapter 6

Knowing What You Want: Finding the Right T'ai Chi or QiGong Class

T'ai Chi's main lesson is to find the most "effortless" way to live. Therefore, when you're looking for an instructor or class to learn T'ai Chi, you don't want to force yourself into a square hole, being the round peg you are. You want to find the class that best suits you. And because T'ai Chi can be learned in many different ways, there's a perfect way for everyone.

This chapter helps you decide what class is right for you by informing you of what's available and providing you with some questions to ask yourself. The clearer you are on what you want from T'ai Chi, the easier it will be for an instructor to fulfill those needs or to point you to another class that can.

Locating a T'ai Chi Venue

Just as T'ai Chi is good for so many different things, it is offered in many different venues. What benefits you seek from T'ai Chi may help determine where you want to study it. Your options include the following:

Businesses. Many company wellness programs offer T'ai Chi classes for employees. Ask your employer. Of course, you may want to study T'ai Chi outside of work or in addition to the company class. Don't limit yourself to taking only the classes at work (however, many company classes are subsidized, so this can be an incentive to do it at work). If you take a work class and enjoy the instructor but would feel more comfortable with a class outside of work, ask the instructor about other classes he or she offers.

Martial arts studios. Many of the "hard" martial arts studios specializing in karate, kung fu, or kenpo offer T'ai Chi classes as well. In fact, a few have offered them for many years. Be aware, however, that martial arts studio classes will often focus on the martial applications of T'ai Chi. Usually, these classes will be more comfortable to someone who is interested in an athletically demanding form of T'ai Chi. These classes may involve a gentle sparring technique known as Push Hands, although Push Hands has many mental and emotional purposes as well.

Even if you are not interested in T'ai Chi's more athletic or martial applications, you should not rule out a martial arts studio until you speak with the instructor. Instructors have their own style, and where they teach may not necessarily indicate how they teach or what their focus is.

Senior centers. Many community centers or senior centers offer T'ai Chi classes geared toward seniors. If you have a chronic condition that limits your mobility or you are rehabilitating from an injury, you may find these classes very helpful. These classes generally progress at a slower, gentler rate than T'ai Chi for the general population.

Being a senior, however, doesn't mean that these are the classes you need. Many seniors want to learn more quickly and are up to more physical challenges. As a senior, you may enjoy a general community class or even a martial arts studio class. You can't judge a T'ai Chi-er by his or her cover. In fact, the more you do T'ai Chi, the younger your "cover" is going to look.

Community center and hospital classes. Many cities' parks and recreation departments now offer T'ai Chi classes, as do many hospitals. These classes are usually for the general population and include students of all ages. Generally, these classes progress through learning movements at a little faster pace than the senior program classes do. However, even the briskest pace is usually quite manageable if you spend a little time each day practicing between your weekly or semiweekly classes.

Church classes. Many houses of worship now offer T'ai Chi classes. T'ai Chi is a health science, not a religion, yet T'ai Chi's promotion of quiet mindfulness is beneficial to anyone's spirituality. Therefore, if your church offers T'ai Chi classes, you may enjoy the instructor's spiritual focus.

Colleges and universities. Usually T'ai Chi is part of the adult continuing education departments of colleges and universities, although many schools now offer accredited T'ai Chi programs. In the continuing education departments, these classes are often introductory courses that give you a sample of what T'ai Chi offers. This tendency occurs because colleges require minimum enrollments to continue classes. Because advanced classes are often too small to sustain through colleges, many quality instructors offer intro programs so students can meet them and then continue advanced study through private studio programs.

Support groups. Many support groups for Parkinson's disease, multiple sclerosis, fibromyalgia, and AIDS (to name a few) may facilitate ongoing T'ai Chi classes for their members. In the Kansas City area, for example, I am working with the local Veterans Hospital to provide T'ai Chi classes specifically geared toward wheelchair practitioners. I am also encouraging hospitals to design rooms with hooks in the ceiling for "climbing harnesses," thereby enabling people with balance disorders to practice T'ai Chi without worrying about falling injuries.

If you are a wheelchair practitioner, you can participate in regular T'ai Chi classes by simply modifying the movements to suit your needs. Interview instructors to find one who can fit your needs. You will need to make your own innovations of the movements if the instructor has no experience with wheelchair students. Also, you may want to take the beginning class more than once because you will have more to cover than your standing peers will.

Sage Sifu Says

Try not to use only your head when choosing a T'ai Chi class. Just because the school looks nice, the credentials sound great, or the instructor has studied for a gazillion years doesn't mean this is the right school for you. When you talk with the instructor, ask yourself, "How do I feel about this person?" That is the most important question.

Also, do not compare yourself to other students in your T'ai Chi class. Some will be more flexible, some will be less flexible, and none of that matters at all. Lao Tzu said that he who does not contend is beyond reproach. You are always perfect, now and after years of practice.

If you have special needs or conditions, you should contact your local hospitals to request T'ai Chi classes geared to your needs. If you have a support group, organize it to encourage the hospital to innovate. T'ai Chi is about forming a life that fits your needs, and creating your T'ai Chi class can be a great T'ai Chi exercise. Have fun and be creative!

Choosing a Class

Choosing your class depends on your needs. What can you afford? What do you seek to accomplish? After you decide on the questions to ask, call around and speak to many different instructors. If they are available, take workshops or sample classes through community education programs. This will give you an opportunity to meet the instructors face to face and experience their instruction before enrolling in a long-term class (although most T'ai Chi classes run for only 6 to 10 weeks at a time).

What Is the Cost?

It's helpful to look at T'ai Chi as if it were health insurance. If you pay now with a little money for the class and some time each day to practice, you will reap the benefits for the rest of your life. You will also likely be more productive and make more money in the future. You'll be more relaxed and do less "impulsive" buying, which will save you money, too. T'ai Chi is a very inexpensive investment with a very high return.

The cost of T'ai Chi classes is often determined by the location and by the quality of the instruction. For example, many martial arts studios have longer contracts, which, of course, require a larger up-front investment. Each studio is different, though, so call and inquire.

No matter what your income level, you will likely be able to find T'ai Chi instruction you can afford. Many T'ai Chi hobbyists offer very low-cost classes through YMCAs or other community centers. Although these instructors may not be as highly trained as those teaching in the more expensive locations, you can still benefit from attending these classes. Also, higher cost does not guarantee higher-quality instruction. If an instructor has studied for many years, he will likely be better than one who has studied for only a year or two, no matter the location.

T'ai Sci

Research shows that stress costs businesses $7,500 per employee per year, driving up our health-care costs. To fight stress-related health costs, some insurance companies and health-care providers now pay for or subsidize the cost of T'ai Chi and/or QiGong classes for their clients. Call your insurance carrier to ask if your T'ai Chi class tuition can be rebated or credited on your premiums. Then be sure to get a receipt from your instructor.

However, to maximize your T'ai Chi experience, you will likely have to pay a bit more. Still, even the highest-quality instruction is usually no more than $10 or $15 per class or $80 to $120 per 8-week session (cities vary in cost). In most cities, this is about the cost of a movie, popcorn, and a soda—not a bad investment for something that can change your life. Also, if you're a member of a senior center or support group, your organization may be eligible for a grant. Such grants may enable you to get very high-quality T'ai Chi instruction at little or no cost to participants.

How Often Should I Go?

Different locations will offer different programs, but one T'ai Chi class per week is the most common arrangement. Each class usually runs from an hour to an hour and a half. Some studios may offer two or more classes per week.

There's nothing wrong with going to several classes a week if you can afford it—as long as you don't do it to the point of burnout. One class per week is often enough as long as you practice at home during the week. In the beginning, you may practice at home for only about 10 minutes a day, but over time, your practice will get longer as you learn more movements.

Eventually, you won't have to think about practicing because you'll look forward to it. Whenever you're having a rough day, or maybe when you want to celebrate having a good day, you may find yourself slipping out to "play" T'ai Chi. You might also want to do T'ai Chi when you get home so you'll be in a better mood to fully enjoy your evening.

Ouch!

Most people don't practice enough, but don't go berserk and burn yourself out, either. Once or twice a day is good for a full session. However, if you're having a tough day at work and want to sneak off for a quick T'ai Chi session in the bathroom or empty boardroom, go for it.

Evaluating an Instructor

There are many things to consider as you look for a T'ai Chi instructor. Degrees or awards your potential instructor holds are not "most" important. More important is whether your instructor's temperament feels good to you. Another consideration is the style of T'ai Chi you want to learn.

Instructor Personality

One good question to ask a prospective instructor is, "Do you still study with other T'ai Chi teachers?" If a T'ai Chi teacher still studies, it tells you she understands the great depth and endless width of the art and science of T'ai Chi. T'ai Chi expands for a lifetime, just as we expand as living beings, always growing and learning.

Sage Sifu Says

Because it's new and slow, at first you may find T'ai Chi a little frustrating. This is not uncommon. Remember to breathe and let go of frustrations you feel as you release your breath. Also, you may catch yourself displacing your frustration on the instructor. Be aware that this can happen, so don't give up on a good instructor for the wrong reasons. The more you can lighten up on yourself, the more the people around you, including your instructor, can lighten up as well.

Second, what is your focus? Are you interested in treating an illness, growing spiritually, or learning the martial applications of T'ai Chi? The answer to this question will help you know what to ask your prospective instructor. For example, if you have a high-stress corporate career, you may feel comfortable with a T'ai Chi instructor who has experienced that lifestyle and can offer you ways to use the tools he teaches in ways meaningful to your life. Or if your desire is spiritual growth, you may seek an instructor who focuses more on that aspect of T'ai Chi. If you have a particular health problem, you may connect well with a teacher who has the same problem. T'ai Chi is multidimensional in approaches and benefits, so any instructor from any walk of life will be good for you if you feel comfortable and accepted in his presence.

What I needed personally as a T'ai Chi student was patience. I needed an instructor who didn't scold and patiently allowed me to grow at my own pace. Of course, the art of patience is at the core of T'ai Chi, so if your teacher isn't patient on a regular basis, that instructor probably isn't living his or her T'ai Chi.

You want a teacher who actually uses the tools she teaches and has benefited from them. You don't want a teacher who's simply teaching because the health club or hospital she works for told her to learn it so she could teach it. If a T'ai Chi teacher is actively using the tools, she is getting better at using them and is growing and expanding as a human being, which makes her better at everything she does, including teaching T'ai Chi.

T'ai Chi instruction is not like a regular job. The instructor should be someone who uses the tools and is immersed in the art of personal growth. This doesn't mean this person is some kind of saint. Don't fall into the trap of thinking the T'ai Chi instructor is "above" the trials and tribulations of normal life. A good teacher is someone who lives all that stuff and is lucky enough to have learned the wonderful tools T'ai Chi offers to make the absolute most out of what life offers. A good teacher is not above fear, stress, and worry, but he is learning how to use T'ai Chi to grow as much as possible, and can communicate to you how he has coped and how T'ai Chi might help you cope as well.

A T'ai Chi teacher doesn't tell you what's right or how to grow. An instructor explains how the growth tools T'ai Chi offers have helped them grow. Whatever truth resonates to you is what you take. A T'ai Chi teacher's life, health, or balance may not even be as good as yours, but it is much better than it would be if he didn't practice T'ai Chi. Therefore, a T'ai Chi instructor can teach a prize fighter how to punch harder and a basketball star how to shoot better, even though the athlete could soundly defeat the T'ai Chi teacher in the sport. A T'ai Chi teacher teaches the tools of growth, but we all grow in our own ways and at our own pace.

As obvious or strange as it may sound, often the best teachers are the ones who make T'ai Chi seem the simplest and easiest rather than hard and complex. We are sometimes led to

In This Chapter

◆ Finding the best place and time to do T'ai Chi

◆ Getting the most for your T'ai Chi buck

◆ Making time for T'ai Chi

◆ On the DVD: examples of what *video T'ai Chi* instructions may look like

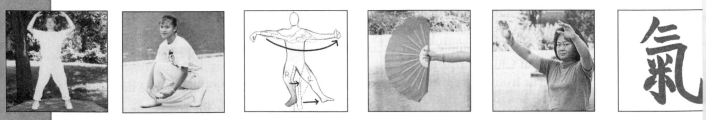

Planning Ahead: Where and When to Practice T'ai Chi

This chapter explains where and when to do T'ai Chi, as well as what to wear. As you read, you will discover that these questions not only are a matter of etiquette or convenience, but they can also affect the health benefits you get from T'ai Chi.

You also will discover the advantages of a large class versus private instruction and video/book instruction versus (or in addition to) live classes. You'll also find tips on how to make time for whatever T'ai Chi program you choose.

Home Practice vs. Class Study

Although practicing at home by yourself on a regular basis is how you realize T'ai Chi's benefits, studying with a qualified instructor—in class or at home via video, if classes don't work for you—is an essential part of the success of your home practice. No matter how many years you study T'ai Chi, you can still benefit from studying in classes. T'ai Chi, like life, is an endless growth process.

Most of us in the modern world want fast answers. We like to take classes or workshops and move on. And sometimes our educational motivation has more to do with getting our hands on a piece of paper that says we know something than with personally being changed by the knowledge.

Therefore, most people rush through a T'ai Chi course to learn a few moves and then think they're done. Of course, you do get some benefit from any exposure to T'ai Chi. Things you learn on the first day can benefit the rest of your life. But why stop there? T'ai Chi can offer you a deep ocean of experience. After 20 years of T'ai Chi practice, I still study with my instructor and enjoy class, book, and video instruction by other teachers. And even though my very first class was beneficial and wonderful, I still find benefits that carry into my home practice in each and every new lesson. Also, as a teacher, I often get new insights into T'ai Chi by learning from other teachers' classes, books, and videos, even those of different styles.

T'ai Chi provides lifelong benefits and should be practiced for the rest of our lives. However, this isn't a marriage contract. Don't feel smothered by this. Drop in and out of T'ai Chi as often as you like. T'ai Chi will always be patiently waiting for you when you come back, like a touchstone or a port in a storm. Eventually, you will do T'ai Chi simply because you feel pretty spectacular when you do. Besides finding classes enjoyable, you will discover that T'ai Chi attracts interesting people, and the social aspect will draw you as well. If self-confidence is an issue, you'll find that most T'ai Chi classes are friendly and low key. However, you can also boost your confidence by learning T'ai Chi from a video program, to help you feel more comfortable beginning live T'ai Chi classes, even a different style. The basics of T'ai Chi often transcend styles. Bottom line: *do whatever it takes for you to enjoy T'ai Chi!*

> **Sage Sifu Says**
>
> If you get frustrated by a class and drop out, don't make it a life sentence. Keep coming back to T'ai Chi. Each class will make you more confident. Repeat the beginner class as many times as you like; there are no deadlines or expectations in T'ai Chi. Relax. Take your time. Play.

Bookworm T'ai Chi

T'ai Chi books are great for helping you understand the philosophy, art, and science of T'ai Chi, and as supplements to classes, or video instruction if classes don't work for you right now. However, a book cannot replace a live instructor or the other benefits of a class or the verbal/visuals of video lessons.

It's difficult to explain in books how the body moves through movements, because books are dependent on still photographs. The ability to see an instructor move and to ask for clarification or hear other students' questions is invaluable. Also, it's easier for instructors to explain things in person in stages while you relax; when using a book, you have to remember facts because the instructor isn't there to remind you.

The DVD with this book will greatly enhance the book's text and illustrated instruction. Also, I accept questions by phone or e-mail from users of my 4-hour *real-time* class, like the T'ai Chi Long Form DVD, *Anthology of T'ai Chi and QiGong: The Prescription for the Future* (see Appendix C for details). Or check my website, www.smartaichi.com, where I'm developing a "frequently asked questions" section. This information may benefit you no matter what style you study.

Video T'ai Chi

If you don't have access to T'ai Chi classes or simply can't work them into your life yet, a video or DVD is the next best way to learn. You can use books to supplement your understanding of what videos teach, too. Using books and videos together can help maximize the benefit of your T'ai Chi practice. As the videos teach visually and audibly enabling your mind to relax, the books round out your intellectual understanding of the movements and exercises.

Consider that the average 8-week introductory T'ai Chi class entails at least 12 hours of instruction. The average T'ai Chi video is 1 hour. As you can see, it's difficult for an instructor to explain a 2,000-year-old art and science that's so rich in benefits in a 1-hour video. Some videos are done in multivolume, several-hour sets, which is the best way to go if you don't have access to or time for live T'ai Chi classes yet. I offer a 4-hour real-time DVD/VHS T'ai Chi Long Form program and a Mulan DVD, which together total well over 5 hours of instruction (see Appendix C for details). The 1½-hour DVD provided with this book is derived from carefully selected excerpts of my fully instructional programs. When the 4-hour *real-time* instructional DVD described in Appendix C is combined with the detailed instruction in Chapter 15 and throughout this book, it is a powerful learn-at-home program.

 Sage Sifu Says

Videos can be great supplements to your ongoing T'ai Chi class, especially if your instructor has produced one or approves one for the class. Be aware, however, that even if a video covers the same style you are studying, it might look different.

Bookstores, magazine ads, and martial arts stores are usually good places to find an assortment of T'ai Chi videos, beyond my programs offered in Appendix C.

The Horary Clock

Acupuncture, Chinese herbal medicine, and T'ai Chi understand that the body has natural rhythms that align with certain organs and functions. You can actually use this "horary" (hourly) clock to treat problems. Each organ has certain hours, called peak hours, that are generally the best for treating that organ:

11 A.M. to 1 P.M.	Heart
1 P.M. to 3 P.M.	Small intestine
3 P.M. to 5 P.M.	Bladder
5 P.M. to 7 P.M.	Kidney
7 P.M. to 9 P.M.	Pericardium
9 P.M. to 11 P.M.	Triple burner
11 P.M. to 1 A.M.	Gallbladder
1 A.M. to 3 A.M.	Liver
3 A.M. to 5 A.M.	Lung
5 A.M. to 7 A.M.	Large intestine
7 A.M. to 9 A.M.	Stomach
9 A.M. to 11 A.M.	Spleen

In Part 3, I introduce some QiGong exercises for specific organs. However, T'ai Chi can generally *tonify* all the aspects of the body and every organ. Therefore, T'ai Chi practice at a peak hour could provide a good therapy. Yet if your peak hour is in the middle of the night, you may prefer a Sitting or Lying QiGong exercise to focus Qi into the desired organ. The Sitting QiGong exercise in Part 3 gives you a great technique to use in peak hours.

Know Your Chinese

In Traditional Chinese Medicine (TCM), the word **tonify** means "to strengthen, energize, and imbue with health." Therefore, it can be applied to Qi, blood, tissue, organs, or processes in the body or mind.

Outdoor vs. Indoor

The single most important thing about practicing T'ai Chi is that you actually *do practice it*. Where you practice is secondary. Don't construe the following recommendation to do T'ai Chi outdoors to mean that you should not practice inside. If you can do T'ai Chi outdoors, do so. However, if you don't feel comfortable doing it outside because of where you live or the weather, then by all means do it inside.

Practicing Outdoors

The purpose of T'ai Chi and other QiGong exercises is to promote the flow of Qi. Qi's life energy flows through us and all living things. Therefore, the Chinese have always advocated performing T'ai Chi outdoors, where you can enjoy and benefit from the Qi of other living things. In fact, TCM teaches that when we do T'ai Chi, our relaxed body and mind benefit from nature's healing energy even more.

Just being in nature has a soothing quality, so if T'ai Chi can magnify this benefit, all the better. German physician Dr. Franz Mesmer, from whom we get the word *mesmerize*, worked with patients suffering from psychotic episodes. Reportedly, Dr. Mesmer would instruct his patients to sit with their backs against a tree whenever they felt an episode coming on. His patients were said to benefit greatly from this "nature therapy." As you practice T'ai Chi in your backyard, the park, or even next to the

plants in your house, you may experience the benefits of this therapy for yourself.

Choosing a Surface

T'ai Chi should be practiced on a level, predictable surface, especially when you are beginning. As you play over the years, you may experiment with more uneven and challenging surfaces. You can perform T'ai Chi on grass, sand, dirt, or pavement. It's good to practice on varying types of surfaces because this gives your mind/body communication even more information for improving your balance.

Try to choose a flat area out of direct sunlight. Soft morning sunlight or evening light is all right, but do not practice in direct sunlight during the hot part of the day. You will discover that practicing T'ai Chi in different light is challenging as well. Doing T'ai Chi in the dimming light of sunset challenges you to use more internal and less external balance references.

Sage Sifu Says

Your balance fluctuates from day to day, yet like a bullish stock market, it is always improving. So on days when your balance is at its worst, don't think you're not benefiting from T'ai Chi. Rather, let go of constantly measuring your progress. Enjoy your loss of balance even as much as you enjoy the T'ai Chi on days when your balance is great.

Practicing Indoors

The benefits of doing T'ai Chi indoors are pretty obvious if it's freezing or smoldering hot, or the mosquito population is in full production. Although outdoors is optimum, you can experience the benefits of T'ai Chi anywhere and at any time. When you're having a tough day at the office, it's great to slip off to the restroom or the supply room to drift into a T'ai Chi getaway. If you practice T'ai Chi at home before work or in the evening, it's often just more convenient to practice inside.

One problem students encounter indoors is space. As you move through your T'ai Chi repertoire, you often will cover more ground than your living room provides. If the next step takes you smack into a wall, just remember where you are, move back a couple steps, and pick up where you left off. Eventually, you won't even think about it. T'ai Chi pours into your living room, just like it easily and naturally flows into your life. Just as T'ai Chi encourages an almost liquid relaxation of mind and body, its use and benefits can seem to pour into every nook and cranny of our lives with much benefit.

Last but not least, when you're doing T'ai Chi indoors, minimize noise around you by turning off the TV and stereo. However, don't let noises *beyond your control* be an issue. Noise is in the ear of the beholder.

Ouch!

When you run out of room doing T'ai Chi, adjust by moving back or forward two steps and then resume. This is "apartment T'ai Chi" for you city dwellers. Don't psych yourself into thinking you cannot practice T'ai Chi because your house isn't big enough. These are not limitations, but opportunities to learn flexibility in mind as well as body.

Large Class vs. Private Class

Surprisingly, learning in a large class has several advantages over more expensive private lessons, although both have their own strengths, depending on your needs.

The Pros and Cons of Large Classes

If an instructor is in great demand, his or her classes will inevitably be larger. Therefore, you will get less personal attention but will benefit from the quality of instruction. On the other hand, you might find instructors in less demand with smaller classes who can provide you with more personal instruction. Decide what your priorities are, and choose a class size that meets your needs.

You can learn very effectively in a large class setting. In fact, being in a large class has distinct advantages. As fellow classmates ask questions for clarification, you can benefit by their inquiries. Also, you will discover that T'ai Chi classes have a group energy. Just as plants emit life energy, so do other people, and as your classmates practice T'ai Chi, you can bask in the glow of their presence—and they in yours.

Usually, an accomplished T'ai Chi instructor will have numerous advanced students who will help as assistants. In a larger class, you can benefit from the expertise these students have to offer. Note that advanced students probably are less than perfect, but so is the instructor. You will learn T'ai Chi in layers, and the advanced students can give you a layer of instruction that the instructor can add to or polish over the months and years.

T'ai Chi classes will benefit you even if you take them for a short time, providing you with tools you can use for the rest of your life. However, it's best to take classes for a lifetime. It is fun, beneficial, and a great way to meet interesting people, so why not? By doing so, you have no deadline or rush to progress at a certain speed. If you practice for a few minutes every day, you will likely learn the forms quite easily. However, if you need to repeat the beginning class again—and again—that's no problem.

Ouch!

Do not assume the instructor is aware of a problem you have with a movement or the class program. Ask questions during class to clarify instruction. However, if you have concerns about the program, discuss it with the instructor after class. Before you stop attending a T'ai Chi class in frustration, discuss your concerns with the instructor. Most instructors want to help you get it—that's why they're there.

If you're in a large class, you may have to move around a bit to see what the instructor is doing. Move to wherever you need to be to see. T'ai Chi is very informal. Usually, in a very large class advanced students will position themselves, in various locations so you can follow them if you cannot see the instructor clearly. If you're not sure what's being taught, raise your hand and ask for clarification. Don't be shy about this. The best T'ai Chi classes are ones in which students interact and ask questions. The least-productive classes are those in which the teacher does all the talking.

The Pros and Cons of Private Lessons

Very few people get private lessons. Part of the reason is that they can be very expensive. A good T'ai Chi instructor usually will begin at about $75 per hour and can go up significantly from there.

However, some people, such as emergency room physicians, have erratic, demanding schedules and are forced to take private lessons. This is a highly effective way to learn the T'ai Chi forms in a very short period of time, because the instructor's entire focus is on you.

Private lessons can also be beneficial to those learning to be instructors, thereby enabling them to learn minute details and background on movements and their purpose.

T'ai Sci

Any malady should be discussed with a physician. However, in addition to your medical doctor, you might want to discuss your condition with a certified doctor of TCM. Using T'ai Chi and QiGong on your own can be a powerful adjunct therapy for a condition you may be treating; however, if used under the direction of a TCM practitioner, they may be even more effective.

Time Out for Class and Practice

To maximize your T'ai Chi benefits, it's best to spend about 20 minutes in the morning doing T'ai Chi or a Sitting QiGong meditation exercise. Then spend another 20 minutes in the evening doing whichever one you didn't do in the morning.

Usually the first response to this suggestion is, "I don't have an extra 40 minutes a day!" If that is your response, ask yourself the following questions:

Do I spend 40 minutes a day watching TV?

Do I spend my morning and afternoon breaks drinking soda or coffee and chatting?

Do I ever spend time eagerly waiting to access the Internet, waiting for the computer to print, or waiting for dinner to bake?

For most of us, the answer to at least one of these questions is yes. If you look, you probably do have an extra 40 minutes a day. So the main difficulty in doing T'ai Chi isn't really having the time, but *deciding* to do it. When we decide to do it, we find that we will make time. Beginning new life habits is one of the single most difficult things people attempt. But T'ai Chi is worth it. Also, remember that if you practice T'ai Chi or QiGong two or three times a week for a few minutes, *that's much better than not doing it at all! Enjoy! Lighten up!*

Sage Sifu Says

Because T'ai Chi practice calms us and clears our minds, it actually creates extra time. When we are calmer and clearer, we are more efficient, we are easier to live with, and we find it easier to relax and sleep. So the 40 or 50 minutes we spend on T'ai Chi and QiGong can save us hours in effort and frustration.

Life Habits Are Hard to Change

T'ai Chi is new for you. You will find that it will take time to get used to doing it every day. Don't punish or scold yourself when you forget. Just enjoy it when you do it. The following example will help you see just how difficult it is to change life habits so you can go easy on yourself as you begin to adapt to a new life with T'ai Chi:

A study of cardiac recovery patients shows just how difficult it is to change. Patients were given a choice of two therapies to follow after their heart attacks. The first was only to take medication and be released within days. Unfortunately, that first choice carried a prognosis of another possible major heart attack within a

few months. The second choice involved staying in the hospital for a much longer period to learn stress-management techniques and new dietary changes, and it offered a much rosier forecast of the patients likely going several years before another coronary. Amazingly, nearly all the patients opted to leave immediately, even though it increased the likelihood of a premature death.

What is ironic about T'ai Chi is that even though it may be difficult to incorporate into your life at first, it will make all other healthful life changes much easier. T'ai Chi is a technology designed to help us change with less effort and stress. Therefore, the longer we practice T'ai Chi, the easier it is for us to change. So if you decide to go on a more healthful diet, stop smoking, or start getting out in nature more, the effort you make to learn T'ai Chi will make all those other efforts to change more "effortless."

T'ai Chi Is Positively Effortless

Studies show that when we change for positive reasons, we are much more likely to change our habits. Therefore, rather than do T'ai Chi because your blood pressure is high or your stress levels are unbearable, do T'ai Chi because it feels good. Don't rush through your T'ai Chi, but make it a little oasis in your busy day. Slow down enough to feel the pleasure of the movement and the stretches. Enjoy how good it feels to breathe deeply and let the whole body relax. This will condition you, day by day, to love the feeling T'ai Chi gives you, causing you to look forward to it and miss it when you don't do it.

Make a Calendar

If you want help remembering to do T'ai Chi, create a T'ai Chi calendar and place it on your refrigerator door. Every time you do your T'ai Chi or QiGong, mark a big X on that day's square. As you begin to get a few days in a row, you'll want to keep that string going. You'll also begin to notice that the more X's you have on the calendar, the better you feel. Your awareness becomes more subtle and pleasant, which will help you make the transition from doing T'ai Chi for the calendar accomplishment to doing it for how it makes you feel.

Ouch!

When you forget to do T'ai Chi, don't scold yourself. Your mind plays funny games to keep from growing and changing. Making ourselves "bad" for not immediately adopting new life habits is one of those games. If you forgot to do T'ai Chi yesterday, just relax and do it now—no big deal. Breathe and enjoy.

Social T'ai Chi

T'ai Chi clubs are increasingly popular in the United States (and worldwide)—as they have been for centuries in China—because even though T'ai Chi is a terrific personal exercise and is thoroughly enjoyable alone, it can also be a terrific social event. T'ai Chi clubs offer a group energy that can heighten the pleasure T'ai Chi provides.

T'ai Chi clubs also are very supportive and encourage T'ai Chi players to practice on their own. When we have a class or a club to get together with, we are much more likely to practice on our own at home. We want to improve our T'ai Chi so we can play more complex T'ai Chi games using mirror-image forms and other games involving several players. Continuing with a T'ai Chi class or club for the rest of your life is a great way to stick with T'ai Chi for the long haul. Social T'ai Chi is also terrific because T'ai Chi practice can extend your life substantially; if you outlive all your peers, you won't be lonely because you'll still have your T'ai Chi club to hang out with.

The Least You Need to Know

◆ If you don't have access to or just can't make it to live T'ai Chi classes, videos (see Appendix C) and books can be very useful.

◆ Treat certain organs by using T'ai Chi and the "horary" clock.

◆ Although outdoor T'ai Chi is optimum, indoor T'ai Chi is great, too.

◆ Large classes can be great if you ask questions. If you use video or DVD instruction, find a presenter who'll respond to questions (such as the author of this book!).

◆ Use a T'ai Chi calendar to get used to practicing. Eventually, T'ai Chi will become an integral part of your life.

In This Chapter

◆ Dressing for T'ai Chi

◆ Preparing mentally and physically for class

◆ Knowing what is expected of you

◆ Learning T'ai Chi lingo

◆ On the DVD: insight into how *classes break down movements* progressively and the *internal massage* quality

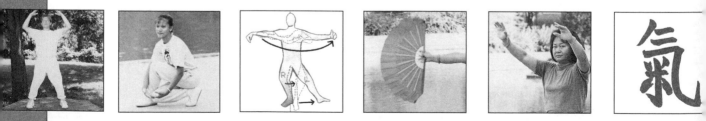

Chapter **8**

Be Prepared: Your First Day of Class

In this chapter, you learn what to wear to do T'ai Chi. Yet beyond fashion concerns, this chapter prepares you mentally, emotionally, and physically for your first day of class. Even those currently involved in T'ai Chi will find these mental and emotional insights into T'ai Chi challenges helpful.

This chapter also provides you with many ways to get the most out of T'ai Chi training by describing class structure, explaining what is expected of you, and clarifying terms you may encounter in class.

Choosing Your T'ai Chi Wardrobe

Ultimately, you can do T'ai Chi in any kind of clothing, but certain clothing *is* suggested for class. Typically, T'ai Chi students wear anything they want. It is helpful to wear something loose and stretchy and to leave jewelry at home; however, the rest is often up to you. The most common T'ai Chi suit is a T-shirt and sweat pants. Spandex or body suits, although not prohibited, are not typically worn in T'ai Chi.

If you practice T'ai Chi at the office, know that longer dresses can make it more difficult for an instructor to see your posture or leg placement, but don't skip class just because you have a longer dress on that day. Also, even though everyone will likely be wearing office clothes, they should kick off their heels. If you go from the office to a studio or community class, or if your company holds classes in an exercise area, bring some sweats and tennis shoes to change into.

Some studios, especially martial arts studios, may require more formal attire. If so, they will direct you to a martial arts supply store that sells the appropriate garb, or the studio may provide them.

What footwear you wear depends on the location. Tennis shoes are fine for most T'ai Chi classes. However, some studios that offer T'ai Chi, such as martial arts or yoga studios, require bare feet. It's not advisable to wear only socks in these studios because socks can be slippery. If you need arch support and attend a class in these locations, you may be able to wear tennis shoes that have never been used on the street or Chinese kung fu shoes. These nonstreet shoes will not damage the floor, but check with the instructor before purchasing them.

Ouch!

Some Chinese masters caution against practicing T'ai Chi barefoot because it opens the feet to "pernicious influences." This sounds sinister, but it may only mean that you could chill if the ground is cold or pick up an infection if the ground is dirty. Conversely, others say it is good to practice barefoot because it connects you to the earth, whereas your rubber shoes electrically isolate you from it.

The only hard-and-fast rule all instructors follow on footwear is that you cannot wear heeled shoes. Heels are hard on your back, make balance difficult, and change the way your whole body moves. If you're doing T'ai Chi at the office, just kick off your heels or bring tennis shoes if they feel more comfortable.

Considering External and Internal Hygiene

T'ai Chi has very few external hygiene rules, but internally, it's good to prepare yourself mentally and emotionally by letting go of some myths about yourself and exercise.

External Hygiene

Unlike most other martial arts, T'ai Chi usually requires no contact between participants. Therefore, hygiene rules are pretty much like those for daily life. You will be fairly close to others, so if your job leaves you a little ripe, you may want to shower before T'ai Chi class. However, if you come to class from the office, there shouldn't be a problem. The only concern might be if you attend class at a studio that requires you to go barefoot. If you go straight from the office to one of these classes, you might think about using some wet towelettes to clean your feet before going into class.

Don't wear heavy cologne or perfume into class because it might be overwhelming to others during the deep breathing you do in T'ai Chi. Also, leave jewelry at home, especially jangly jewelry.

Internal Hygiene

Cleansing the clutter from your mind, heart, and body is the most important thing you should do before attending your first—or one hundredth—T'ai Chi class.

In the long run, T'ai Chi will help relieve allergy problems, but if you have heavy allergies and are heavily medicated, it may be helpful to lighten up on the medications before T'ai Chi if your medications make your balance more difficult or make it harder to focus. However, never adjust your prescription medication without your doctor's approval.

If you haven't tried acupuncture for your allergies, now might be a good time to try it. It can be a terrific nonpharmaceutical way to alleviate allergy symptoms with great results. Acupuncture treatments cannot harm you, but they can enhance your clarity or balance.

T'ai Chi and Massage Therapy

T'ai Chi is meant to loosen the mind and body and increase internal awareness (see the *Moving QiGong Warm Ups Excerpt* on the DVD for more on internal awareness). Tension disconnects the mind from the body. Therefore, you may find it very complementary to begin massage therapy before your first T'ai Chi class and to continue massage therapy for the rest of your life. Most good T'ai Chi teachers will advocate massage therapy as part of your T'ai Chi training, just as many good massage therapists will recommend T'ai Chi to their clients. You also might find that massage therapy is helpful in relieving chronic problems such as allergies.

Sage Sifu Says

As T'ai Chi teaches the body to move and change more easily and effortlessly, it provides a model for the mind and heart to change more easily. As you continue with T'ai Chi, you may discover you eat more healthfully, drink more water and less soda, get better rest, adopt habits such as regular massage therapy, and spend more time with people who make you feel good about yourself.

Resistance to Change

T'ai Chi helps us change. Our minds and bodies get accustomed to the way we have always done things, even things that are not really good for us. Therefore, on a subconscious level, parts of us resist good changes that T'ai Chi fosters because we don't want to let go of the way we've always been. Part of us likes to be a "couch potato" and doesn't like the way T'ai Chi is getting us more involved in an active life. Resistance to change may manifest itself in many ways and may …

◆ Cause you to scold yourself, to tell yourself you are too clumsy, too uncoordinated, too slow, or too tired to do T'ai Chi.

◆ Tell you T'ai Chi is for other people who are better, smarter, stronger, or more coordinated than you are.

◆ Tell you the teacher doesn't like you or T'ai Chi is dumb and useless.

◆ Tell you it would be much more fun to watch TV and eat potato chips tonight than going all the way out to your T'ai Chi class.

◆ Tell you, "You're already too far behind; don't go back there," if you miss a class.

If you hang in there long enough, however, you will discover that after nearly every T'ai Chi class, you will feel much better than you did before going. If you become conscious of the voices of "resistance" and see them as the debilitating illusions they are, you will be more likely to stick with T'ai Chi.

"Wrongness" Is Our Culture's "Resistance"

Your T'ai Chi progress will be held back by something that affects our entire culture. If you understand this, it will take a great deal of pressure off you and your instructor. Most Western students are obsessed with learning the T'ai Chi movements "perfectly," and this causes them stress, which slows their ability to learn and enjoy T'ai Chi. In fact, we often convince ourselves that our attempts to learn are so "imperfect" that it is pointless to continue with our study.

Ouch!

Students often obsess on remembering each detail the instructor tells them; some even bring a pad and pencil to class. Don't do that. Relax. Good instructors will repeat important things over and over. Let yourself enjoy the class. Don't make T'ai Chi class another "important," "serious" thing in your life. Let it be playtime.

T'ai Chi will show you on a very basic level that you are never "wrong." You are growing and learning how to do things better and better each and every day of your life. T'ai Chi is simple enough to use the very first day of practice, but its richness is so subtle that you can refine your T'ai Chi movements for the rest of your life. Therefore, you do not need to "perfect" the first movement before learning the second. You learn a layer of the movements, and learning that layer changes who you are and how you function. Your new and improved self can then learn the movements at yet a deeper, more subtle level, and so on for years and years. T'ai Chi leaves you in an endlessly blooming state of perfection.

Attending Your First Class

When entering your first class, you probably aren't sure what it will look like, how to treat the instructor, or what is expected of you. So let's look at these expectations one at a time.

Mainly, you will be expected to relax and enjoy yourself. You will also have a little homework, but as you'll see, this could be the best homework you ever had.

How to Address Your Instructor

You have several possible options for addressing your instructor. The safest way to find out what is right for the class you enroll in is to simply ask the teacher how he or she would like to be addressed. The formal Chinese term for T'ai Chi teacher is *Sifu* (pronounced *see-foo*), meaning "master of an art or skill." However, many T'ai Chi classes in the West are very informal. Most instructors simply go by their first name.

If a Chinese teacher asks you to call him or her Sifu, this is not because of an ego trip. Actually, this is a great compliment. This means they consider you a worthy student, and that is an honor.

Class Structure

T'ai Chi is informal, and each class is different. Some classes begin with a Sitting QiGong exercise, using chairs forming a circle. For this relaxation exercise, the instructor will likely lead the group through an imagery exercise as they sit quietly with their eyes closed. Other classes will not use chairs and may begin with a standing relaxation exercise, also with the students' eyes closed. Still other instructors may begin the class by leading students in warm-up exercises without first practicing a QiGong or relaxation exercise.

Ouch!

Your main goal in T'ai Chi class should be to relax and breathe. By not trying too hard, you learn more easily. Students who frustrate themselves by mentally repeating that they "can't get it" usually prove themselves right. If you really can't learn the movement, just follow the other students as you breathe and relax. You'll feel good after class, and you can repeat the session again—and you'll be the expert in class the second time around.

Once relaxation exercises are done, the physical class structure will probably have students staggered throughout the room, facing the instructor. The instructor usually faces the class, which forms lines throughout the room, giving each student enough space to swing his or her arms without striking another student. However, smaller, more informal classes may form a circle. An instructor may alternate facing the class or demonstrating the moves with his or her back to the class. He or she might also move around the room to give students different angles to see from.

If you're in a class that's formed in lines facing the instructor, find a place where you can see what he or she is doing. Many large classes will have advanced students to help, and you can watch them if you can't see the instructor. If you can't see what's going on, ask questions or change places. Be clear about your needs. The teachers want to help you understand the movements, but in a larger class, they may not know you need further explanation. Don't be afraid to speak up.

The following list gives you an idea of the process a T'ai Chi class might go through; however, each instructor has his or her own format:

◆ Sitting or Standing Relaxation Exercise (if your class performs this).

◆ T'ai Chi warm-up exercises—gentle, repetitive movements that prepare you physically and mentally for T'ai Chi (many warm-ups are moving QiGong exercises and are discussed in detail in Part 3).

◆ After warm-ups, the instructor may teach individual movements to practice, or if she teaches by exhibition, she will begin performing the entire T'ai Chi set and you will be expected to follow along.

◆ Your homework is the movements themselves, although it is highly recommended to begin using the QiGong relaxation exercises at home for your own health and pleasure.

T'ai Chi usually does not require anyone to sit or lie on the floor; however, some instructors may have warm-up or cool-down exercises that require it. If you are unable to do so because of an injury or physical limitation, discuss alternatives with the instructor.

> **Sage Sifu Says**
>
> You can get all the benefits from T'ai Chi without straining. You don't have to memorize all the terms, do the movements exactly like your teacher does, or read any certain books. T'ai Chi's amazing benefits will come to you by simply breathing deeply, relaxing your mind, and playing T'ai Chi in class and every day at home. Play T'ai Chi every day, and everything else will take care of itself.

How Are T'ai Chi Movements Taught?

T'ai Chi forms involve a series of choreographed martial arts poses that flow together like a slow-motion dance. How these movements are taught can vary. Some classes are taught by example, meaning the instructor will lead the group all the way through the entire T'ai Chi form and the students mimic until, over time, they remember all the movements.

However, many classes are taught for different levels. In these classes, the movements are broken down into one or two movements per class. If you are an average learner, these classes are preferable. It's much easier to learn one movement at a time and practice it all week than it is to try to assimilate an entire T'ai Chi form. It's easier to memorize movements in smaller bites. Realize your learning will be much easier if you don't miss classes, because for each class you'd miss, that would make the learning bites get larger. View the lesson excerpts on the DVD to get a feel for how movements may be broken down in classes.

To help you get the most out of your classes, review the following points on how T'ai Chi is taught or might be studied:

◆ Warm-ups and relaxation techniques are usually repeated weekly, although if you practice these every day on your own, you will be all the better for it.

◆ You must learn and practice the actual T'ai Chi movement of the week on your own that week.

◆ Each week a new T'ai Chi movement will be added to your growing form or repertoire.

◆ The form will get longer and longer each week until you learn the entire form. The DVD's *Long Form Lesson 7 Excerpt* contains excerpt lessons from my multihour real-time program (see Appendix C for more info) relating to 5 consecutive movements of the 64-movement Long Form. Viewing this will help you see how your form will grow week by week as you add a new movement each week.

◆ Long forms of 20 minutes take between 6 and 8 months to learn.

◆ Short forms of 10 minutes may take 2 to 6 months to learn, depending on the instructor and the form.

◆ Advanced students often repeat beginning or intermediate classes for years to refine their performance of the T'ai Chi forms.

◆ Advanced students may serve as assistant instructors in class.

◆ As an advanced student, you may be asked to assist new students learning the forms for the first time. T'ai Chi, like all martial arts, is based on a mentoring system. As an assistant, you'll usually teach the first of the following three stages of T'ai Chi instruction.

◆ T'ai Chi is taught in three stages:

1. The movements are learned.

2. The breath is incorporated into the regimen by learning an inhalation or exhalation that's connected to each movement.

3. A relaxation element or awareness of the flow of energy through the body is

learned. Although the first step offers many benefits from the first day, the benefits get richer and deeper with each level you learn.

> **Sage Sifu Says**
>
> Normal T'ai Chi exercises can be easily adjusted to conform to your living room's size. Also, the more advanced Sword or Fan forms some styles teach, although more challenging, can easily be done indoors, too. For example, you can use retractable swords and leave them retracted when you're practicing indoors. The bottom line is, you can always practice T'ai Chi, no matter what style or where you are.

You Mean There's Homework?

T'ai Chi class exposes you to the movements, but then you must practice those movements at home. There are two ways to look at this: either as another burden on your life's full plate or as a chance to take a break and let all the weight of the world roll right off your shoulders.

The very first movement you learn on the very first day of class is a fantastic QiGong relaxation exercise that, if you do it in the right frame of mind, can help you begin to dump stress. If you do the T'ai Chi movement only to prepare for the next T'ai Chi class, it won't be that relaxing. However, if you breathe deeply and let every muscle of your body relax, allowing the burdens of the week to roll off your shoulders each time you practice the movement, it'll feel great! Refer to the *Long Form Lesson 1 Excerpt* on the DVD to see how the first movement can be used as a *relaxation therapy*, even as you learn it, by including deep, full breaths. Learning in this spirit can make all the movements become relaxation therapies even as you learn them (more on deep breaths in the DVD's *Moving QiGong Warm Ups Excerpt*).

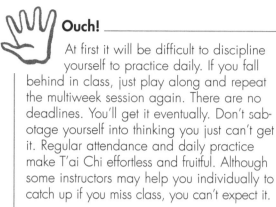

Ouch!

At first it will be difficult to discipline yourself to practice daily. If you fall behind in class, just play along and repeat the multiweek session again. There are no deadlines. You'll get it eventually. Don't sabotage yourself into thinking you just can't get it. Regular attendance and daily practice make T'ai Chi effortless and fruitful. Although some instructors may help you individually to catch up if you miss class, you can't expect it.

To learn T'ai Chi, you will need to practice at home. But we learn T'ai Chi because it feels good, so why wouldn't we want to practice something that makes us feel good?

T'ai Chi Etiquette

Most instructors are happy to get questions during class. The rest of the class, or at least some of them, are probably facing the same uncertainties or challenges you are. A good instructor has been studying many years and may not remember all the challenges new students have, so your inquiries help him *help you* as well as the other students in class.

If your questions are criticisms of the format or structure, it would be best to offer them to the instructor personally after class. The instructor may not be able to fix it, but he may explain why it is done the way it is.

Knowing Your Martial Terms for T'ai Chi

Because T'ai Chi was originally a martial art, an introduction to some martial arts terms may be helpful. When you learn T'ai Chi, your instructor may use these or similar terms to describe the T'ai Chi movements.

Understand that any one of these martial arts movements can be done any way that you need to do it for your own comfort. So if you have an injury or condition that limits your movement, do it in a way that feels comfortable to you. Never strain yourself to do something that doesn't feel right; just modify it a bit, kick lower, or reach less. As you play T'ai Chi in a way that feels good, over the days, months, and years, your kicks will get higher and higher.

A T'ai Chi Punch Line

Many of the movements in T'ai Chi have martial arts applications and were patterned after the movements of creatures or images in nature. Therefore, T'ai Chi movements serve practical self-defense purposes and simultaneously are soothing natural motions that encourage the flow of Qi through the body just as Qi flows through all of nature.

Punches

T'ai Chi has punches. They're not hard, grunting punches, but instead soft, relaxing punches. There are generally three types of punches used. Both punches illustrated in the following figures begin with your fist by your hip, with the palm side of the fist turned up toward the sky. The first is a common T'ai Chi punch and begins with the fist at waist, palm turned in toward the body, with no rotation of the fist as you punch. The other two are slightly more complex and, therefore, are shown in the following figures. However, then you do a full twist as you send it out to punch in front of you, so the fist ends up with the palm facing down to the ground.

The second punch is a Half Twist Punch. This begins with the fist near the hip with the palm turned up. When you throw the punch out, the fist rotates only a half turn, leaving the knuckles lined up in a row, top knuckle toward the sky and pinkie knuckle toward the ground.

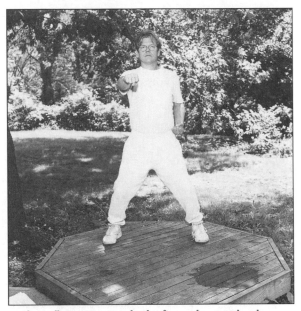

In the Full Fist Turn Punch, the fist ends up palm down.

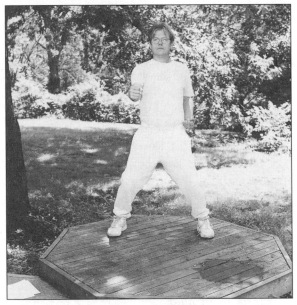

The Half Twist Punch is more common in T'ai Chi, with the knuckles ending up vertical.

Punches are generally not thrown out in big, circular haymaker punches like John Wayne threw. They come straight out from the hip like a piston, with the elbows tucked in. The elbows usually don't extend out from the sides, but stay in near the body.

Because of the many Western movies we've seen, most Westerners also try to punch with the whole upper body, actually leaning into the punch. However, in T'ai Chi and all martial arts, you do not normally lean into the punch. When the punch is complete, your head will still be posturally aligned above your dan tien.

Although there may be exceptions to how punches are thrown in various T'ai Chi forms, usually the rule of not leaning forward is always observed. However, there are times when the fist may circle around rather than punch straight out from the hip. In Part 4, you will see an example of this in the Box Opponent's Ears movement.

Blocking

There are three types of blocks: In Blocks, Out Blocks, and Up Blocks. Their names explain whether the arm is blocking in toward the center of your body, out away from the center of your body, or up away from the body. One other less-used block is the Down Block, which looks like an Out Block in reverse. An example is seen in Part 4's "Wind Blowing Lotus Leaves" movement.

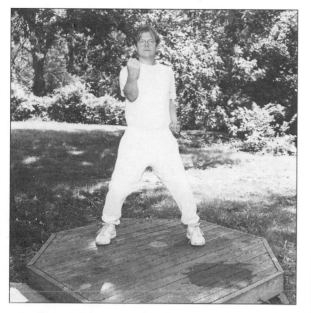

An In Block begins with the fist near your ear; then your arm is pulled in a circular motion across the front of your body.

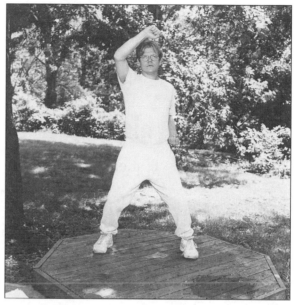

An Up Block begins with the fist palm facing your face; then your palm is twisted away up to the sky, blocking up and away.

Kicks

T'ai Chi generally uses three kicks: Side or Separation Kicks, Crescent Kicks, and Front Kicks. Examples of these kicks can be viewed in Part 4, where the side kick is called "Separation of the Right Foot (and Left Foot)," the Crescent Kick is called "Wave Hand over Water Lily Kick," and the Front Kick is called "Front Kick."

The Least You Need to Know

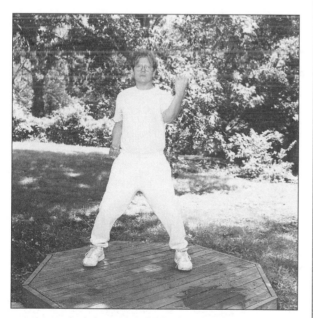

An Out Block begins with the fist near your groin; then your arm is pulled in a circular sweep up across your body to block outward.

◆ Before your first T'ai Chi class, ask the class instructor what you should wear.

◆ T'ai Chi can encourage healthful lifestyle changes, such as massages or drug-free treatments for health problems.

◆ Practicing T'ai Chi makes life changes easier.

◆ In a T'ai Chi class, your instructors will tell you what is expected of you.

◆ Practice T'ai Chi not only to learn and remember the movements, but also because it feels good!

In This Chapter

- ◆ Understanding the importance of T'ai Chi posture

- ◆ Learning how T'ai Chi protects your joints

- ◆ Discovering how T'ai Chi's moves teach effortless living

- ◆ Knowing that breath is the beginning of everything

- ◆ On the DVD: *Locating your Dan Tien and Vertical Axis, Sinking into the Horse Stance,* and the organ massage aspect

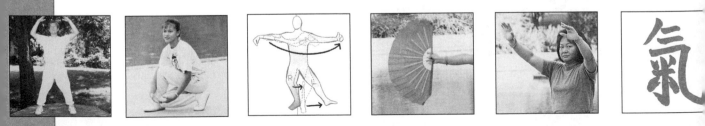

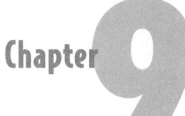

Chapter

Saddle Up: Horse Stance and Other Terms

This chapter explains the core concepts that will ensure a rich T'ai Chi experience for you, whether you are beginning classes or a video instruction program. You will discover the basic concepts of T'ai Chi, how its movements are to be performed, why they are performed that way, and how to breathe when performing them. By understanding that T'ai Chi is very different from Western exertion exercises, you won't make it harder than it is, and by relaxing into it, you unlock its full, effortless potential.

T'ai Chi Posture Is Power!

I introduced the dan tien in Chapter 2. In T'ai Chi, we move from the dan tien by first sinking into the Horse Stance. This is how we sink our Qi, which makes us more solid, more balanced, and more down to earth physically, emotionally, and mentally.

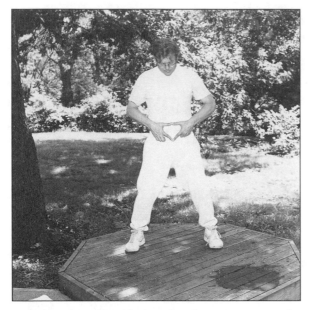

Make a triangle with your thumbs over your navel and with your forefingers extending downward. Your fingertips will meet at the level of your dan tien. Refer to the DVD's *Locating your Dan Tien and Vertical Axis* sections.

Where Is the Dan Tien?

Where the dan tien is located on the outside of the body only tells its height, for the dan tien is actually inside the body. Here's how to find your dan tien inside:

1. With your fingers forming a triangle as described in the previous figure, point your fingers as if they could extend inside your body.

2. Your fingers are now pointing toward your dan tien; however, the dan tien is near the center of your body, so it only can be felt on the inside.

3. Now tighten your sphincter muscles, as if you were pulling up your internal organs from within, and then immediately relax. Repeat this over and over until you experience a subtle tugging sensation inside, just beyond where your fingers are pointing to your upper pelvis or lower abdomen.

4. The place where you feel that subtle tugging feeling is where your dan tien is. That isn't your dan tien itself—that was a muscle tugging—your dan tien is an energy center.

5. Dan tien only can be experienced as energy, tingling, or other light sensations. This is where all powerful movement or action comes from, and cultivated awareness of the dan tien with T'ai Chi makes any action you take more powerful, with less likelihood of injury.

Know Your Chinese

Although the *dan tien* usually refers to an energy point below the navel, there are actually three dan tien points, all near the center of the body: one below the navel, **Qi Hai;** the second at heart level, **Shan Zhong;** and the third at eyebrow level, **Yin Tang.** Each dan tien is an energy center where certain energies are focused or supercharged into the system.

The Horse Stance and Dan Tien Ride Together Again

The dan tien is the basis of the Horse Stance. The Horse Stance is the basic stance for all martial arts, including T'ai Chi. It aligns the three dan tien points, *upper, middle,* and *lower,* to give you the best posture and most effortless movement.

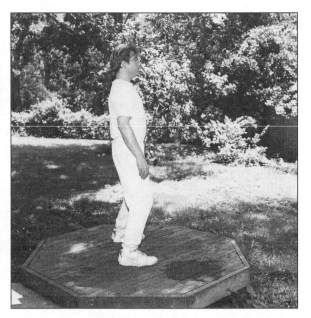

Note that the head is drawn upward toward the sky, as if a string were pulling from the center of the head. The chin is slightly pulled in, and the tailbone or sacrum is dropped down. This has the effect of lengthening the spine.

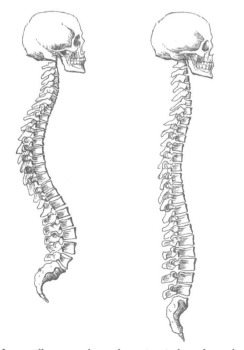

This figure illustrates how the spine is lengthened as you drop into the Horse Stance, although this is an exaggeration.

Ouch!

The lengthening of the spine that occurs as you sink into your Horse Stance is not a "forced" position. Do not "stand at attention"; rather, allow the muscles around the backbone to let go, enabling you to relax into a lengthened posture. Refer to the DVD's *Sinking into the Horse Stance* section for more on the Horse Stance.

The Vertical Axis and You

Many lower-back injuries are caused by poor performance posture. T'ai Chi encourages you to maintain good posture and reminds you when you get sloppy. To achieve proper posture, align the three dan tien points over the soles of the feet, with the weight slightly more to the heels than the front.

As you practice T'ai Chi's slow, gentle forms, your back may experience discomfort whenever you forget posture and let your butt creep out too much. However, when done correctly, the slow, gentle, low-impact nature of T'ai Chi will alert you to correct your posture or any other poor physical habits long before real damage occurs. This is what sets T'ai Chi apart from other training. In fact, you often don't become aware of problems in high-impact sports until the doctor is telling you not to play that sport *ever again*.

Everything and the Sinking Qi

T'ai Chi is about sinking. This isn't like heaviness as in a ship sinking, but more of a weightless release of muscles, allowing the skeleton to effortlessly hold the weight of the body. Let your relaxed shoulders sink away from your neck as you sink into your movements. It's as if you were swimming through an atmosphere of effortlessness as you move through your forms. The DVD's *Sinking into the Horse Stance* section provides a visual support for these instructions.

A T'ai Chi Punch Line

An advanced T'ai Chi student went to study with a grand master in China. The grand master told him to stand on one leg and said, "Keep standing, I'll be back." The grand master returned 15 minutes later and reached down to squeeze the student's calf muscle on the leg he was standing on. The master scoffed, "Too tight! Why is your leg so tight? Keep standing, I'll come back and check later."

Sinking Your Weight

Each T'ai Chi movement is associated with an inhale and/or an exhale. When you move and exhale, you allow your body to sink into a feeling of effortlessness. As you transfer your weight from one leg to the other, relax the entire weight of the body down into the weight-bearing leg. The Chinese call this "sinking your Qi." By practicing this in T'ai Chi, you will move more effortlessly and your balance will improve. This also promotes blood and energy circulation through the body and encourages less joint damage by removing chronic tension from your daily movements. Tight muscles make tighter joints. The DVD's *Long Form Lesson 1 Excerpt* provides a visual image of how the breath is related to "sinking" into the movement.

Don't Tear the Rice Paper!

If you ever watched the TV series *Kung Fu*, you may have seen Kwai Chang Cane walk across the rice paper for his graduation ceremony at the Shao Lin Temple. This looked very mystical, but it was actually a very practical test.

The purpose of the test was to discover whether he was pivoting the foot that was carrying his weight. In most T'ai Chi, you do not pivot the weight-bearing foot because this can destabilize your balance and, more important, can cause knee damage. Styles that do pivot on weight-bearing legs do so rarely and take certain precautions to prevent injury. These pivots are not recommended for arthritis sufferers.

Ouch!

To pivot a weight-bearing foot with no damage to your knee, lift your dan tien at the same time, so as to relieve pressure on your knee. If you have knee problems, I recommend not performing these types of pivots or modifying the form to be safe for you.

T'ai Chi movement is a process of "filling" and "emptying" each leg of Qi, or weight. The position of the dan tien over a leg determines that it is full and the other leg is empty. You "fill" the opposite foot by shifting your dan tien over that opposite foot. Then your "empty" foot has no weight on it and can be pivoted with zero damage to the knee. The DVD's *Long Form Lesson 1 Excerpt* provides a visual example of how only the emptied foot is pivoted. Chapter 15's *shadowing illustrations* also clearly explain this for all the long form's movements in that chapter.

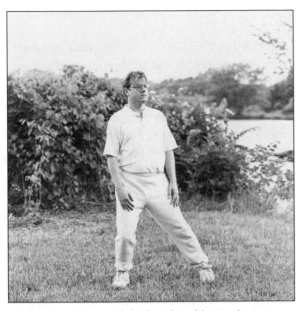

The vertical axis of the head and heart dan tien points lines up over the lower dan tien. This axis moving over a leg fills that leg with Qi, or weight. As you let your breath out and relax your body weight onto a leg, you sink your Qi into that leg.

Active Bones Under Soft Muscle

T'ai Chi is unlike any exercise you have ever done because it is done best when it's done easily. T'ai Chi's way will also provide a model for practicing the art of effortlessness in everything you do. When viewing the DVD's T'ai Chi exhibitions, notice how *effortlessness* seems to be the T'ai Chi player's goal.

T'ai Chi Is Not Isometrics

Most Western exercises involve some type of force or strain. T'ai Chi does not. The more effortlessly you are moving, the better you're doing it. You may catch yourself subconsciously tightening muscles because we have been taught that exercise must cause strain. Also, at first your balance may not be very solid, and you will tighten your leg muscles a lot to hold

you steady. This is normal, and over time you'll find that you can relax your muscles more and more. As you get used to proper posture, using the vertical axis alignment, you'll need less muscle tension to hold you up. So don't be discouraged if T'ai Chi doesn't feel so "effortless" at first. We are learning how to move effortlessly, by first becoming aware of how tight we are and then using QiGong breathing techniques taught in Part 3. Soon we begin to "let go" of needless effort as we move through T'ai Chi movements *and life*.

> **Ouch!**
>
> Becoming more comfortable with your forms and using proper posture with the vertical axis allows you to relax more as you move. At first you will notice yourself losing balance as much as or even more than before you started T'ai Chi. This is not unusual. Before, you probably held your balance by holding your body tightly. Now you are learning to balance while loose.

When doing T'ai Chi warm-ups, allow your mind to let go of thoughts and center on your effortless breath. Then enjoy the sensations of the muscles loosening as you move. On each breath, think of letting the muscles beneath the muscles let go, letting go of each other, and letting go of the bones beneath. As we relax our muscles, the bones moving beneath provide a deep-tissue massage and the body can cleanse itself of toxins. Also, the relaxed abdominal muscles allow a gentle massage of the internal organs, which tonifies them and improves their function. View the DVD's *Moving QiGong Warm Ups Excerpt* for a visual image about relaxed internal *massaging of the organs*.

Don't force yourself to go as low or deep in your stances as your instructor. You have the rest of your life to get lower. Right now, just focus on breathing, relaxing, and letting the muscles relax on the bones, again by allowing the entire body to relax as you exhale. The DVD's *Mulan Style "Ouch!"—Mulan knee bend caution* discusses this in relation to the Mulan Style. Chapter 15's instructions also deal with this.

> **Sage Sifu Says**
>
> Don't fall into an "all or nothing" trap of self-sabotage. For example, if you have a knee problem that prevents you from rotating your knees the way the instructor does, or if you have asthma that prevents you from breathing as deeply or effortlessly as you would like, that's perfectly fine and natural. Do what you can in a way that feels good to you.
>
> Just because T'ai Chi and QiGong often help people lessen their reliance on pain or asthma medications doesn't mean you *must* give up your medication. On the contrary, use what works and helps you live better. Yet ironically, over time, T'ai Chi and QiGong may reduce your reliance on the very medications that help you feel comfortable enough to move and breathe through T'ai Chi.

Always keep the knees bent in T'ai Chi and QiGong. The depth of that bend depends on what feels good to you. (Refer to the DVD's *Moving QiGong Warm Ups Excerpt* about bending your knees.) Someone with knee problems may bend his or her knees only slightly at first, whereas someone more athletic may bend more. Do not let competitiveness cause you to go any deeper than what feels good. You won't win a prize, and you'll enjoy the class less because you are straining too much. The relaxed bend of the knees allows the rest of the body to be more loose and flexible, especially the hips.

Easy Does It

T'ai Chi is a mind/body exercise that integrates your mental, emotional, and physical aspects. Therefore, as you learn to move more effortlessly, you will notice that emotionally and mentally you find ways to move through life with less and less effort. This doesn't mean you'll get less done. You'll probably get more done because someone with calm emotions and a relaxed mind is much more creative than someone who is in constant mental or emotional turmoil.

> **T'ai Sci**
>
> Some doctors believe our central nervous system is affected by the rhythms of our breath. Because the central nervous system regulates all other organs, a restriction in a freely moving respiratory system could lead to disease. The goal of T'ai Chi is to foster unrestricted breathing. By doing so, T'ai Chi may improve central nervous system function, which may reduce the incidence of disease.

As you study T'ai Chi, be aware of any patterns you have that make learning T'ai Chi more difficult. You may find that you push yourself very hard, straining at every movement. Or you may discover that you are hypercritical of yourself, or perhaps you sabotage your progress by avoiding practice and skipping classes. All these patterns are probably something you do in all aspects of your life, not just in T'ai Chi. By learning how to "play" T'ai Chi in a process of effortless learning, without strain, self-judgment, or self-sabotage, you will discover a new way to learn T'ai Chi and create a new, more effective way to learn in all your life's endeavors. You will become more successful and self-actualizing by becoming clearer and more self-aware of unconscious patterns that inhibit the realization of your dreams.

Round Is Cool

In Chinese, the word for "round" is roughly equivalent to the American slang word *cool.* The Chinese felt that roundness was calming and comforting, and T'ai Chi is filled with images of roundness. In practicing T'ai Chi, we often move our hands over imaginary orbs or spheres of energy that, over time, become tangible enough to feel. This practice, although at first a little alien, eventually becomes very soothing. It helps us become attuned to our sensations. It is like practicing "feeling." Practice makes perfect, and this is no exception. Refer to the DVD's *Long Form Lesson 1 Excerpt* for a visual on this idea of *roundness* as part of the T'ai Chi movements.

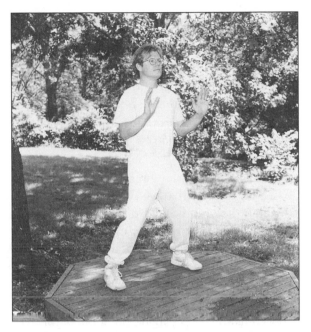

After the hands slide up and over the giant pearl, they descend along the backside until coming to rest in front of your chest, as if you were about to push someone.

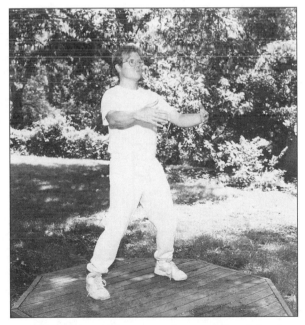

In this Moving QiGong exercise, your hands begin at groin level and circle up as if stroking a huge 3-foot pearl in front of your torso. Move your hands up, over, and down the back of the pearl.

Breath Is the Beginning of Everything

The essence of T'ai Chi is the breath. While doing T'ai Chi, you inhale or exhale with every movement. There is nothing more effortless in the entire universe than the release of a full breath. (Refer to the DVD's *Moving QiGong Warm Ups Excerpt* for more on T'ai Chi breathing.) Therefore, T'ai Chi's ability to weave exhales with the relaxation of sinking your Qi into your weight shifts creates a powerful habit. This habit of relaxed breathing through everything we do is simple and yet may change the way we live the rest of our lives. But again, the reason to do it is because *it feels good.*

Postbirth Breathing

There are many QiGong breathing exercises. In fact, all QiGong exercises are breathing exercises, when you get down to it. However, among all of them there are two main forms of breathing: *postbirth breathing*, which is pretty normal, and *prebirth breathing*, which takes a little more getting used to.

The names of these breathing forms may be based on the fact that we drew breath in through the umbilical cord before birth, and we draw air in through the upper body afterward. This is reflected in the way we draw air into the body during QiGong breathing, depending on which type we are doing.

With postbirth—or normal—breathing, the abdominal muscles expand out a bit as you breathe in to the abdomen; then the chest expands as the tops of the lungs fill. They then relax back in as you exhale, emptying first the chest and then the lower lungs. This is how T'ai Chi and many QiGong exercises are done. However, some QiGong exercises employ prebirth breathing.

Ouch!

Rapid expansion of the chest cavity may not efficiently oxygenate the body. However, QiGong's relaxed abdominal breathing can be highly effective in increasing circulation of blood and Qi.

During postbirth breathing, do not force the breath, but rather allow the body to relax as the breath enters. The following figure illustrates postbirth breathing, along with the DVD's *Moving QiGong Warm Ups Excerpt:*

1. Breathe into the lower lungs as the abdomen relaxes slightly outward.
2. Allow the lungs and upper chest to fill as well.
3. As the body relaxes with the exhale of breath, the upper chest deflates first.
4. Then the abdomen relaxes in, completely expelling the air from the lungs.

Repeat this for 10 or 15 minutes if you like, with wonderful results for mind and body.

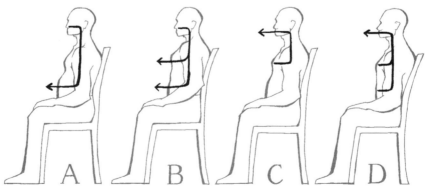

Four-step postbirth breathing.

Prebirth Breathing

Prebirth breathing is just the opposite of postbirth breathing. As you inhale, draw your abdominal muscles in gently, and allow them to relax as you exhale. (Each breathing method has different qualities and is discussed during the moving exercises in Parts 3, 4, and 5.)

In prebirth breathing …

1. Slightly draw in your abdomen, especially your lower abdomen, as you inhale.

2. Then, when you exhale, relax your abdomen back out.

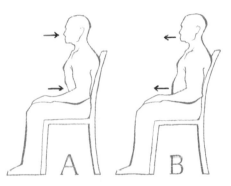

Two-step prebirth breathing.

Prebirth breathing involves a bit of training and some cautionary notes. It is advisable to practice normal postbirth breathing only during your exercises, unless you're training with an experienced QiGong instructor.

A T'ai Chi Punch Line

The Chinese believe that prebirth breathing moves our Qi through the lower dan tien. This energy is associated with cell regeneration and sexual or procreative energy. Therefore, it is believed that prebirth breathing heightens the regenerative ability of our life energy and actually slows the aging process.

The Least You Need to Know

◆ Your posture is your power.

◆ Sinking Qi improves your balance.

◆ T'ai Chi practice protects your joints.

◆ Roundness is the image that permeates QiGong and T'ai Chi.

◆ Proper breathing techniques are the most powerful health tool you have.

In This Part

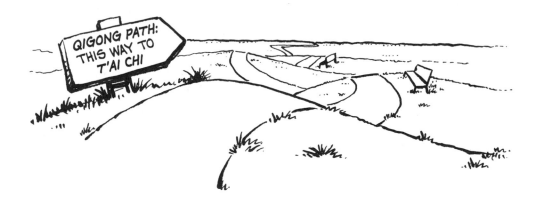

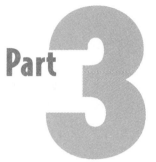

Part **3**

Starting Down the QiGong Path to T'ai Chi

Part 3 details how QiGong can ease the way for us to fit into a new world developing around us in these rapidly changing times. Practical exercises for young, old, and everyone in between will help you breathe the breath of life and have some fun doing it.

In this part, you will also learn some QiGong history and see why some QiGong is different from T'ai Chi. Learning QiGong will make your T'ai Chi experience much richer. It is said that medicine cures, but the best medicine prevents. To that end, you'll learn not only about the personal healing powers of QiGong, but also how you can share your Qi, or life energy, with others.

This part also alerts you to some common challenges you may encounter as you begin exploring your inner self with Sitting QiGong. The Sitting QiGong exercise in Chapter 11 will get your Qi overflowing. In fact, it will lead you through an explanation and exercise that may actually change the way you view the universe you live in. Chapter 12 exposes you to the beautiful and wonderful feeling of Moving QiGong exercises, or Dong Gong. There are thousands of them, so in Chapter 12 you will be able to only dip your toe into the ocean of what's out there. The T'ai Chi warm-up exercises in Chapter 13 are QiGong exercises that not only calm the mind, but also prepare the body for T'ai Chi. These exercises alone can have a wonderful impact on your day.

In This Chapter

- ◆ Understanding why breathing is so important

- ◆ Finding out how QiGong and T'ai Chi differ

- ◆ Reading up on the history of QiGong

- ◆ Surviving and flourishing through QiGong challenges

- ◆ Discovering the healing art of External QiGong

- ◆ On the DVD: *full abdominal breathing* and T'ai Chi's *smoothing-out-tension-blocks* quality

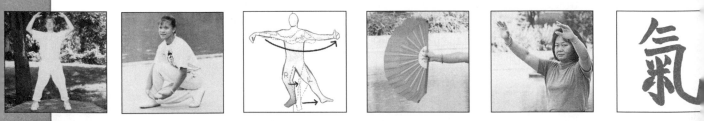

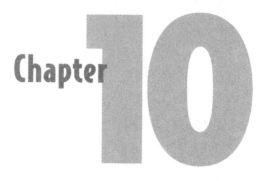

Chapter 10

Introducing QiGong

The purpose of QiGong is to let go of energy blocks by relaxing the mind, body, and emotions. All the many thousands of QiGong exercises share this goal, including T'ai Chi forms, which most consider to be one of the many forms of QiGong.

QiGong differs from standard meditations but shares many of their healing potentials. QiGong can be used as therapy for specific conditions as well as a general tune-up. Also, we can actually treat another person with the life energy QiGong fills us with.

There are two types of QiGong: active QiGong, or Dong Gong, and passive QiGong, or Jing Gong. Active QiGong involves obvious movement, like T'ai Chi, or other Moving QiGong exercises. With passive QiGong, the external body is still, but the awareness is directed and felt in various areas of the body, by breath, imagery, or both.

We encounter many challenges when beginning QiGong practice. By realizing that these are common, we can begin to move past them and get all the benefits QiGong offers. These challenges to QiGong practice represent challenges we face in all aspects of our lives and personal growth. Therefore, by learning to move through these challenges in QiGong, we begin to untie knots in many other parts of our lives as well.

Let's Do Some Heavy Breathing

Many ancient cultures have recognized the breath as our connection with the life force, or Qi. In Chinese, the character for Qi, or life energy, is the same character used for air, as in breath. In Latin, the *spir* of *spir*it or re*spir*ator means "to breathe." Spirit is the *breath of life*, or life energy, which is another word for Qi. So in both the East and West, breath was and is recognized as the key to life's energy. Therefore, if you breathe shallowly, you're cheating yourself out of a lot of life.

Know Your Chinese _____

Literally translated, *Qi* means "air" or "energy," and *gong* means "work." Literally translated, *QiGong* means "breath work" or "energy work."

Many T'ai Chi classes begin with Sitting QiGong exercises that require us to breathe deeply. When we begin, we sometimes might find this difficult because our lungs might have lost capacity from lack of use, or our back and chest muscles are tight with tension. This will change; as your rigid muscles relax, you will soon discover your lungs finding new capacity. The *Moving QiGong Warm Ups Excerpt* on the DVD gives visual insight on full abdominal breathing and shows you how to begin to *loosen up* your chest, back, and torso muscles to facilitate breathing. You'll find that Moving QiGong enhances and supports Sitting QiGong, and vice versa, and all will support your coming T'ai Chi experience.

Sometimes we're just embarrassed to let other people hear us breathe. Maybe it's because we think of hearing deep breathing only during sex or other intense feelings, and we're taught not to show our feelings in public. After a few classes, most people get more comfortable with each other and get comfortable with the idea of breathing. Then the tentative group transforms into *a wild bunch of breathing bohemians!*

If you forget everything about QiGong except to remember to breathe deeply when you're under stress, you will find great benefit. Of course, that's only the beginning—the key to the door of what T'ai Chi has to offer—so don't stop there.

A T'ai Chi Punch Line _____

A corporate executive arriving promptly for a QiGong class informed the instructor, "My doctor said QiGong would be good for my heart condition, so I want to learn QiGong. But I heard about all that weird breathing you do. I want you to know, I am not into the breathing thing." The instructor responded, "We'd better hurry and get you into it before it's too late, because I don't do CPR."

QiGong first teaches us to feel good about ourselves and to follow what our bodies want and need, like breathing deeply, *even in public.* In fact, QiGong practitioners get to where they can even yawn in public. I know that may seem pretty risqué now, but after learning QiGong, even you will be able to yawn unashamedly in public. And this ability will reflect an even deeper ability to believe in yourself enough to do what your body tells you it needs, whether it's more rest, better foods, regular gentle exercise, or a good, solid yawn, even in the middle of a department meeting.

A T'ai Chi Punch Line _____

A Chinese T'ai Chi master was asked, "Why do we do T'ai Chi?" His answer was, "To burp." He meant that T'ai Chi makes us aware of what the body needs and self-assured enough to satisfy those healthful needs. A yawn is a form of deep release, both physical and mental. To deny that release is not a healthful habit. Yawn away!

T'ai Chi vs. QiGong: What's the Difference?

T'ai Chi's goal of relaxing the mind and body to encourage the flow of energy through us makes it QiGong. However, not all QiGong is T'ai Chi (because some QiGong is sitting or lying, and all T'ai Chi is moving and standing). The mental strain of trying to figure out whether you are doing T'ai Chi or QiGong will limit your ability to get the benefits, so forget about it. As you practice T'ai Chi and QiGong exercises, the differences will become obvious. *Doing* is the best way of *seeing*.

Above all, don't sweat it. The following chapters will show you clearly what the difference is, and after Parts 3 and 4, you'll be an expert on the tenets of both T'ai Chi and QiGong. Remember, much of T'ai Chi and QiGong are interchangeable and synonymous anyway. As stated before, the premise of all Traditional Chinese Medicine (TCM), of which T'ai Chi and QiGong are integral parts, is that energy flows through the body, and when that energy flow gets blocked, we are likely to get sick. So QiGong's goal to allow the mind and body to release the past and fears of the future to live a more flowing, healthful life is also the goal of T'ai Chi.

QiGong is a form of meditation; however, it can be more as well. QiGong can actively be used to treat a specific organ or an area of pain and discomfort by directing Qi to that area.

Like other meditations, such as zazen or transcendental meditation, QiGong allows the mind to empty of active thought and be passively aware. In zazen, this state of mind is achieved by not thinking about anything, but just letting thoughts drift through the mind without fixing or holding on to them. In transcendental meditation (TM), a *mantra* (a verbal utterance used in meditation) or perhaps a *mandala* (a visual meditation tool) is used to take the mind out of the problem-solving mode and into a state of free flow, whereby it "observes" rather than "thinks about" things that flow through the mind.

QiGong combines this passive awareness, or "letting go," with an active healing intention. If we're treating a headache, for example, once we think about the energy filling the muscles in our heads, we have to let that thought go and then just experience how nice it feels as Qi's healing energy, or light, relaxes the head. We observe the healing release in the tight muscles, and in a way, the passive observation of our own healing becomes a mantra or mandala.

T'ai Sci

In the *Chinese Medica* (the book of collected Traditional Chinese Medical therapies), there are about 7,000 different breathing exercises, all gentle, all pleasant, and all QiGong. In traditional Chinese hospitals, physicians may prescribe a QiGong exercise to help heal a problem, much the same way a Western doctor might prescribe a drug (of course, QiGong exercises have only *good* side effects). Many Western doctors are now beginning to prescribe T'ai Chi and QiGong as well.

A T'ai Chi Punch Line

The ultimate source of Chinese medical knowledge is The Yellow Emperor's *Classic of Internal Medicine* (200 B.C.E.), which prescribed QiGong for curing and preventing illness. According to this ancient book, true medicine cured diseases *before* they developed. T'ai Chi and QiGong can be very effective at doing just that.

A Brief History of QiGong

QiGong is believed to be more than 2,000 years old. Its roots are with ancient Chinese farmers who observed that nature's balance makes things strong. Moderation, flexibility, and constant nurturing filled crops with the life force, or Qi. These ancient observers developed exercises that mimicked that healthful way of cultivating life energy.

Welcome Back to the Future

What many Western hospitals are now considering as cutting-edge treatments for cancer, for example, can be found in the 800-year-old *Taoist Canon*. At the Simonton Cancer Center, mental imagery exercises are successfully used to help cancer sufferers live nearly twice as long as their peers who do not use imagery techniques. The *Taoist Canon* wrote of thousands of visualization techniques meant to heal various conditions.

Know Your Chinese

The ***Taoist Canon*** (1145 C.E.) held all the early writing on QiGong, although at that time it was known as *Tao-yino*. (*QiGong* is a fairly modern term.) Taoist philosophy emphasizes being attuned to the invisible laws of nature. QiGong, or Tao-yin, was viewed as a way to connect with that deeper part of ourselves that knows what's best for us.

Is Your Mind Half Full or Half Empty?

Here in the West, we have no trouble understanding and accepting that our mind can make us sick. We know that worry can cause an ulcer or that chronic anxiety can lead to a heart attack. However, we have a big problem accepting just the opposite: that our mind can also heal us.

So the world has come full circle, and what was ancient treatment in China is now the cutting edge of modern healing in the West. *Welcome back to the future.*

Know Your Chinese

QiGong has had other names in the past, such as *tu gu na xin,* "expelling the old energy, absorbing the new," and *tao-yin,* "leading and guiding the energy." Actually, the term *QiGong* is a fairly recent way of saying "energy exercise." Refer to Ken Cohen's brilliant book *The Way of Qigong* for rich explanations of Chinese medical terminology.

It's an "Is the glass half full or half empty?" kind of thing. We know our stress can cause our shoulders to tighten and our breath to get shallow and constricted, leading to hypertension and maybe a headache. But the concept of using our minds to heal us is often thought of as a "weird" idea. Ponder this: we all know that recalling an argument we had a week ago or even a month ago can cause our muscles to tighten, our breathing to shallow, and our blood pressure to skyrocket. *Now, that is strange!*

So if something as abstract as a week-old memory can wreak havoc on our health, it makes perfect sense that the mind can have a healing effect on itself today. Unlocking its grip on worry and tension, the mind can allow each cell to bathe in the radiant glow of health.

Bored? It's QiGong Time!

If you're wondering when to do QiGong, the short answer is, anytime you need it. In fact, as you practice energy work more and more, you'll find that, in a way, you *always do it.* As you open more to the feeling of energy flowing rather than being squeezed off by stress, you will automatically sit back and breathe yourself open each time stress begins to close off your flow of Qi.

I always remind students that after learning QiGong, they need never again be bored. Any time you catch yourself getting anxious in a line or in a waiting room, you now can just mentally kick back and practice these wonderful exercises instead of stressing out.

Although you can practice QiGong with great results at any time of the day, TCM has found that the energy flowing through your body is different at different times of the day. Just as Chapter 7 explained how T'ai Chi can be performed at different times of the day for different effects, so can QiGong exercises. (Refer to Chapter 7 to see the times and related organ systems.)

T'ai Sci

Western medical research has discovered that the immune system follows certain rhythms and is weakest at about 1 A.M. and strongest at about 7 A.M. This may partially explain why when you are sick, your cold or flu symptoms keep you from sleeping at night, and then suddenly in the morning you are ready to sleep well. Ancient Chinese doctors were not only aware of this general pattern, but also began to distinguish similar cycles in specific organs.

Mental Healing and QiGong Challenges

QiGong helps heal us mentally, emotionally, and physically, but the beginning of healing entails *becoming more aware*. This can present challenges for the novice because when we become more aware of our mental, emotional, and physical discomforts, we often think this means T'ai Chi and/or QiGong doesn't work. Many of us think a mind/body exercise such as T'ai Chi means "instant and permanent nirvana," and when we discover that we have to "feel" discomfort such as tension before we know to let it go, we may mistakenly think the tools "don't work."

Remember, this new self-awareness is part of a healing process, and you will get enormous benefits from your practice if you stick with it.

Bliss vs. Discomfort

T'ai Chi, QiGong, and other mind/body fitness exercises are sometimes mistakenly seen as "escapist," whereby we can use them to run away from our problems. Although T'ai Chi and QiGong can sometimes seem like a soothing vacation from our problems, they also help us heal or release the source of those problems.

For example, when doing Sitting QiGong exercises or meditations, you may feel your shoulders getting very tense. Remember, the exercise is not making you tense. The exercise of sitting mindfulness is helping you become aware of a pattern or habit you have of holding tension in your shoulders. Now that you're aware of it, you can practice the release and relaxation systems presented in Chapter 11 to begin to let that pattern go.

As you practice T'ai Chi and/or QiGong, you may experience tension or even anxiety. Do not let that stop you or make you think you're doing it wrong. The emergence of these feelings is an opportunity to begin releasing them, using your new tools of breath and life energy. Over time, your practice will "smooth out" those tension blocks, and you'll experience the sense of soothing flow as the T'ai Chi players obviously are enjoying in the *Exhibition of the T'ai Chi Long Form* and *Exhibition of the Mulan Style Basic Short Form* sections of the DVD.

Trying Too Hard to See the Light?

If your QiGong exercises make you feel intensely anxious or tense, it's usually because you are trying too hard to make the tools work. Ironically, the harder we try to relax, let go, and make light or life energy flow through us, the more we squeeze it off.

Life energy flows effortlessly through us when we let the mind and body let go. This is what QiGong teaches us to do. Furthermore, QiGong practice will teach you how to let your conscious mind work with the effortless power of life energy. This will take practice. You'll catch yourself trying too hard to feel life energy or trying too hard to make muscles relax. Always remember that the Qi, or life energy, is completely effortless. Your mind or thoughts can direct your Qi to tense shoulder muscles, but once that thought is directed, you can and must let your mind relax, letting go of the outcome.

Chi, I'm a Healer?

That's right, you are a healer, *master.* After practicing the Sitting QiGong exercise in Chapter 11, you will feel the Qi flowing out of your hands. Medical studies have shown that this energy can help people heal. Many nursing schools in the United States now teach a form of External QiGong called Therapeutic Touch (TT) and are finding great success with everything from anxiety reduction to facilitating healing. If someone you know has a headache, you can usually get some results even if you're a novice. Whether you completely heal the headache or not, the sufferer will likely get some relief, or at the very least, his headache won't last as long as it normally would.

Know Your Chinese

Wai Qi Zhi Liao is the term for External QiGong. Modern Therapeutic Touch (TT) used in many Western hospitals is a form of External QiGong.

In the following figures, you will see one form of an External QiGong exercise you can begin practicing today. After completing steps 1, 2, and 3 and before proceeding to step 4, ask the recipient to describe to you how she feels. Your experience with these tools is the best teacher of what they offer you and others.

1. As you let your Qi flow through your hands into the receiver's heart, slowly bring your hands over her shoulder and down, keeping her arm between your hands so your Qi can flow into her arm.

2. Bring your hands back up to her heart, and repeat three times.

3. Shake off your hands between each brush down to let go of any stress or heavy energy you might have brushed off on the receiver.

4. Repeat this entire process after moving to the other side so the recipient's left and right side are both brushed down.

Many other healing exercises exist for various purposes. These are general cleansing treatments that will benefit anybody. However, the recipients have to feel comfortable with the process, because if they feel tense it won't work as well. Many nurses simply place their hands on patients to comfort them and then let their energy flow into the patients without their conscious awareness of it. This allows the patients to relax.

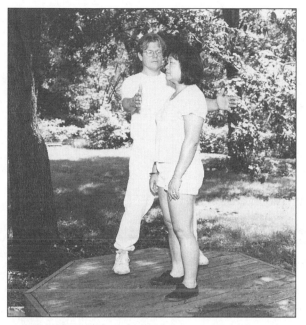

The giver of energy stands to one side of the receiver, with his hands extended over the recipient's heart.

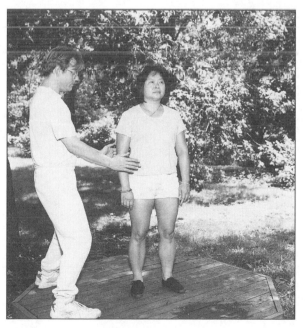

Then he slowly brings his hands over the recipient's shoulder and down her arm to allow the giver's Qi to flow from his hands into the recipient's arm.

Try to do much more of your own Sitting QiGong (Chapter 11) for *self-healing* than you do working with others. Encourage others to learn their own QiGong practice rather than depending on you for relief.

The Least You Need to Know

◆ If you breathe, the rest is easy—*all of it.*

◆ T'ai Chi is one form of QiGong, but there are thousands of QiGong exercises that are not T'ai Chi.

◆ QiGong is an ancient/modern healing art.

◆ Discomfort is information, not an enemy. Rooting out blocked areas and feeling *dis-ease* helps avoid future disease.

◆ You are a healer and a master, and understanding this involves "letting go" of self-imposed limitation.

In This Chapter

- ◆ Seeing and feeling Qi

- ◆ Remembering that we are made of energy

- ◆ Experiencing how Sitting QiGong lights you up

- ◆ On the DVD: a *smooth, loosening T'ai Chi flow* that *Sitting QiGong* exercises help prepare you for *internally*

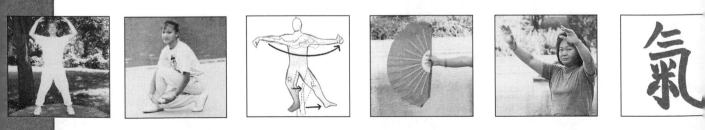

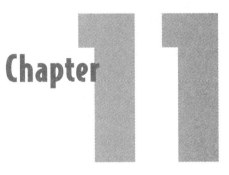

Chapter 11

Sitting QiGong (Jing Gong)

We can measure the Qi flowing through our bodies in many ways. A common way to see energy flow is through Kirlian photography. This chapter provides some examples of how Kirlian photography captures images of our energy.

QiGong practice isn't about pretending to be energy; it is about feeling what we really are, which is energy. Actually, the entire universe is energy. This chapter ends with an exercise of Sitting QiGong, which will allow you to actually feel the nature of your energy and how life energy, or Qi, feels as it flows through your body. You'll love it!

A Word About Energy Medicine and QiGong

Previous chapters explained how Traditional Chinese Medicine (TCM) works by unblocking or directing the energy flowing through the body. QiGong and T'ai Chi also work to balance and unblock that energy.

However, QiGong is also about realizing that the body isn't a solid entity, but instead an open, moving wave of energy. QiGong will actually help you realize your energy nature by providing quiet sitting exercises that enable you to feel it. Over time, you'll begin to feel your energy aspect in your T'ai Chi practice as well. Some of the instructional figures in Chapter 15 include notes on energy flow during T'ai Chi, and when you view those *figures/instructional notes* while watching the DVD's *Exhibition of the T'ai Chi Long Form*, you can get a feeling of the T'ai Chi player's loosening *flow of Qi* as he or she enjoys the T'ai Chi forms, and which Sitting QiGong helps prepare you for *internally*.

The Sitting QiGong exercise presented at the end of this chapter enables you to feel the Qi or energy that moves through your body. Before I get to that, however, I'd like to show you how the process works. Then, when you do the exercise, you can let your brain—and skepticism—relax and get out of the way. The energy flows more easily when you are *effortless*. So don't worry about memorizing any of these facts. Rather, sit back and be entertained by the fascinating insights into who you really are.

> ![hand] **Ouch!**
> Some studies identify cynicism as our greatest health risk. Being constantly suspicious of the world around you triggers unhealthful stress responses. Keep an open mind and relaxed body as you learn about your energetic nature.

Kirlian Photography: Seeing Qi Is Believing

There is actually a way to take photographs of the energy aspect of our bodies. (You may have heard this energy referred to as *aura*.) Kirlian photography has been around since the 1950s, but it received a lot more attention as we in the West learned about Qi and QiGong because it seems to be able to take pictures of Qi, or at least aspects of Qi.

When a Kirlian photograph is taken, the person, or leaf, or any living thing rests on a photographic plate, and a mild electrical current is run through it. Then the camera takes an image of the energy or Qi of the plant or person.

Phantom of the Aura

When Kirlian photography was first introduced, skeptics argued that the photography captured nothing more than the electricity running through the plant or person's hand or whatever was photographed. However, this all changed with the discovery of the "phantom

effect." The following figure illustrates the phantom effect, seen on a leaf.

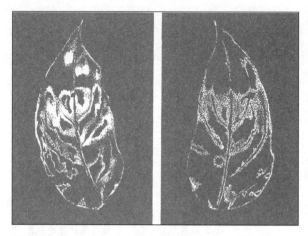

This illustration represents the "phantom effect" as it appears in a common Kirlian photograph of a leaf.

In these front and back images you see a leaf, but what's amazing is that the top part of the leaf you see in the figure *isn't really there!* The top quarter of the leaf was torn off before the photo was taken. So what looks like the top part of the leaf is actually the Qi, or energy aspect, of that missing top. You can see where the leaf was torn but still see the veins and edges going up. This discovery changed not only the way people viewed Kirlian photography, *but also the way science looks at what we are made of.*

The T'ai Chi Zone, Do-Do-Do-Do, Do-Do-Do-Do ...

Eating right, getting enough rest and exercise, and practicing T'ai Chi and QiGong can positively affect your energy flow, whereas behavior shown to be detrimental to health can negatively affect Qi flow. The following figure illustrates how our behavior affects our Qi, or energy. This is important for understanding the benefits of the Sitting QiGong exercise we will do later.

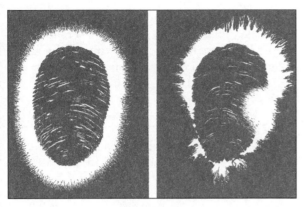

Kirlian photographs illustrate how our behavior affects our Qi, or energy flow, through our body and beyond.

The figure shows a woman's fingertip and the energy flowing through and around it. The image on the left shows this woman's fingertip in a normal state; the Chinese would call that Smooth Qi, or a healthful state. However, the image on the right is the same woman after she drank a cup of coffee and smoked her very first cigarette. The energy went wild! In fact, notice that in some places there seems to be no energy.

We all know how smooth Qi feels, as on those days when you wake up and everything just clicks the way it's supposed to. Every paper wad you throw lands right in the center of the trash can. In basketball, it's called being *in the zone*. We all know how it feels when we are there, in the zone, but we might not know how to get there.

T'ai Chi and QiGong offer a way to get into the zone. As we practice our T'ai Chi movements every day, day after day, we find ourselves spending much less time frazzled and wired, like in the second image. And we find ourselves more and more in the calm center of smooth Qi, like in the first image.

> **T'ai Sci**
>
> *The Tao of Physics* shows how the modern subatomic physicists' view of reality is often very close to the view held by ancient Chinese mystics. By going within themselves in QiGong meditation, these mystics somehow began to understand what modern physicists understand about the energetic nature of reality.

Mind over Qi

The following figure is very important in preparing you for the upcoming Sitting QiGong exercise because it illustrates how the mind can direct energy. In this figure, you see two sets of hands; both belong to the same man. In the image on the left, you see his hands in a normal state. However, in the image on the right, you see his hands when he's consciously thinking of *sending energy* out through his hands.

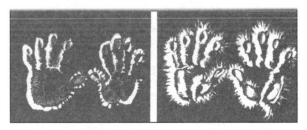

Kirlian photographs illustrate how our energy or Qi flow can be directed by thought.

When the man was thinking of *sending energy* out of his hands, he wasn't grunting and straining. He simply relaxed as he *let it happen*. I mention this before you start the Sitting QiGong to remind you not to "try."

This is an important point because we often think that anything worth doing must be hard. We want to put our "shoulder to the wheel," our "nose to the grindstone," and "furrow our the brow" to get something done. However, the energy work, or QiGong, doesn't work that way. The more you try, the more the muscles tighten up and the less the energy flows through you.

So as the man was sending energy out through his hands, he just thought of it happening and then relaxed and enjoyed the feeling as he let it flow out. You may experience what he felt during the Sitting QiGong exercise.

Know Your Chinese

Twenty-five years ago, I smoked about two packs of cigarettes a day. It was nearly impossible for me to sit still for 20 minutes to do Sitting QiGong—because in Sitting QiGong we begin to become conscious of the energy disruption our habits cause. However, over time, as my energy flowed more smoothly, I scaled back on my smoking and eventually replaced the need for cigarettes with the pleasure of my renewed energy flow. You don't have to quit smoking to enjoy QiGong, but over time, QiGong may help you cut back or eventually quit when the time is right.

The Sitting QiGong is a very effortless process. When it begins, I'll invoke images, such as a soothing flow of relaxation or light energy pouring over your head and face, relaxing all the muscles. When you read this or hear it on an audiotape (you may find it helpful to record the Sitting QiGong in your voice and then listen with your eyes closed rather than reading), you will want to imagine the shower of lightness or relaxation pouring over you. But then let go of the image and just enjoy the feeling of effortless relaxation spreading through your head and facial muscles as the lightness spreads through them. (See Appendix C for my audio and visual resources that teach forms of Sitting QiGong verbally in real-time guided visualizations.)

Researchers have found that if you think of the image, let go of that mental image, and then let the lightness flow through, you will be more able to feel the pleasure of that flow.

T'ai Sci

Harvard Medical School did studies on several relaxation response techniques and found that one thing is necessary to get the most out of any of the exercises: you have to adopt a state of mind called "passive awareness" or "effortless concentration." This means you can't force the experience of QiGong.

$E = MC^2$ Means You Are Only Energy

It's easier to relax and let your Qi flow through you if you know that everything in the universe—*including* you—is only made out of energy. Einstein's famous $E = MC^2$ equation means E (energy) equals M (mass) times C (speed of light squared). Don't get an algebra attack, though, because all it means is that all things, including you, are made of energy.

Actually, we are mostly just empty space. To understand just how spacious we all are, consider the following: if you could take an atom out of anything in the universe, like one of your body's atoms, and blow it up to the size of a football field, the nucleus of that atom would only be the size of a BB in the center of that football field. The electrons that revolve around it would be like dust motes 50 yards away in the end zone. So everything between the BB and the dust mote 50 yards away is energy field, or empty space.

In fact, imagine if you could take all the atoms of *all the human beings on the whole planet* and somehow smush all their atomic particles together, getting rid of the empty space or energy fields we are made of. All the humans on the entire planet's smushed-up atomic particles would add up to just one grain of rice. That is it!

The best image to illustrate that we are mostly open, permeable space is found in something called a "particle chamber." (You might have seen one in your local children's science museum.) A particle chamber is a big glass box filled with ammonia mist. A plaque on the chamber explains that there are cosmic particles falling through space, through the roof of the building, through your skull, your body, your shoes, and right into the earth as you sit here reading this. However, the particles are too small to be seen with your eyes. So the chamber's ammonia mist wraps layers of ammonia around the particles and shines bright flood lights on them, making them big enough to see. When you look inside the particle chamber, you see a blizzard of these particles—the same blizzard that's flowing through us all the time.

I mention all this to set the mood for the Sitting QiGong exercise because it reminds us that we are not a solid, impenetrable mass. We are mostly empty space, and the Qi or life energy can flow through our skulls and brains just as easily as it flows through the air around us.

The only thing that can limit the Qi flow is a thought limitation. So if when I invoke an image of a relaxing flow of energy pouring through your head, you think, *Hold on there—my head is solid mass*, your muscles will tighten up a bit. This tightening will restrict the flow of energy that flows through you.

QiGong and T'ai Chi do not make energy flow through you. The energy flows through you every moment you are alive. Yet as we age, we often squeeze off the flow of life energy, turning it into a dribble rather than the river of life that flowed through us when we were kids. T'ai Chi and QiGong work by allowing your

mind and body to let go of fears, tensions, and grudges that squeeze off our energy flow. This Sitting QiGong exercise is about letting go effortlessly with every breath. The energy flows by itself.

Ouch!

Don't feel as though you have to sit perfectly still while doing the Sitting QiGong exercise. If you need to fidget, roll out your neck or shoulders, scratch an itch, or yawn constantly, let yourself do it. Let your body be as loose and comfortable as possible. However, don't let your mind be distracted by having your eyes open. Close your eyes after reading each point, giving yourself time to experience the effects of each suggestion.

Getting Started with Sitting QiGong (Jing Gong)

In this exercise, you will begin to feel your flow of Qi, or life energy. The Qi will be referred to as "light" because the Qi flows right through you, like sunlight seems to soak right into your bones on a nice spring day.

Remember not to try. You are not *supposed* to see or feel anything. We are just going to have a nice, relaxing experience. So as I offer images, read them and then close your eyes and let yourself feel the result. You may want to tape-record yourself reading this exercise and then do it with your eyes closed. Also, you will find my energy-work audio tapes or a CD available for purchase in Appendix C. These will guide you through this and other Sitting QiGong exercises, enabling you to sit back with your eyes closed throughout the entire exercise.

Sage Sifu Says

To get better results and enjoy a wonderful experience, complete this exercise from beginning to end all in one sitting. This may take about 20 minutes. To only read this is not enough to understand Sitting QiGong. You must let your mind and body go through the different levels of relaxation to actually "feel" the results. Otherwise, it would be like only reading about water and having never felt water.

The Qi will move through you with no effort; the words in this exercise only initiate the process; then you can sit back and enjoy as the light or Qi moves to where your thought effortlessly directs it, as you close your eyes to experience each instructional byte.

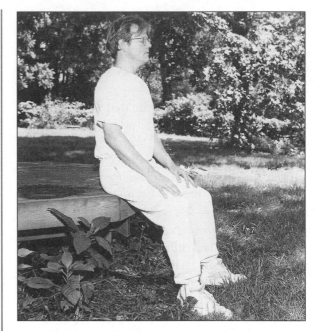

Sit with your feet flat, your palms flat on your thighs, and your back straight but not rigid.

This exercise is best done sitting upright in a comfortable chair that supports good posture. Your feet should be in solid contact with the floor. Also, if your arms and legs are not crossed, the energy flows easier. When you see spaces between text divided by … (an ellipsis), give yourself a few seconds to assimilate and feel the experience *with your eyes closed* before reading on.

1. Begin by placing your feet flat on the floor, with your palms flat on your legs. Let your eyes close comfortably and naturally. This exercise is broken into sections, so you can open your eyes to read a section and then close them for a few moments to let yourself experience, or feel, the responses.

2. All T'ai Chi or QiGong exercises begin by simply becoming aware of the breath. Notice how your lungs fill and empty. Let your chest and back relax so your lungs can fill from the bottom all the way up to the top. Notice how, as you release the breath, your lungs empty from the top, or the chest, and then empty all the way down into the abdomen as the abdominal muscles pull in slightly.

3. Let your mind relax as the muscles in your head, neck, shoulders, chest, and back relax. As the body relaxes, the breaths become not only deeper, but also more effortless. Allow your awareness to relax and ride on the rhythm of that breath, as if the whole body was being breathed by the air. Let the whole body relax as you release each breath.

4. As you feel the body let go of the breath, feel the brain let go of your thoughts and worries of the day. Just as the deep exhales or releasing yawns allow the muscles to let go, the exhaled breath can let go of mental tensions. Likewise, the muscles within and around your heart can hold on to fears or emotions. So as you release each breath, yawn, or sigh, allow the heart to release emotions, the body to release the muscles, and the mind to let go of worries. Each breath is a deep letting go on all levels.

5. Notice that as you let out each breath, it feels as though the atoms of the body are actually expanding away from one another. That's because they are! When we get tense, the body's atoms actually squeeze together, tightening us up. So as we breathe and allow the body to open, the atoms and cells relax away from one another … feeling as if the wind could blow right through you.

6. Now think of the sun directly above your head. Just by thinking of an orb of light ness above your head, you may experience a subtle lift or lightening throughout your mind, or your presence. This Qi, light, or subtle energy vibrates at a higher, more silken rate than the body's vibratory rate. Therefore, you may experience a feeling of lightness, or loosening, and a deep letting go throughout your entire being. Good.

7. Let that sun open and release a shower of clear, washing light, or silken energy, to pour over your head and body, and through your feet down into the earth below. Let go of that image and open to the feeling of deep release as you are washed by that silken energy. Like a water hose spraying through a screen door, just let the body open and be washed through, as you release each sighing exhale.

Ouch!

Whenever you notice that your breathing is very shallow or that you are holding your breath, make it a point to breathe deeply. Let the body relax open, allowing air down into the bottom of the abdominal region of the lungs, and let the whole body relax that breath out, as if the breath were breathing you. Do not force—just let.

8. Be aware as a feeling of lightness expands through the tissues of the body. Notice the light spreading through the muscles in the top of your head. As the cranial muscles relax, they release their grip on the skull, allowing that permeating lightness to expand through the scalp. Expanding through the sides and back of the head, the entire scalp is lighted, as light flows out through every follicle and every hair on the head. Feel the scalp relaxing around the root of every hair.

9. Now allow the light to expand into the muscles at the base of the neck, then down and throughout the connected muscles in the shoulders and upper back. As they let go of their grip on the bones, experience the airy lightness permeating between muscles and bones … a deep letting go.

10. Feel as the energy expands up the back of the head and over the sides … feel the hinges of the jaw relax.

11. Now allow this energy to expand over the forehead, over the brow, down the bridge of the nose, and into the temples. Don't try to feel anything or make anything happen; just effortlessly observe as the light expands into the left eye socket … and then the right. Experience all the tiny optical muscles letting go.

12. Perceive the illumination expanding through all the soft tissue of the face, nose, mouth, and lips.

13. Experience an airy radiance expanding up through the nose into the deepest recesses of the sinus cavity. Feel that opening release as the sinuses fill with light.

14. Now into the ears: feel the deep skeletal muscles in the sides of the head let go as the silken energy expands into the inner ears, allowing a deep letting go in the sides of the head.

15. As the inner ears relax, the Eustachian tubes open, allowing the soothing energy to flow down into the mouth. As the mouth fills with light, the upper palate, upper jaw, gums, and even the teeth seem to lighten, loosen, and let go. And now the lower jaw.

> **Sage Sifu Says**
>
> Do not rush through this. Be sure to close your eyes between each instruction point, allowing yourself to sit back and savor the experience of each image. Don't rush through it. Enjoy. Breathe. Breathe.

16. As you become aware of any saliva gathered in your mouth, swallow it and experience the energy expanding down your throat, through the neck, and into your chest, shoulders, and back.

17. The heart itself can begin to lighten. If you catch yourself trying to feel or make something happen, let all that go. Be willing to feel absolutely nothing as you passively observe the lightness expanding through your heart and chest, permeating all the fibrous tissues of your lungs.

18. This allows every beat of the heart to carry lighted oxygen to all the extremities of the body; in fact, every cell begins to be lighted as the energy moves through the liquid systems of the body. Let the body open to that lightness, even in the tightest places.

19. Allow the light to expand through the abdomen, lighting the stomach … the liver … intestinal tract … kidneys … and lower back.

20. Now think of the sun above your head again. Think of it opening and releasing an even greater flow of light over and through the body. After you think the thought, let go of it and experience the feeling of expanded release … as the bones themselves begin to lighten, the deepest skeletal muscles begin to release their grip on the bones.

> **Sage Sifu Says**
>
> The light or Qi heals and lifts without any effort on your part. Let go of those tight head muscles, and enjoy the feeling of release.

21. As the skull becomes permeated with light, the soothing energy expands right into the brain, illuminating the left frontal lobe and then the right frontal lobe, and expanding into the forebrain, above and just behind the eyes, into the midbrain and temporal lobes, and on into the brain stem, or old brain, in back.

22. Experience as all the billions of brain cells open to that silken effortless radiance. It's as if the brain were a muscle we've held clenched very tightly for a long, long time. And now as we allow the light to expand through the brain, we are finally

allowing that muscle to let go, to expand open, and to light.

23. Now let the energy expand through the spine to the entire nervous system. Any nervous tension on the frayed nerve endings can now be released into that silken healing lightness now passing through all the nerves to the farthest dendrites in the skin.

24. Experience the light flowing down to the tip of the tailbone and radiating out, filling the pelvic bowl and expanding on down through the legs and feet. Now think of the feet opening to allow this river of cleansing energy to pour right through into the cleansing pull of the earth.

25. Let the whole body open to be washed through as the feet release any loads or heavy tensions down into the earth's cleansing pull.

26. As you allow yourself to be washed through by this radiant cleansing shower, you may become aware of blocks in the flow. Tight spots, tensions, anxiety, feelings of restlessness, or thick drowsiness may appear. Any discomfort you feel is due to a block in the flow of energy. Note where you may feel those blocks or discomforts. Take a deep breath, and as you close your eyes, let the breath out. Think of the light expanding in the center of that tightness or blockage. Experience the opening release.

27. This enables the light to expand in the center of the blockage, allowing that area to open. Release the blockage into the cleansing shower that pours through you to wash away the blockage and release it out through the feet into the earth. Breathe and release yet a bit deeper with every exhale, as if the bones themselves could let go of the load they carry.

28. Sit in this cleansing downpour for a while, enjoying the release. As any thoughts, worries, or tensions surface in your mind or heart, release them into the cleansing shower of washing light. Breathe, release, and enjoy.

29. Now think of the feet closing. Instantly that happens, with no effort. By closing the feet, you may experience a sensation of back-filling energy on the soles of your feet as the light fills the feet and the field around, like a silken cocoon of light, coming up over the feet, ankles, knees, legs, and torso, and spilling over the top of your head to fill the field around you.

 Sage Sifu Says

Our thought directs energy, and once directed, it moves there without any effort on our part. Having our eyes closed allows us to experience this within ourselves, to enjoy the cleansing release. This is effortless. The light, or Qi, moves with no effort. After you think the thought, let it go, and sit back and enjoy your responses.

30. With the eyes closed, lift your hands in front of you, as if you were holding a giant beach ball between your palms (see the following figure). Think of the palms and fingers opening, and effortlessly the back-filling energy in your body now flows out through your palms and fingers.

31. Take a few deep-cleansing breaths to release all the muscles in your upper body, even though your hands are raised. It's the letting go that allows the energy to flow through more powerfully.

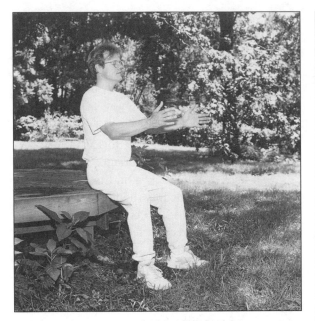

Be sure to let the upper body relax, even though the hands are raised. Slowly move them together and, with eyes closed, open to experience the sensations of Qi in your hands.

32. Slowly begin to move the palms of your hands toward one another, opening them to the experience of the energy you've begun to gather, not only within and around you, but between your palms as well. Move them toward one another until they are almost touching … and experience.

33. Good, now slowly move your hands apart until they are about 3 or 4 feet away from one another, feeling the difference as they move apart. (Repeat moving the hands in and out two more times.)

34. Now gently place your palms back down on your thighs. With each releasing breath, let all that go, relaxing a bit more into your chair with each exhale.

35. As you let go of that experience, reopen yourself to the down-pouring light washing over and through your head and body. With the feet closed, the body is saturated with light. Allow it to spill over the top of your head, quickly filling the field around you.

36. Soon it will feel as though you are floating within a limitlessly expanding ocean of light. With every exhale, allow yourself to be floating more effortlessly within it. Sit back and enjoy this feeling.

37. In doing so, you can begin to feel any remaining loads or heavy energy squeezed within the muscles or other tissues being magnetically lifted up and out of the body in all directions.

38. You can literally begin to feel burdens being lifted up and off of the shoulders just by breathing and being willing to let go. Any worries and concerns are lifted off the temples or brow, again just by being willing to let go and then observing the release. The deep facial muscles release tensions they've held on to throughout the day.

Sage Sifu Says

After learning and regularly practicing the soothing exercise of Sitting QiGong, you will become very adept at it. So when waiting in line at the supermarket, rather than being bored or anxious, just pretend to be staring at the latest tabloid scandal and open yourself to a soothing flow of life energy as it fills and permeates all the areas where your body is holding on to tension.

39. Now any heaviness or angst around the heart begins to be lifted up and off your chest. As the body continues to release these loads, you become aware of your entire being filling with a limitless permeable lightness, refreshing and absolutely effortless.

40. This process of release, cleansing, expanding, and enlightening will continue throughout the day. Even when you're not consciously aware of it, the rhythm of breathing and the willingness to let go will allow you to be lifted into the lightness of this ocean of silken energy. Here your stresses and loads can continually be released into the cleansing light, and your cells and surrounding field will be bathed in its effortless healing.

41. Let yourself sit within this ocean of light, assimilating and soaking in the light. Let go. There is no need to hold on to the light, for the more we let go, the more there is.

42. After assimilating the light for a few minutes, very slowly and very gently, when you're ready … open your eyes.

The Least You Need to Know

- Qi, or life energy, is scientifically observable and measurable.

- QiGong is effortless. It's one of the easiest and most fulfilling things you can do.

- Practice Sitting QiGong every day to supercharge your strength, calm your attitude, and improve your health.

- Use QiGong to program each cell in your body to let go of stress at the earliest indication of blockage.

- QiGong programs your mind and body to radiate health.

In This Chapter

- ◆ Understanding mindful movements and mindless exercise

- ◆ Practicing Bone Marrow Cleansing

- ◆ Becoming elegant with Mulan Quan

- ◆ Learning to make walking a meditation

- ◆ Tonifying kidney function with Carry the Moon

- ◆ On the DVD: *Mulan Lesson Example—Tupu Spinning Moving QiGong Warm Ups*

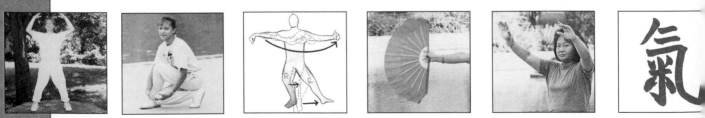

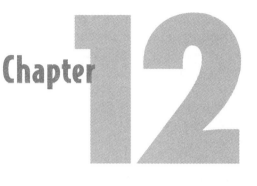

Chapter

12

Moving QiGong (Dong Gong)

The Sitting QiGong presented in Chapter 11 is a prerequisite for the simple, yet powerful Moving QiGong exercises in this chapter. Remember, "mindfulness" is the act of observing, experiencing, and perhaps enjoying rather than analyzing the world around us *or within us*. Sitting QiGong's effortless mindfulness of truly experiencing yourself from the inside is a big part of how Moving QiGong works its magic.

In this chapter, you will experience how Moving QiGong can help treat illnesses and organs. QiGong can enhance immune system responses by cleansing the bone marrow of stress.

The following Moving QiGong exercises promote elegance and grace in your movements, while also promoting a calm and peaceful state of mind. The very helpful 1½-hour DVD in this new, third edition includes a video *exhibition* of the *Tupu Spinning Exercise* in this chapter. Do not use the DVD insert for instructional purposes, but rather, always use this chapter's text and photo references in their proper sequential order (the same applies to other chapters in this book). The DVD's valuable lesson excerpts were carefully chosen from my two *real-time* fully instructional DVD programs, which together contain more than 5 hours of content. Obviously, all that would not fit here in its entirety. Therefore, the carefully selected video excerpts powerfully enhance the text and illustrated instruction. (For information on my fully instructional multihour *Mulan* and *T'ai Chi Long Form* DVD programs, see Appendix C.)

Mindful Movement vs. Mindless Exercise

Like Sitting QiGong, the goal of Moving QiGong is to let the mind initiate physical, mental, and emotional releases throughout the body. The more we let go, relax, and open, the more easily and healthfully the energy flows through us.

Much exercise is not very thoughtful. We strain and pound our joints and tissue running on pavement or in other high-impact exercises without paying much attention to the toll it can take on the body. Nor do we give much thought to the toll this takes on our mind, as we often listen to loud music or watch the news while scurrying through our exercises. Studies have shown that loud noises and excessive TV watching can actually elevate damaging stress responses.

Moving QiGong, like T'ai Chi, is different. When you practice these exercises, let yourself take a break from the rat race, the noise, and the endless demands of the day. Practice QiGong in silence, hearing only your breath and the motion of your body. Let your mind be filled with the experience of letting go of *everything*.

Bone Marrow Cleansing

Some Moving QiGong exercises, such as the Bone Marrow Cleansing, have a specific purpose. As you go through these gentle motions, the energy is encouraged and allowed to flow through the body, even the bone marrow, to cleanse this tissue of frantic energy. The tissue can function at a higher, clearer level when not burdened by old stress.

Sage Sifu Says

Many centuries ago, before modern microscopes, Chinese health professionals understood that blood and bone marrow were associated with the immune system. They studied exercises such as Bone Marrow Cleansing not by viewing another's cells with a microscope, but by practicing the exercise and then observing their own internal health responses.

What follows are the instructions for a Bone Marrow Cleansing QiGong exercise. These instructions are broken into sections. Each section is followed by a photograph that captures a key step in the exercise.

1. Bone Marrow Cleansing begins with the feet about shoulder width apart and the knees slightly bent. Your hands are relaxed at your sides.
2. Bring your hands up in front as if lifting a 1-foot ball to chest level, and then letting the hands come together at the sternum.

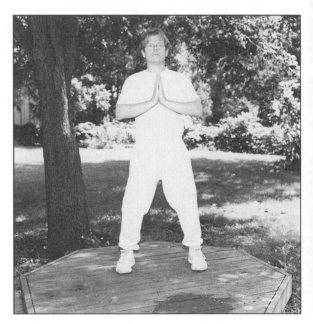

Hands at chest in prayer position.

3. Lower your hands now back down to your sides and then slowly raise your arms out to the sides.
4. Turn the palms outward. Think of opening the body to absorb the energy of life from the universe. Allow the body and mind to become open and porous.

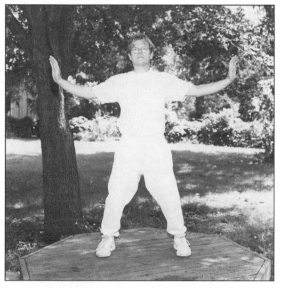

Arms out to sides, palms turned outward to universe.

5. Allow your arms to slowly descend to your sides.

6. One hand now floats up and outward away from the body until eventually it is above your head, with the palm turned down toward the top of your head. Meanwhile, the other hand drifts to settle so the back of your hand is on the small of your back.

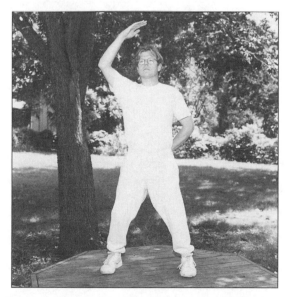

One hand overhead with palm down, and the other hand with back of hand on small of back.

7. As the palm above your head turns palm down, allow the energy to pour over and through the head and body. As the hand descends down in front of the body, the body fills with energy, washing through the bones and bone marrow, cleansing the body of any toxins, which are carried right down into the earth through the feet.

8. Repeat this on the other side, each hand now doing what the other did before. Repeat on both sides three times.

9. Then, with both arms relaxed at your sides, begin lifting both palms up toward the sky.

10. Push your hands up toward the sky above your head, then turn the palms over to face downward.

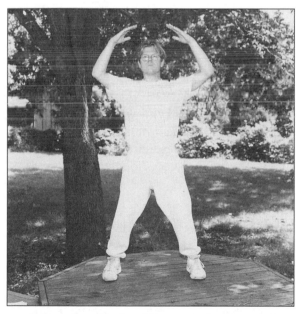

Palms above forehead down, similar to Grand Terminus.

11. As the palms float down in front of the body, let the energy pour through the bones and other tissues, carrying any impurities or dense energy right out through the feet into the earth.

A T'ai Chi Punch Line

Sometimes in classes, students express their concern for the environmental repercussions of releasing their heavy or toxic energy down into the earth. Look at this like our physical human waste, which becomes fodder or nutrients to the earth. Heavy energy the body releases is transmuted and lifted back into a healing force, just like trees breathe our carbon dioxide to create new oxygen. All things balance.

The Elegance of Mulan Quan

Mulan Quan warm-ups incorporate several lovely Moving QiGong exercises. These promote elegance in movement and carriage but have healing effects as well.

Spread Wings to Fly

Spread Wings to Fly is a Moving QiGong exercise that specifically helps with upper limb disorders and loosens tightness in the shoulders. This is a wonderful exercise to perform during breaks at work to release job tension.

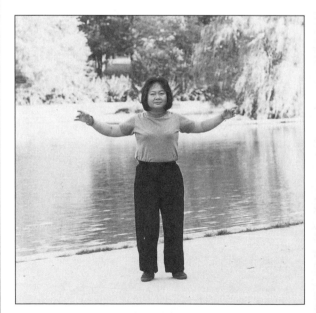

Ouch!

Although all Moving QiGong is likely an excellent addition to any physical therapy you may be involved in, you should use common sense and not force yourself into positions you are not ready for. Always consult your physician or physical therapist before beginning any new exercise program.

1. Begin with your hands out in front of your chest. Relax your shoulders and breathe naturally, with the tip of the tongue lightly touching the roof of your mouth.

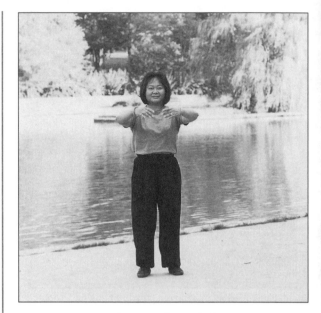

Hands out in front of chest.

2. Begin a long, slow inhalation of breath as you gently pull your arms back around to your sides (as shown in the following figure) until the shoulder blades touch in back, while simultaneously turning your head slowly to the left.

Arms back until shoulder blades touch.

3. Begin exhaling as your arms slowly circle back down and around (rolling out the shoulder sockets) to the start position in front of your chest, while turning your head back to the front.

4. Repeat the entire process, with your head turning to the right this time.

5. Repeat the process, alternately turning your head to the left and then the right until completing eight forms (four with the head turning to the right, and four with the head turning to the left).

Tupu Spinning

Tupu can be therapeutic for movement limitations of the back, buttocks, legs, knees, and ankles. View the *Mulan Lesson Example—Tupu Spinning and Stretch* on the book's DVD as you read the following instructions. Do not use the DVD for instructional purpose, but as support for the text instruction, where you can practice all the warm-ups in their proper sequential order. The DVD, excerpted from my multi-hour *fully instructional* DVDs (see Appendix C), will help you get a feel for the text instructional patterns throughout the book, not just the ones supported by the DVD.

Sage Sifu Says

It is very difficult to fully comprehend how to perform QiGong by reading it from a book. If live classes are unavailable to you, check out one of the many fine QiGong videos available. The Mulan Quan QiGong described in this section is available on the *Mulan Quan Basic Short Form* video listed in Appendix C.

1. Begin by forming fists held at your waist, with your elbows tucked in and your knees slightly bent. Breathe normally and easily, yet fully.

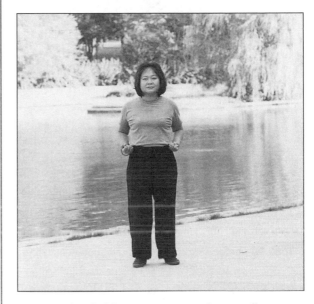

Form fists held at your waist with your elbows tucked in and knees slightly bent.

2. Inhale as you extend the right shoulder forward and as your right hand pushes out in front of your body. Simultaneously, your left shoulder and elbow pull back as you turn your face to look back over your left shoulder. Exhale as you reverse this, pulling your right hand back to square off your shoulders, thereby returning to the start position.

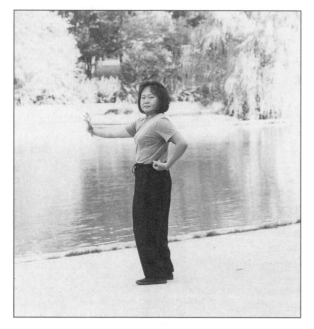

Look left, extend right arm out, left shoulder pulling back.

3. Switch, extending your left shoulder out as your left hand pushes, and your right shoulder pulls back as you look back over your right shoulder.

4. Repeat on both sides four times each.

Bring Knee to Chest

This movement not only feels great; it also helps with any pain in the legs and buttocks and is therapy for functional disorders of the leg involving bending and extending.

1. Begin with your hands relaxed at your sides, your knees slightly bent, while breathing easily and naturally.

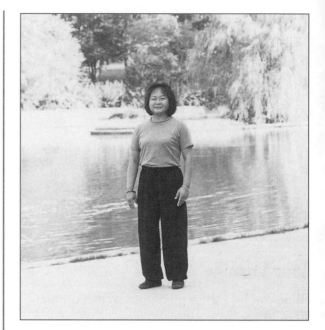

Hands at sides relaxed, knees bent.

2. Now begin inhaling as you step forward with your right leg, shifting your weight to the right leg as your arms swing upward and back in great round arcs.

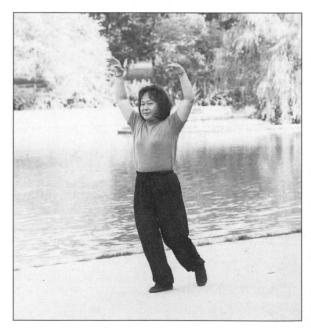

Step forward with your right leg, swing arms backward.

3. As the arms' arcs begin to swing down and toward the front, the left leg begins to lift.

4. Lift your left knee in front, pointing the toes of the left foot down, and wrap your hands around your knee to help it stretch up gently.

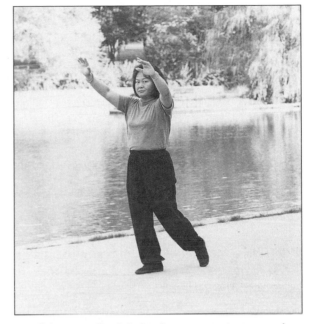

Left leg steps back behind as arms swing up and over.

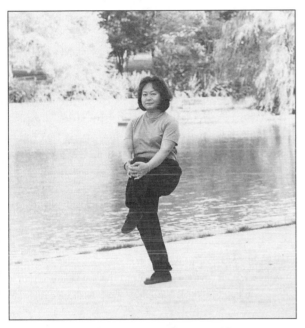

Lift left knee, wrap hands around knee.

5. Now exhale. As the left leg is released, the arms begin to swing down and back.

6. Place your left foot behind you, and shift the weight back onto the left leg as your arms swing from the back over the top toward the front.

7. Allow the right leg to come back even with the left as your hands descend, returning you to the start position.

8. Repeat with the left leg stepping out this time. Repeat the entire process alternating sides (four times on each side).

Zen Walking in the Old Soft Shoe

Zen meditations involve a mindfulness that simultaneously allows your mind to let go of the worries of the world while attuning yourself to the world in a clear and healing way. Zen walking is a common T'ai Chi exercise. It teaches us how to let our movement fill our minds, while improving our balance and dexterity. Follow these instructions to Zen-walk like the masters, and remember to breathe easily and naturally when Zen walking.

Sage Sifu Says

Just as Zen walking makes a meditation or relaxation therapy out of simple walking, we can expand this ability throughout our lives. T'ai Chi and QiGong's teaching of mindful awareness of the subtleties of life can help us make anything we do a meditation, whether it's washing dishes or paying bills. In doing so, every moment becomes more healthful, pleasant, and meaningful.

1. Place the heel of one foot outward at a slight angle, while maintaining balance over the back foot.

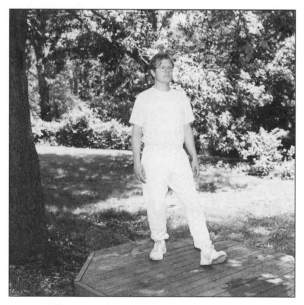

Zen walking resembles the way Groucho Marx used to walk.

2. Slowly shift your dan tien, or weight, up toward your front foot, while slowly rolling the foot down onto the ground.

3. The back foot stays flat until your vertical axis, or dan tien, is settled over the front foot. Now let your heel lift up, then the foot, and now bring that foot up near your weight-bearing foot before placing it out

in front at a slight angle, just like in the beginning.

4. Repeat many times, all the way across your living room or backyard. The goal is to Zen-walk enough that you forget about everything in the world except the soles of your feet, the ground they contact, and the shifting tissue in your body.

Carry the Moon

As discussed in Chapter 3, QiGong can treat specific organs, or systems, in the body. Carry the Moon is great for keeping the spine supple and can also tonify kidney function. It has been said that this may also help reduce premature baldness. This may be because, as with all QiGong and T'ai Chi, it promotes circulation, but in the case of Carry the Moon, especially in the scalp.

Ouch!

Although QiGong may help with premature hair loss, it works best as part of an overall healthful lifestyle. So if you are in a high-pressure job you hate, aren't getting enough sleep, and are smoking too much, the benefits of QiGong will be limited. QiGong practice may help you sleep better and eventually quit smoking. Therefore, QiGong should be viewed not as a cure-all, but as a stairway to a more healthful lifestyle. Realize that even with a job you hate and not enough sleep, you're still better off doing QiGong than not.

1. Begin by letting your hands and head simply hang loosely over as you bend effortlessly forward. Do not try to strain, as if attempting to touch your toes. Just let yourself hang comfortably, with your hands at about knee level or higher. Breathe naturally and easily.

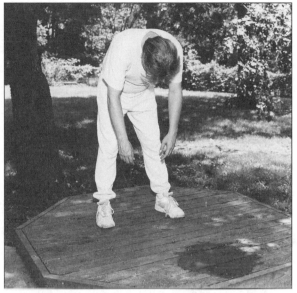

Leaning over with hands hanging down to about knees.

2. Form a circle using the thumbs and forefingers of both hands. As you slowly rise up, the hands ascend above your head.

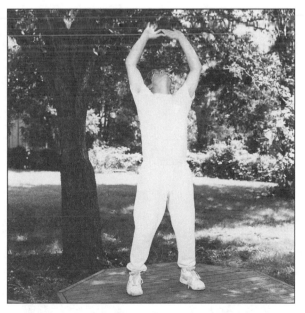

With hands above head forming a circle between thumb and forefingers, looking through it.

3. Let the hands go up and slightly back behind as you gently arch your back to look up through the circle your hands form.

4. Hold this position as you breathe effortlessly and naturally for a few moments; then let yourself hang forward again, and begin again. Repeat several times.

The Least You Need to Know

- Sitting QiGong prepares you for Moving QiGong.
- Breath and mindfulness are important in QiGong.
- QiGong can improve all organ functions.
- QiGong's circulation promotion may help slow premature hair loss.
- Use QiGong as a launch pad to a healthier you.

In This Chapter

◆ Using warm-ups to calm and center

◆ Loosening the body and the mind

◆ Healing your joints while perfecting your balance

◆ Cleansing your tissues and your mind

◆ On the DVD: *Sinking into the Horse Stance* and *Moving QiGong Warm Ups*

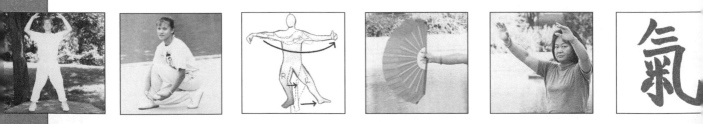

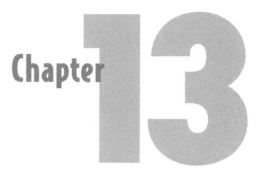

Chapter **13**

Warm-Up Exercises

T'ai Chi warm-up exercises are meant not only to warm the muscles and other tissues, but also to center the mind. You cannot listen to the radio or watch TV while warming up for T'ai Chi.

Of course, there are exceptions to every rule: when you get to the "Let the Dan Tien Do the Driving"; the "Filling the Sandbags, Sinking the Qi"; and the "Deep-Sinking Your Qi" sections of this chapter, you'll be encouraged to view the related DVD sections. (These valuable excerpts on the book's DVD are extracted from two of my DVD programs that total more than 5 hours of content, Carefully selected sections were extracted to augment this book's text and photo instruction. For information on my multihour *real-time* fully instructional DVD programs, see Appendix C.)

Unlike the way many of us were taught to "stretch" out our muscles when warming up by using straining stances, T'ai Chi warm-ups start from the very center of our being. We begin by becoming self-aware of that center and then relaxing ourselves from the deep skeletal muscles outward. We prepare ourselves for fluid and effortless movement by allowing our body to relax around our breathing lungs, and then all the muscles relax on top of the moving skeleton.

Each warm-up is a form of QiGong and promotes health and healing on many levels. These warm-ups are a beneficial exercise program even without T'ai Chi, but T'ai Chi offers so much more.

Dan Tien Takes Us for a Ride

When we start our Sitting QiGong, warm-ups, or T'ai Chi movements, our minds are usually scattered. We are thinking about what we need to do at work, what we need to do to prepare dinner tonight, and so on. So the first task of warm-ups is to center our minds, and the center of our being is, as you know, the dan tien.

Breathing Our Way to Center

There's nothing more calming and centering than hearing and feeling your own breath. Therefore, all T'ai Chi–related exercises begin by simply closing your eyes and feeling the rhythm of your own breathing:

- Let your eyes close easily and naturally as you stand comfortably with your feet fairly close together and knees slightly bent.
- Notice how your lungs fill and empty. Think of breathing into the bottom or abdominal part of the lungs and then letting the top or chest area fill.
- As you breathe, allow the muscles in your head and torso to let go. This allows the breaths to become not only deeper, but also more and more effortless, almost as if the breath were beginning to breathe you.

Sage Sifu Says

When doing all T'ai Chi warm-up exercises, let your eyes close so your awareness can relax within. Enjoy the sensations of loosening and breathing. Breathe fully, but don't force yourself. Breathe easily and naturally.

- Let your awareness or mind relax, riding on the rhythm of your own breath.
- Now think of breathing down into the dan tien area. You can experience the slight expanse of the upper pelvic muscles as you breathe in, and how those muscles relax in as you release the breath.
- You may experience a feeling of air expanding down into that area. Of course, the lungs don't go down that far, so you are feeling the Qi, or your awareness, expanding through your dan tien area.

Also refer to the DVD's *Moving QiGong Warm Ups Excerpt* for a quick video tutorial on abdominal breathing.

Let the Dan Tien Do the Driving

The breathing exercises help your awareness expand in the dan tien area, which prepares you to let the dan tien be the movement. This may sound a little odd at first, but after playing the following exercises for a while, it'll be quite natural and will dramatically improve your focus, balance, and movement. The first two T'ai Chi warm-up exercises employing hip rotations help you practice this. See the *Moving QiGong Warm Ups Excerpt* on the DVD for an exhibition of the first of the following warm-ups and more on *letting the dan tien doing the driving*.

Sage Sifu Says

If you are in a wheelchair or have an injury or condition that requires you to sit, let the most inner part of your upper pelvis go into motion and be aware of that motion, allowing the body to relax as much as possible around that motion. If you are paralyzed, let the internal rotation begin in the center of the body at the lowest point your physical awareness begins.

1. With your feet close together, let the dan tien, or hips, begin a counterclockwise rotation, sort of like a hula-hoop motion. If you were looking down at a clock face beneath your feet, you would be going counterclockwise.

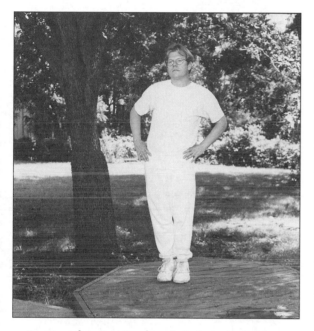

Feet together, rotating hips in hula-hoop fashion.

Notice that the dan tien begins to move effortlessly like a gyroscope in motion, allowing you to let your muscles relax while the dan tien moves the skeleton underneath. The shoulders do not move too much; most of the motion is in the dan tien, or hip area. However, don't be rigid about this. The goal is to get loose.

2. Repeat the counterclockwise hip rotations 32 times, if that feels good to you, and then repeat 32 times in the opposite direction, clockwise.

Close your eyes as you rotate the dan tien. At first this may challenge your balance, but you'll get better. With your eyes closed, your awareness can go within. You will notice areas of the body loosening as

you rotate and breathe. Think of letting the muscles let go of bones and other tissue, allowing the body to just generally loosen on top of the skeleton. You will notice the lower-back vertebrae loosening as the muscles around them begin to let go. You will also notice this loosening spreading up the back through the lumbar region, up through the dorsal vertebrae between the shoulders, and into the neck and the back of the head. Basically, anywhere you let your light of awareness shine within, your body, mind, or heart can begin to loosen as you breathe effortlessly and move effortlessly in these dan tien rotations.

Ouch!

If your balance is too unstable on the first set of rotations with your feet close together and eyes closed, open your eyes, but soften your focus so your awareness can still go inside. You'll find that when you move to the second exercise of rotations with your feet shoulder width apart, your balance will be more secure.

3. Now repeat the hip rotations both ways (first counterclockwise and then clockwise), with your feet about shoulder width apart and knees slightly bent. Relax and enjoy the sensations of movement. With the feet farther apart and eyes closed, you will notice that you can very tangibly feel the top of the femur or hipbone rotating in the hip socket. Slow the rotations, and you will feel the hipbone rotating all the way around the inner rim of the hip socket.

Enjoy the deep-tissue massage the rotating bones give, as the deep hip muscles begin to let go of the tensions built up there. As you breathe and let muscles relax on top of the moving skeleton, you can enjoy this loosening through the back, legs, and the rest of the body.

The enjoyment of this internal loosening helps us almost "see inside ourselves." Practicing this pleasant internal vision is a powerful health tool. By becoming aware of how good effortless motion feels inside, we also become aware of tensions or "diseases" at a very early stage before they actually become diseases.

Know Your Chinese

We are a very shallow-breathing society. You may catch yourself breathing very shallowly or even holding your breath as you move. Let your lungs fill effortlessly all the way down to the abdominal region and up to the top. Allow the entire body to relax that breath out, as if every cell of the body were letting go at the deepest level with each breath. Each breath lets us practice living effortlessly. There is nothing more effortless than the release of a breath.

Lengthened, Not Stretched

In T'ai Chi warm-ups, we don't strain to stretch out our muscles. We allow ourselves to "lengthen" until we begin to ease up against strain. The tension we become aware of indicates a block. Then we take a deep breath, and as we exhale, we allow light, or Qi, to fill the area of tension or restriction, which lets the block begin to let go. You can actually feel the lightness or release spread effortlessly through a tight or restraining muscle as you let out the breath. Our mind's awareness of the block directs the Qi, or energy, into the center of the block as we let the breath relax out of our bodies.

1. With your fingers interlaced, extend your hands up over your head.

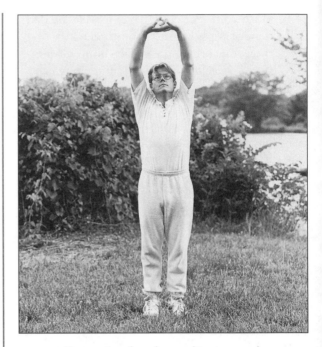

Fingers interlaced, stretching upward.

2. Don't stretch, but allow your body to be effortlessly lengthened, as if the hands were being lifted up toward the sky.

3. As you release each sighing exhale, think of letting the muscles beneath the muscles let go.

4. Enjoy the feeling of effortless release through the back, shoulders, neck, and head, and down into the hips and legs. As you breathe and let go, the entire body gets a bit of a stretch.

5. Now stretch out to either side, but rather than thinking of stretching, think of the hands being drawn out and upward toward the sky out to the left and then the right. First the hands are drawn outward and up off to the right side of the body, and then easing back upward and over to the left side.

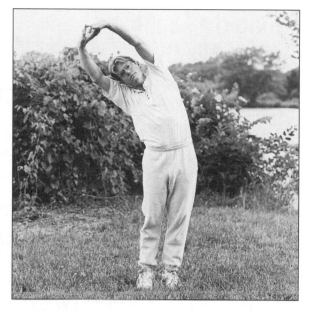

Hands extended, but now stretching over sideways.

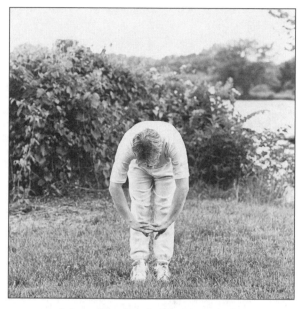

Back bent flat, with hands hanging down.

6. Go back and forth. Do not stretch so far to the side that you feel a big strain. Rather, go just far enough that you can savor the sensation of the muscles stretching across the back, between the shoulders, and through the neck. Again, as you loosen, the entire body gets a bit of a soothing, effortless stretch.

7. Now lengthen straight up again before stretching out and forward. The back should be fairly straight, bending from the hips and letting the arms just hang down.

8. Do not strain to touch your toes. That's not the point. The point is to feel an effortless lengthening through the upper body as you simply let go.

9. Enjoy that feeling of effortless elongation through the shoulders, neck, and back of the head. Notice that with each releasing exhale, you can let go even more. With each releasing breath, the muscles in the head can let go even more, showing you that relaxation is not a destination, but an endlessly enriching process of letting go.

10. Slowly and gently straighten back up to the original position, with hands interlaced high over the head.

11. With your eyes closed, take a deep breath. on the sighing exhale, allow the hands to descend to the sides so slowly that you can feel the air passing between the fingers. As the hands arc down from above the head out to the sides and the breath relaxes out, experience the different muscle groups letting go through the head, face, jaw, neck, shoulders, torso, arms, legs—even into the hands and feet.

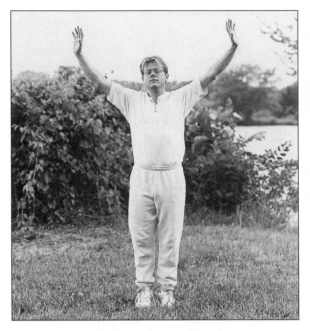

Hands descending to the sides.

12. Let each exhale trigger a deep letting go from the very center of your being, as if the bones themselves could let go. Let every cell in the body relax those breaths out.

13. As you stand with your eyes closed, let go of all the muscles with each breath, and also let go of the heart. Just as the muscles release tensions with each sigh or yawn, the heart can let go of tensions or loads it has squeezed in the heart muscle or muscles around the heart.

14. Think of the brain or mind letting go. Just as the cranial muscles let go of their grip on the skull, the mind can release worries and mental tensions with each releasing breath.

15. Realize that each breath can trigger a deep cleansing on many levels—mental, emotional, and physical. With each exhale, experience a deep letting go.

Filling the Sandbags, Sinking the Qi

Settling down into the Horse Stance is sinking your weight down into both feet as if you were sinking down into a saddle on a horse. The tailbone drops as the pelvis tilts slightly up, and the head is drawn upward toward the sky, while the chin is pulled slightly in. This causes the spine to lengthen, which is great for the back, releasing a lot of the pressure daily stress puts on it. Moving from the Horse Stance not only improves posture and balance, but it can also preserve your joints and make you more powerful.

Refer to the *Sinking into the Horse Stance* section of the DVD for a video supplement of this settling into the Horse Stance instruction.

Moving from the Horse Stance

After you settle in the Horse Stance, let the dan tien flow back and forth from one leg to the other. Picture yourself sitting on an office chair with wheels, rolling from side to side. Or as if you were sitting on the back of a park bench, sliding your bottom from side to side. Notice that the head and shoulder never lead the way, nor do the hips stick out from side to side. The upper body stays stacked above the dan tien as it flows back and forth.

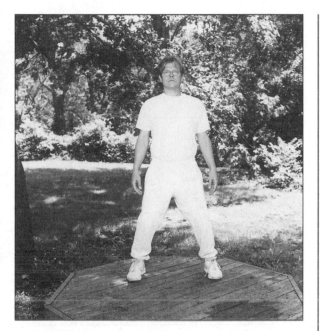

Note that while in Horse Stance, the knees are slightly bent and the upper body is stacked above the dan tien, erect but relaxed and not rigid.

As you become aware of discomfort or tension—the fatigue you may feel in the muscles above the knees, for example—play the following game.

1. Let yourself feel the tension or discomfort, wherever it is in your body.

2. Experience how it feels and where you feel it.

3. Now, as you let the next breath out, think of letting the light, or Qi, expand right in the center of that feeling.

4. Let your awareness sit back and enjoy whatever responses you experience. Often you will experience a lessening of the discomfort or even a pleasure of the expanding lightness.

Ouch!

Do not feel as though you must do all T'ai Chi warm-ups. Only do whatever warm-ups fit your abilities. However, you may be able to modify exercises to fit your ability. If you are in a wheelchair or must sit while performing T'ai Chi, develop upper-body stretches you can perform.

Sinking the Qi

In T'ai Chi, the upper body does not lean; it stays stacked up above the dan tien, just like in the Horse Stance. The dan tien flowing toward one leg fills that leg with the Qi, or energy (or the weight of your body). Simultaneously, the leg the dan tien moves away from is emptying of Qi, or weight. In T'ai Chi, you rarely ever pivot a leg that has weight on it because it makes your balance precarious. More important, it damages the knees to pivot feet that bear weight. So this Moving from the Dan Tien exercise teaches you to shift your weight from one leg to the other. This simple exercise is the most important T'ai Chi warm-up because this is what T'ai Chi is. All of T'ai Chi's elaborate forms are based on the dan tien moving from one leg to another.

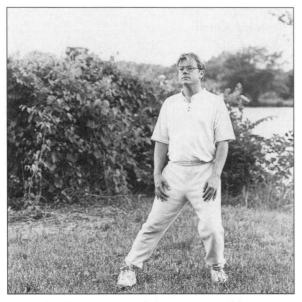

Flowing upper body to the other side.

Deep-Sinking Your Qi

If your mobility permits and you feel adventurous, you can practice a Deep Sinking of the Qi exercise. Also refer to the *Deeper/Expanded Moving QiGong Warm Ups Excerpt*, in the *Moving QiGong Warm Ups Excerpt* on the DVD, for a video supplement of the instructions here. The DVD is not to be used as an instructional, but to supplement the step-by-step text and photo instructions in this chapter in their proper sequential order. (For information on my fully instructional real-time multihour DVD programs, see Appendix C.)

Note that as the dan tien drops deeply down into one leg by bending that knee, the back is not bent over. As always, you do not bend, but you keep the upper body stacked up above the dan tien.

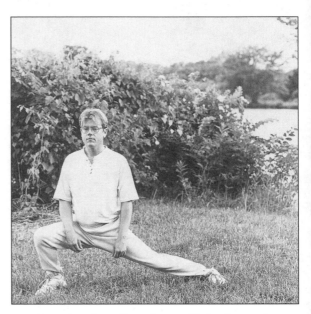

Deep bending of one knee with back straight.

The Chinese Drum's Kaleidoscopic Sensations

The Chinese Drum mimics the motion of those little toy drums with the two swinging beads. When the drum is turned from side to side, the beads twist and drum alternately on each side. This is how your relaxed arms and hands will gently strike your body, as you follow these instructions:

1. Stand up with your feet about shoulder width apart and knees, as always, slightly bent. Gently turn, swinging your arms out. The lead arm swings across the back to strike the flank or lower back, as the trailing arm swings across the front of the body to strike the shoulder.

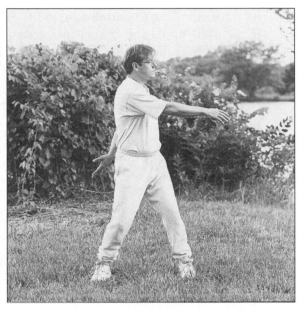

Turning and arm swinging out from body.

2. As the hands strike the shoulder and flank in back, close your eyes and enjoy the physical contact. The gentle slapping begins to massage the muscles as you turn back and forth, alternately slapping each flank and shoulder in turn.

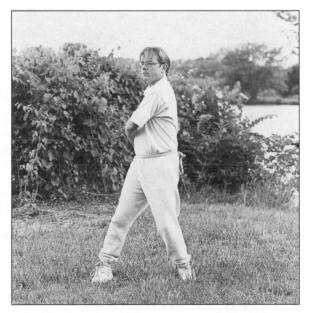

Hands striking body in back and shoulder.

3. Let your mind release any analytical or problem-solving thoughts, and simply open to the pleasure of the motion.

4. With each turn and releasing breath, allow the body to let go even more.

5. Let the mind relax into the pleasure of that letting go, allowing the mind to experience the tens of thousands of sensations throughout the body.

6. With your eyes closed, you can attune yourself to the sensations of the pads of the feet shifting on the floor, the interactions of bones and muscles throughout the body, and the releasing pleasure of each breath. Feel the wind on your skin as you turn through space.

7. Even with your eyes closed, patterns of light and shadow flow across your eyelids, and sounds both internal and external flow over and through you.

8. Do not try to hear, feel, or see. Rather, let your mind relax and allow sensations, images, and sounds to pour over and through your mind the way clear mountain water pours over a waterfall.

Let the mind give up straining to function or reaching out to the world, but rather allow the world to flow to you in a soothing experience of effortlessness. Think of your mind releasing its grip on the dock of logical thought and floating down a river of kaleidoscopic sensation, carried on the beauty of existence, savoring the ability to breathe, flow, and experience sensation … effortlessly.

Deep-Tissue Cleansing Leaves You Radiant

QiGong provides many deep-tissue cleansing exercises, and the following is only one of them. It contains two parts that should be practiced gently and, as always, with awareness of your own mobility range.

Flinging Off and Breathing Out Toxins

Most of the tensions we carry around are energy we've squeezed in our minds, our hearts, and the muscles in the body. You know this is true because on days when you feel heavy and weighted down by the world, if you get on a scale, you don't weigh any more than usual. Therefore, we can simply fling off much of the loads we lug around.

1. Begin with your hands above your head and then simply swing them gently outward and downward, flinging off the weight of the world you've held in your body.

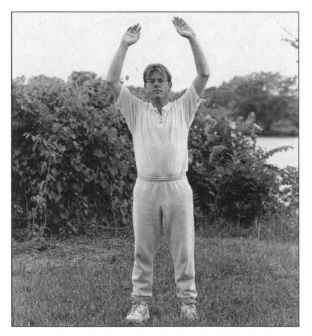

Hands up high, ready to swing out and down.

2. Think of letting the bone marrow itself release the load it's holding on to, which, of course, it can release.

3. As the hands fling toward the ground, think of the hands and feet opening to release that load to fly out of you into the cleansing earth. As your hands swing out and down, exhale deeply to facilitate the release.

4. Breathe in as you raise the hands back up over the head, and again release all as you swing the hands out and down again. Repeat several times.

Elvis Impersonations Cleanse the Soul—Baby!

This tissue-cleansing exercise looks very much like an Elvis impersonation.

1. With your feet about shoulder width apart, eyes closed, and knees slightly bent, just shake. Gently let the arms and entire body go liquid and shake. Do not jolt the joints, but allow a liquid rippling to wave through every muscle and joint.

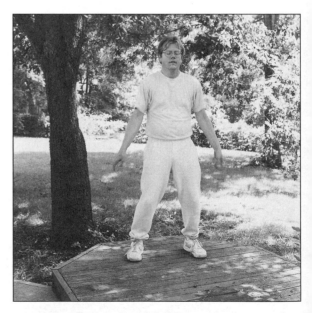

Let yourself go as liquid and limp as you can, with your eyes closed, enjoying a loosening throughout your being.

T'ai Sci _____
Blood lactates, or lactic acids, accumulate in the deep skeletal muscles during times of anxiety. Studies also show that these acids produce anxiety. Therefore, T'ai Chi and warm-ups like the Elvis Impersonation or Tissue Cleansing allow the body to release these long-held anxieties and to cleanse itself of them.

Experience the skeletal muscles jiggling on the bones, from the top of the head to the pads of the feet. It's very slight and very subtle, but as those muscles loosen, they begin to cleanse the body of deep toxins. Think of the brain and heart loosening as well, letting worries, angst, and tensions evaporate out of the body with each yawn or sighing exhale.

2. Have one last good series of shakes while taking in a nice, full breath. On the long sighing exhale, stop shaking and just feel the body awakening. Notice how every cell fills with an effortless lightness, clear, clean, and alive. Wherever you notice remaining tension or block, with each releasing breath, allow the light to expand in that area as if the body were expanding endlessly outward, releasing any heavy loads to evaporate in that endless lighted expansion.

The Least You Need to Know

- The dan tien makes all movement effortless.
- Let warm-ups loosen your entire being and be almost a sensory amusement park.
- Moving from the Horse Stance is the most important warm-up exercise.
- The Chinese Drum cleans your mind and body.
- Doing warm-ups with your eyes closed helps the mind relax within.

In This Part

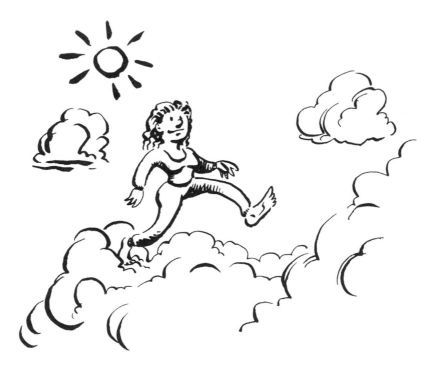

Part 4

Kuang Ping T'ai Chi: Walk on Life's Lighter Side

Part 4 introduces the Kuang Ping Yang Right Style's 20-minute long form, augmented by this edition's new DVD, which provides a noninstructional video exhibition of the entire form. Chapter 14 helps you prepare mentally for the physical experience presented in Chapter 15. You will learn how T'ai Chi movements aid certain organs and what T'ai Chi has in common with the ancient Chinese *I Ching*, or *The Book of Changes*. Chapter 15 illustrates the 64 postures of the Kuang Ping Yang Style's forms in detailed sketches that help you analyze and study each move individually, as well as how they flow together. The text accompanying the images further details how movements are performed.

In addition to the example lessons for a few of the more complicated movements taught in Chapter 15, the DVD shows you the very first movement, to help you better understand how the illustrated/text instructions in Chapter 15 work. The insert gives overviews of several styles from several of my instructional videos. Carefully selected excerpts bring life to the instructional methods in Chapter 15 in a big way. The video excerpt explains the text/illustration methods on selected moves. That understanding will be useful to moves taught in Chapter 15 that wouldn't fit on the insert DVD.

Many of these forms can be seen performed in other styles of T'ai Chi as well. So the explanations of the benefits each movement provides and the T'ai Chi principles and insights explained can also benefit those practicing other forms. As you learn and practice T'ai Chi, you will constantly ask yourself one recurring question: *How did I ever get along without this?*

In This Chapter

- ◆ Uncovering T'ai Chi's ancient roots

- ◆ Learning how T'ai Chi became a philosophy of life

- ◆ Absorbing the advantages of the T'ai Chi long form

- ◆ Finding out why the Kuang Ping Yang has 64 movements

- ◆ Discovering how the historical roots of medicine and T'ai Chi intertwine

- ◆ Understanding the Kuang Ping Yang Style is *just one of many* wonderful T'ai Chi styles available

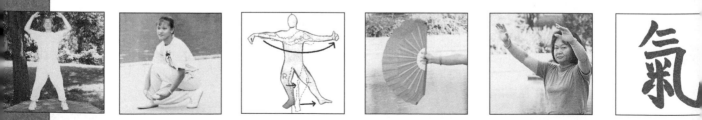

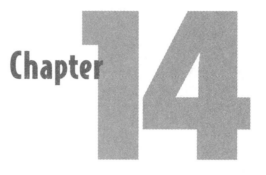
Introducing the Kuang Ping Yang Style

The Kuang Ping Yang style of T'ai Chi has a rich and colorful history, as do all the ancient styles. (See Chapter 6's "T'ai Chi Styles" for background on the other *wonderful* T'ai Chi styles.) The history of T'ai Chi is a great way to better understand its benefits and why it is so perfect for our modern, harried lives.

This chapter discusses the roots of all T'ai Chi and explains how Kuang Ping Yang and the more extant Yang style became different. You also learn why some styles offer shortened versions and why Chapter 15 offers a long form. Understanding some of T'ai Chi's historical or ancient tenets may actually help you get many more and endlessly richer benefits from its practice. The more your mind believes in your therapy, the more powerfully it heals.

The Snake and the Hawk

According to legend, T'ai Chi was born from an observation of nature. A martial arts master observed how a snake slowly evaded a crane's attack by moving away each time the crane's sharp beak struck. What may have been mortal combat became a gentle exercise that left the exhausted crane flying off for easier prey.

This example of yielding to the brute force of the world has created not only a powerful martial art, but also an extremely healthful philosophy for surviving the stressful onslaught of an accelerating future. If this crane's attacks are compared with today's rapid changes, we may be much smarter to bend and yield to that change than to dig in our heels and fight it. The snake's yielding was much less stressful than a head-to-head fight with the larger, sharp-beaked crane.

Ouch!

If the idea of learning a long T'ai Chi form that may take 8 to 12 months to learn is daunting, remember, the journey of a thousand miles begins under one's own feet.

The Shao-Lin Temple: Where It All Began

The Shao-Lin Temple that was featured on the famous television series *Kung Fu* is actually where T'ai Chi began. Around 400 C.E., an 18-movement stretching exercise that eventually grew into T'ai Chi was taught to the monks by a man known as Ta Mo. The purported founder of modern T'ai Chi, however, was a monk named Chang San-feng, who lived about a thousand years later. It was Chang San-feng who is said to have watched the snake yield and avoid the crane's harsh attacks.

From the Temple to the West

The Chen family, founders of the Chen style of T'ai Chi, created one of the earliest family styles. The Chen style was taught to a young martial artist named Yang Lu-chan, who was the founder of today's Yang style.

Know Your Chinese

Chinese names begin with the family name. Therefore, *Yang Lu-chan*, founder of the Yang style, would be called Lu-chan Yang in the West because Yang is his family name.

The Yang family taught a style of T'ai Chi while residing in the city of Kuang Ping. Here, the founding master Yang Lu-chan's eldest son, Yang Pan-hou, was made an offer he couldn't refuse: to teach T'ai Chi at the imperial court and become the emperor's personal teacher. Yang could not refuse the emperor, so he decided to create another version of the family style to teach him, one that was different than the Kuang Ping Yang style. It's worth stating here that *all the various Yang styles* (and other styles) can be powerful health and wellness techniques.

This Kuang Ping Yang style was passed down from Yang Pan-hou to his student Wong Jao-yu, who taught master Kuo Lien Ying. Kuo Lien Ying eventually migrated to the United States and taught this to students, who have since spread this style all across the United States, just as other masters spread the other wonderful styles of T'ai Chi throughout the world.

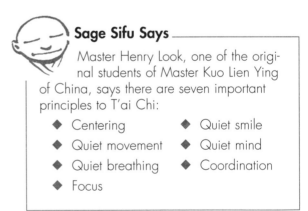

Sage Sifu Says

Master Henry Look, one of the original students of Master Kuo Lien Ying of China, says there are seven important principles to T'ai Chi:

- Centering
- Quiet movement
- Quiet breathing
- Focus
- Quiet smile
- Quiet mind
- Coordination

This can be about as difficult to sort out as the cast of a soap opera, so don't worry about these details. It's just important to remember that the tools you are about to enjoy are the fruits of centuries of study. I include these stories not to confuse, but to acknowledge and to thank these people for making available all that T'ai Chi has to offer in its various forms and styles.

T'ai Chi Becomes a Philosophy

Around 1500 C.E., the Taoist philosopher Wan Yang-ming began to blend the gentle centering philosophical concepts of Taoism into the equally centering physical concepts of T'ai Chi. This gave practitioners a real way to live a more healing, nonviolent life—not just preaching it or thinking about it, but actually training their mind and body how to live that way through T'ai Chi's gentle mind/body fitness program. The modern styles now widely practiced—Yang, Chen, Wu, Mulan Quan, Sun, and others—all incorporate the beautiful personal growth concepts of Taoist philosophy. This book is *not* meant to favor any one style, but to celebrate *all T'ai Chi styles.*

 A T'ai Chi Punch Line

T'ai Chi styles have been created with the same fluidity to the world's demands that T'ai Chi encourages its practitioners to have. For example, the Wu style was created by Wu Quan-yu, a palace guard in the Imperial Court who designed a system of T'ai Chi that could be performed in the restrictive clothing of an imperial palace guard's uniform.

The philosophy of T'ai Chi is based on the idea of the balance of nature, both internally in our health systems and externally in our relationships with the natural world. Therefore, you will see nature imitated in many of the following Kuang Ping Yang T'ai Chi long form names, but also in other styles' form names as well:

◆ Wave Hands Like Clouds
◆ Wind Blowing Lotus Leaves
◆ White Crane Cools Its Wings
◆ Retreat to Ride the Tiger

The poetic quality of these names does more than just remind us how to perform the movements. On a subliminal level, they make us feel more at home in the natural world, somehow more attuned to our connection to the whole of life.

T'ai Chi movement names can also help us remember our multidimensional nature. We are all physical and mental beings, of course, and T'ai Chi integrates these aspects of ourselves well, but it connects our minds and bodies with our spirit or energy nature as well. This connection is reflected in movement names:

◆ Strike Palm to Ask Blessing
◆ Focus Mind Toward the Temple

T'ai Chi reminds us that we are part of the universe and that, in fact, we are made of the same energy stars and everything else are made of. T'ai Chi is meant to open us to the limitless supply of energy within us, in the earth we walk upon, and from the universe our world hurtles through. That universal connection is also reflected in movement names:

◆ Step Up to Form Seven Stars
◆ Grand Terminus

Grand Terminus, the final movement, opens us to the limitless energy of the universe around us.

Short Forms vs. Long Forms

Today several short versions of the original long forms of T'ai Chi exist. Although these shortened versions serve useful purposes, such as enabling a student to acquire a practice system more quickly, there may have been a reason for the average 20-minute length of some of the long forms. The value of a 20-minute-long form is now borne out in modern medical research.

Sage Sifu Says

Most short forms of T'ai Chi take between 5 and 10 minutes. If you practice a short form, simply loop it so you can exercise for 20 minutes and get more benefit. However, if you ever get an opportunity to learn the long form of your style, do it. The complexity of 20 minutes of different movements keeps your mind in a state of relaxed focus, even more than repetition of the same movements does.

We now know the original ancient forms, which usually took a minimum of 20 minutes to complete, were that length for a good reason. In his groundbreaking book *The Relaxation Response*, Dr. Herbert Benson notes that a 20-minute relaxation response exercise seemed to evoke the optimum benefits. Apparently, the mind uses the first few minutes of a relaxation therapy to just wind down; the remaining time truly allows the deep alpha state relaxation these therapies are known for. It is highly advisable, therefore, to take the time to learn a long form of T'ai Chi.

T'ai Sci

Some T'ai Chi movements look very similar to modern physical therapies. For example, Dropping the Duck's Beak, which is an extension of the fingers bending down to touch the thumb, is the same as a Carpal Tunnel prevention exercise used in many corporations. Could it be the therapy for modern repetitive stress disorders had been discovered centuries ago?

Why Sixty-Four Movements?

The more extensive Yang form names 108 movements, and the Kuang Ping Yang style long form claims 64 movements, yet they both average around 20 minutes to perform.

There may be more to the Kuang Ping's 64 movements than just chance. The number 64 has profound philosophical meaning. The Chinese classic *I Ching*, or *The Book of Changes*, is an ancient text of divination and philosophy that attempts to explain how the universal forces of yin and yang ebb and flow, combine and disintegrate, and rise and fall to create the dance of existence. The central premise is that all things are in a constant state of change, including our lives and us. T'ai Chi's goal is to help us flow with the change and not be compulsively attached to the old *or the new*, using what works and discarding what is no longer useful. As if you were a surfer riding the changing waves of life, let go of old waves as they recede, to ease onto the mounting power of the new wave.

The *I Ching* uses Trigrams, or figures with three lines (shown in the following figure) to symbolize the changes in life. When two Trigrams are combined, 64 possible combinations are obtained. These 64 hexagrams are said to represent all possible states of change in the universe. Therefore, Kuang Ping Yang's 64 flowing movements symbolize—and in some ways physically help us to flow through—all the possible changes and challenges of life those changes entail.

Ouch!

It is not important to mentally calculate what movement or direction benefits what system of the body. It is more important to simply allow the mind and body to enjoy the exquisite pleasure of effortless breath and movement as you do T'ai Chi. Rest assured that each aspect of your mind, heart, and body is being nourished and healed by the life energy T'ai Chi practice promotes.

That Kuang Ping Yang style T'ai Chi forms involve 64 movements may have deeper reasons than we know. The complexity and powerful healing qualities T'ai Chi offers are only now beginning to be discovered by modern science. Perhaps many other details of how and why T'ai Chi does what it does will be uncovered in years to come.

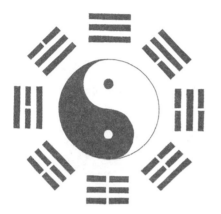

Trigrams are combinations of three lines, which can be broken in half or remain whole, making eight possible combinations.

T'ai Chi and Chinese Medicine

As I discussed in Chapter 3, Traditional Chinese Medicine (TCM) uses the Zang Fu system of understanding how organs interact. Each of these organ systems is represented by one of the five elements of the earth, according to ancient Chinese physics:

Metal	Lungs and large intestines
Wood	Liver and gall bladder
Water	Bladder and kidney
Fire	Heart/pericardium/small intestine/triple warmer
Earth	Spleen and stomach

T'ai Chi movements are described with this same system, and the motion of the body that T'ai Chi promotes may have a healing effect on those systems. The directions of movement each correlate to one of the earth elements:

Movement Directions Relative to the Body		Movement Directions Relative to Earth	
Metal	Advance	Metal	West
Wood	Retreat	Wood	East
Water	Left	Water	North
Fire	Right	Fire	South
Earth	Center	Earth	Center

The 64 postures of the Kuang Ping Yang style take about 20 minutes to complete. The movements flow in an unending progression from one to the next until the final movement, the Grand Terminus. The movements move the body outward and backward in all the directions previously described. There is also a meditative quality to that motion that cannot be described or conveyed in print.

Chapter 15 provides detailed sketches of each of the 64 Kuang Ping Yang style movements, numbered in sequence. It also explains many of the benefits of each movement, complete with pointers on correctly performing them and cautionary notes to help your T'ai Chi experience be both healthful and profound. If live classes don't work for you, you may want to check out my 4-hour *real-time*, classlike, *fully instructional T'ai Chi Long Form* and *Mulan Basic Short Form* DVD programs listed in Appendix C. Valuable excerpts from those programs are used on this book's 1½-hour DVD to greatly enhance this book's instructional value.

The Least You Need to Know

- ◆ T'ai Chi teaches us to yield when life attacks and advance when opportunities open.
- ◆ Twenty-minute-long forms have advantages over short forms.
- ◆ The 64 Kuang Ping movements ease the mind and body through changes.
- ◆ T'ai Chi movements have healing abilities we've yet to completely understand.
- ◆ *All forms* of T'ai Chi can offer profound healing benefits.

In This Chapter

◆ On the DVD: *Exhibition of the T'ai Chi Long Form* and detailed lesson excerpts

◆ Learning the Kuang Ping Yang T'ai Chi long form

◆ Adjusting T'ai Chi to fit your body

◆ Breathing through life's challenges

◆ Using T'ai Chi to help prevent repetitive stress injuries

◆ Relaxing into "complexity" and tapping into universal, limitless energy

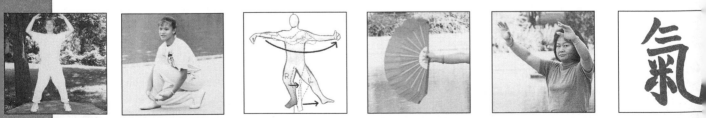

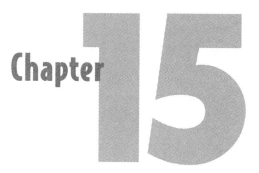

Chapter 15

Out in Style: Right Style, That Is

No matter what style T'ai Chi you practice, this book will greatly enhance your experience by offering you value that you may not get otherwise, by fleshing out how and why each movement can benefit you, and by understanding the internal mechanics of posture, weight shift, and Qi flow.

Because T'ai Chi is constant movement, the 1½-hour DVD that accompanies this new edition gives you visual support for this chapter's already unequaled illustrated and text instructions. *Only* use this chapter's text and illustrated instructions in their proper order for T'ai Chi instruction, *preceding T'ai Chi practice with the warm-ups in Chapter 13*. The DVD with this book provides visual enhancement of select movements and is meant to enhance this chapter's text and illustrated instructions—*not* to replace them.

The DVD includes many excerpts from two of my acclaimed *real-time, fully instructional* video programs that together total more than 5 hours of content. All of this *obviously* could not be included in this book's 1½-hour DVD in its entirety. Therefore, I've carefully chosen valuable sections from my fully instructional programs to bring a sense of detail, timing, and flow to the text and illustrated instructions.

In Appendix C, you can learn about my world-acclaimed DVD programs, which the excerpts for the DVD with this book were taken from, including my 4-hour fully instructional DVD program, *Anthology of T'ai Chi and QiGong: The Prescription for the Future*. Its detailed, easy-going instructionals for all the 64 movements, in this chapter in a *step-by-step* lesson-based, *real-time* format, as well as its QiGong breathing tutorial instructing you when to breathe in and out with each movement, *Moving QiGong Warm Ups*, and Sitting QiGong instruction make it a valuable supplement to the superb resources already in this book and its 1½-hour DVD. The *multihour* programs described in Appendix C are the closest thing to live, personal classes *in the comfort of your own home*.

Ouch!

The DVD's *Exhibition of the T'ai Chi Long Form* exhibits all the movements taught in this chapter. Remember, it is an "exhibition," *not an instructional*. Do not *physically* follow it through without first learning each movement step by step in its proper order, by using the detailed instructions in this chapter's text and illustrations. (Refer to Appendix C for *fully instructional* video information.)

The explanations and instructions you find in this book—and now with the new 1½-hour exhibition DVD—are unparalleled and provide profound added benefit to the at-home user or to those in live classes. Each movement is broken down in a series of sketches to help you see both external and internal aspects, as the exhibition of this *T'ai Chi Long Form* on the DVD brings the illustrated instructions to life. Also on the DVD you'll find several example lesson excerpts that break down certain movements. These are not intended to be instructional in themselves, but to support their corresponding instructional figures in this chapter, to help you familiarize yourself with the "patterns" of this book's illustrated and text instructional techniques. In this way, you'll be clearer on all the text movement instructions, beyond just those that have video supplements on the DVD.

The movement sketches and their accompanying text in this chapter include the following:

◆ **Directional arrows.** Arrows show how your limbs or body move from the previous "ghost image" position into the current position, taking all the guesswork out of how you get from one pose to another.

◆ **Markers.** "L" and "R" are marked on the figures so you can see at a glance whether the left or right side of the body is depicted.

◆ **Shading.** The leg the weight is on, or the *filled leg*, is shaded to a darkness level reflecting just how much weight is shifted onto it. When both legs are shaded, weight is evenly distributed.

◆ **Posture line.** This is a line indicating your *vertical axis* or postural alignment centered over the dan tien.

◆ **Emphasis.** Occasional *italicized* text explains what *sensations* and *internal awareness*, releases, and benefits you may be experiencing *within* as you go through the motions.

◆ **"Ghost" images.** Most of the sketches have a ghost image indicating what the previous posture was, helping you see transitions.

Begin by viewing the *Exhibition of the T'ai Chi Long Form* and the detailed instructional lessons or lesson excerpts on the DVD, while viewing the corresponding illustrated drawings in this chapter and reading the associated instructional text. This will make all the illustrated instructional cues more tangible as you progress through the instruction for all the 64 movements in this chapter.

Some of the more complex instructional figures in this chapter were selected to have corresponding video excerpts with support video on the DVD. They include figures for movements #1, #6 through 8, and #15 through 19, but you'll see "Sage Sifu Says" notations by those figures, indicating they have video support. This combination helps make *all* of this book's text and illustrated lessons unequaled in user-friendly clarity.

A couple sketches also reflect how the Qi, or life energy, flows outward through the hand or the foot. This is shown only in a few figures because too many graphics would be distracting. As a general rule, when you are physically moving an empty foot to a new location on the floor, you take an *in-breath*. When the weight (vertical axis) is shifting over/into/onto a leg and foot, *the breath is being exhaled as you sink into the leg*, allowing Qi to flow down through your relaxed "filling" leg and out the extending arms and hands. This illustrates why the practice of Sitting QiGong is such a critical element to a powerful and effective T'ai Chi form (no matter what style you do), as it enables you to practice "feeling the Qi," or relaxation flowing through your arms and body.

The Kuang Ping Yang style long form takes approximately 20 minutes to complete. Before beginning the movements, to understand why the vertical axis and filling illustrations are so important to your T'ai Chi practice, try this simple exercise:

1. Standing comfortably in the Horse Stance, close your eyes and breathe while relaxing the entire body and standing in your proper vertical axis with the head stacked up above the lower dan tien.

2. Lean your head forward, noticing how the muscles tighten to hold you up. As the head goes back into vertical axis alignment, notice how effortless the stance becomes. The same thing happens when you lean back slightly.

Moving in vertical axis posture makes everything more effortless. (Refer to the *Locating your Dan Tien and Vertical Axis* section of the DVD for more explanation.) Practicing T'ai Chi with this awareness of effortless versus effortful movement easily and naturally changes the way you move through life. T'ai Chi, and life, should be mostly effortless—and strangely,

when it is, this is usually when we are getting *the most accomplished.*

As you go through this exercise, note that the movement names offer two tools: they evoke healthful and soothing mental/sensual images to calm the mind and heart, and they offer visual mental images to help you remember how to move. Part of the calming effect results from T'ai Chi's left brain/right brain integration of "feeling" and "thinking." Before you dive into learning the movements using the following text and illustrated instructions, if you haven't already, pop in the book's DVD and view the entire *Exhibition of the T'ai Chi Long Form* while flipping through the pages of this chapter, to get a general feel for the motion of T'ai Chi movement.

 Sage Sifu Says

Look at figures for Movement #1, and view *T'ai Chi Long Form Lesson 1 Excerpt* on the DVD (excerpted from my 4-hour DVD; see Appendix C). Pay attention to the motion arrows, shading, posture lines, ghost images, and text instruction to see how the illustrated instruction in this chapter works. Repeat viewing to get a feel for the patterns. Familiarizing yourself with the patterns helps with all the instructional figures, not just the ones with video supplements.

Strike Palm to Ask Blessings, #1

Breathe in deeply and lift your palms as if circling them up in front of you over a large 3-foot ball, shifting your weight toward the left foot.

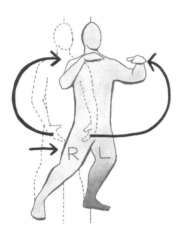

As the palms pull back over the sphere, ending up in front of your chest as though you were going to push something away, the weight shifts back to the right foot, sinking the Qi, or filling the right foot, as palms drop to the sides of the hips.

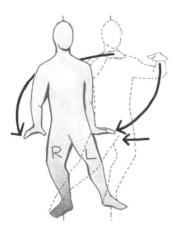

From palms down position, palms pull out and behind a bit to rotate out the shoulders. As your empty left foot comes out in front, place

your left heel lightly on the ground. Continue circling your arms around in front of the body as if hugging a large tree, and the left heel touches just as your palms meet. The left palm is lateral as in the sketch, while the right palm is vertical. Although the movement is called Strike Palm, the palms don't actually strike; pretend there is a soft energy sphere the size of a honeydew melon between your relaxed, rounded hands.

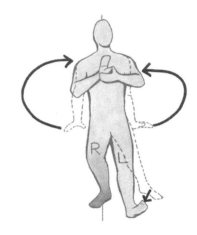

Grasp the Bird's Tail, #2

From completed Strike Palms, reach with your arms up and out to the right as your left toe reaches out to the left and back.

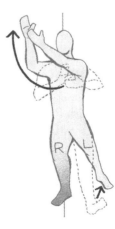

With your right hand palm down on top of your left hand palm up, stroke the bird's tail as your arms pull down and back. Your weight shifts back to the left foot behind.

Your hands stroke down to the groin, releasing the bird's tail. Turn your palms away from your body with your elbows at your sides while your hands continue to circle up in front of your face. Your right foot pulls back, touching your right toe near the left instep.

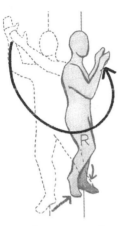

Now turn your dan tien and torso to the right at a 45-degree angle (front/right), while your arms follow around and in front of your chest, ready to push out diagonally to right.

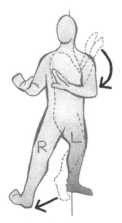

Sage Sifu Says

Strike Palm, Grasp Bird's Tail, and Single Whip are all wonderful for loosening the daily stress from tight shoulders.

Single Whip, #3

Step out with your right heel, pushing your hands forward as the weight shifts onto the right foot (rolling onto the heel first and then the rest of the foot goes flat). Notice how Qi flows through the relaxed body, out your pushing hands, and down through the filling right leg into the earth. At first you simply relax and exhale; then over time, a feeling of "empty flow" will settle through you, and in time you'll perceive a soothing flow of energy.

Your arms stretch out to your right side, as the fingers on the right hand bend down, touching your right thumb (forming a duck's beak).

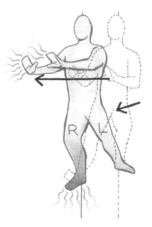

Your left fingers stroke the inside of the right arm. Your left palm pulls across your body in a great half-circle toward the left side as the body follows, turning at the dan tien.

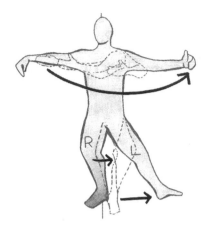

Your left palm continues over to the left side, as if circling a globe on its axis, until your palm is near your shoulder …

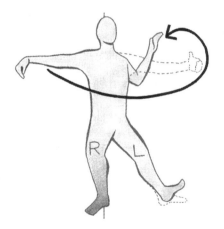

T'ai Sci

T'ai Chi's a uniquely right-brain/left-brain experience. Your analytical mind follows detailed forms, while your sensory mind enjoys a sense of being carried through motions, almost being massaged by the process effortlessly. Book instruction is left brain; video/class is more right brain.

… and then your left hand pushes the imaginary globe away to the left, while the weight sinks onto the left heel and then the rest of the left foot. Again, note how the Qi or life energy flows through the relaxed body, out the hand, and down the leg into the earth.

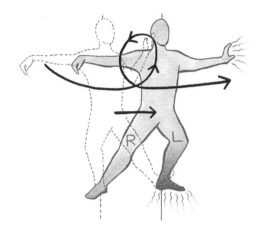

White Crane Cools Its Wings, #4

Your weight shifts to the left leg as the torso turns to the left. The left arm drops down to your side, the palm facing the ground, as the right arm circles from behind up above head.

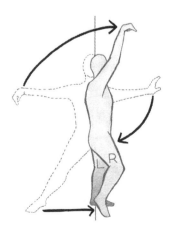

T'ai Sci

Place the tip of the tongue lightly against the roof of the mouth while performing your movements, and fully fill and empty the lungs from bottom to top on each breath, allowing the torso to "relax" around your breathing. Studies show that long, relaxed abdominal breathing oxygenates the body much more effectively than rapidly inflating the chest.

Note that the following two sketches show the same pose, so you can now see it from a front angle as well. The right arm comes straight down as the right foot sticks out a few inches in front.

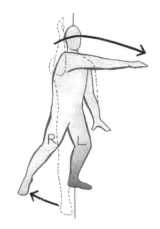

Now shift the weight to the right foot as the right elbow pulls across in an elbow strike, allowing the sinking dan tien to pull the elbow strike across.

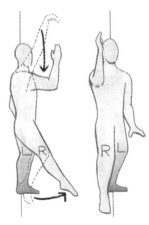

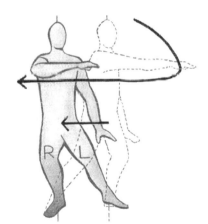

Step out to the right side with your right toe, as the right elbow circles to the left side, to prepare, by winding up, for upcoming elbow strike. (Both your palms are face down, in their respective positions.)

Lift the left foot and place it out in front, as the left hand moves slightly to the front.

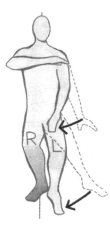

Sage Sifu Says

Remember that the "ghost" images in most of the instructional sketches represent the previous posture and are included to help you see *transitions between positions*.

Brush Knee Twist Step, #5

The left hand extends out 45 degrees to the left of front, as the left foot steps back behind slightly. The right forearm twists a bit so the "back" of the right hand is facing the chest, and the palm faces out.

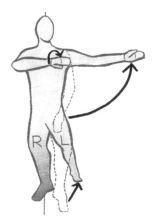

Now the weight sinks back into the left foot as the left arm brushes to the center of the body, as if slapping an imaginary wall in front of you. Exhale and allow the body to relax as the weight, or dan tien, sinks back on each Brush motion.

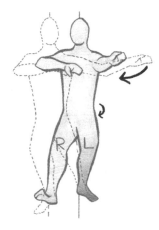

With the weight back on the left foot, the right empty foot steps slightly back as the right hand extends out 45 degrees to the right, and the "back" or left hand is placed in front of your heart.

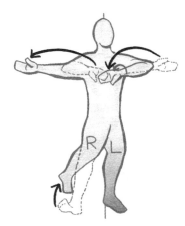

Just as you did on the left side, now shift your weight back to the right, brushing the right hand toward your center.

Repeat once more on both sides, as in the first four figures of Brush Knee Twist Step (Movement #5). As you finish the last brush, shift to your right foot and brush across your body with your right hand.

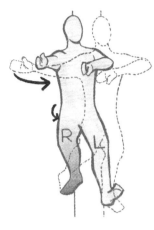

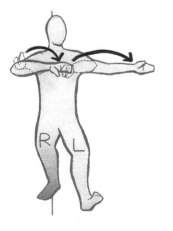

Ouch! _____

If any of the movement descriptions cause pain, alter them to suit you. For example, if you have a bad knee, share some weight on the empty foot as well.

Move the left hand out 45 degrees to the left, but do not move the left foot this time.

Brush the left hand across the body, and let the left arm circle out in front as the right hand forms a fist by the right hip.

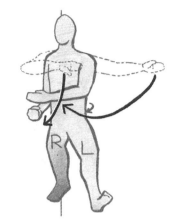

Now shift your weight 60 percent onto the left foot, and throw the right-fisted punch out in front beneath the left arm, circling out in a defensive posture, or parry.

Sage Sifu Says _____

Look at the figures for movements #6 through #8, and view the *T'ai Chi Long Form Lesson 4 Excerpt* on the DVD (taken from my 4-hour DVD; see Appendix C). Pay attention to the motion arrows, shading, posture lines, and ghost images on the figures, and relate the video to the book's instructional patterns.

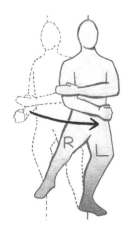

Apparent Closing, #6

From the Parry and Punch position, the palms turn down; then your hands open and come back to the temples as your weight shifts back onto the right leg and the left foot rolls back on its heel.

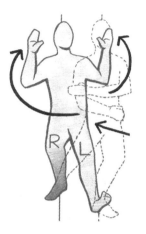

Push out as the weight rolls forward onto the left leg. Step through with the right foot and then shift your weight to the right leg as you push out to point with flat hands.

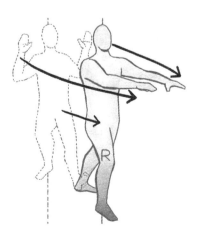

Push Turn and Carry Tiger to Mountain, #7

Carry Tiger to the Mountain, as other movements, reminds us of our connection to nature as we mimic the grace of noble beasts.

With your weight on the right foot and your hands pushed out flat, your weight comes off the left foot until only the toe is touching as your pushing hands circle flatly (as if on a table top) to the left as the left foot pivots on the toe.

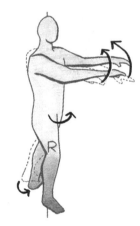

At ¾ of the hands circling to the left, your weight begins shifting to the left foot as the empty right foot pivots on the toe.

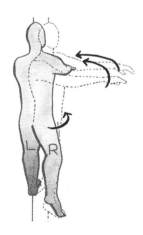

With the 180-degree turn complete, your weight settles back on the right foot. Only the left heel touches, as your left toes come up off the floor and your right fist rests over the thumb of your open left hand in front of your abdomen. Note the two figures in this sketch depict the same posture, only shown twice so you can now view it frontally.

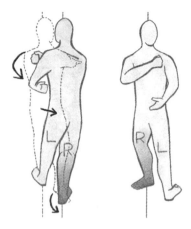

Spiraling Hands to Focus Mind Toward the Temple to Parry and Punch, #8

This movement encompasses the spiritual image of Focusing Our Mind Toward Our Temple, which is the heart, while providing a protective shield for the vital/vulnerable areas of the body.

With your hands open, the palms should be parallel to one another and pointing straight as the left heel lifts (your weight is still on the right leg) and the left heel lightly retouches the ground.

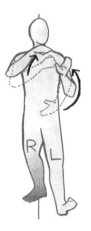

Your weight slowly shifts up to the left foot as your hands begin a clockwise corkscrew downward. (Keep your hands relaxed at the wrists so they pivot facing straight.)

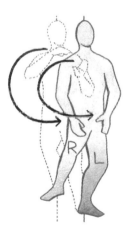

As your weight shifts completely to the left foot, your hands begin the upward part of a clockwise rotation, lifting the right foot up from behind, as if a string were attached from your hands to your feet, and reaching the top as the right heel touches the ground in front of you.

Remember not to "bob up" as you shift up into the front leg. In T'ai Chi, you always stay "down" in a slightly bent knee stance.

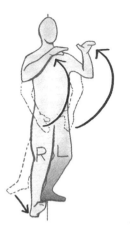

Repeat this stepping/shifting/spiraling hands with the right foot out this time, and repeat left foot out, and then right foot out (for a total of five times stepping forward on this Spiraling Hands Movement, alternating feet each time, of course).

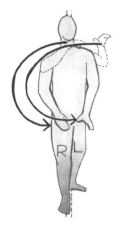

However, on the fifth step, which is with the left foot out, do not shift your weight to the left foot. Leave it out and empty as the hands corkscrew one last time all the way around.

Then allow the right hand to fall to your side, forming a fist as the left circles in front to parry.

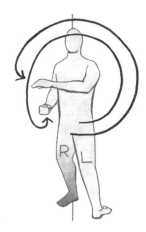

Now parry and punch, with your weight shifting about 65 percent onto the left foot.

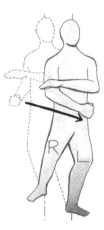

Fist Under Elbow, #9

With your weight still mostly on the left foot (in the punch parry position), drop your right fist down under your left elbow.

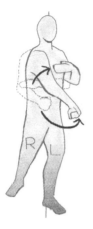

As your right fist is pulled up with the palm facing your chin, the left parry hand drops to the palm up position to rest at the left hip.

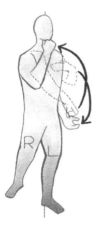

Repulse the Monkey, #10

Repulse the Monkey can be a powerful martial arts tactic of blocking an incoming blow, yielding to the opponent's force, and allowing that force to carry the opponent off to your side. However, it also fosters a

very healing exchange of energy that Traditional Chinese Medicine (TCM) calls Long Qi when the open palms pass one another in front of the heart chakra, an energy center called the middle dan tien. According to TCM, this has a supercharging effect, opening the body to the healing force of Qi, and practitioners feel this sense of opening release through that area of the body each time they practice.

Without moving your legs, the left hand (palm up at your waist) begins an outside arc up to the left ear, as if stroking out and away over a large orb at the side of the body.

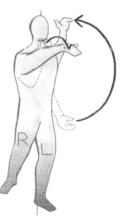

Now the right hand, palm up, pulls back to the right side of your waist, while the left hand, palm facing front, pushes outward from your chest; simultaneously, weight sinks back into your right leg.

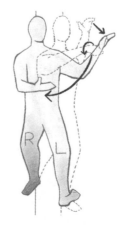

Now the weight shifts back to the right leg. Notice how your relaxed torso and body allow Qi to flow out of your relaxed left shoulder, arm, and hand as it also flows down and through your sinking back into the right leg.

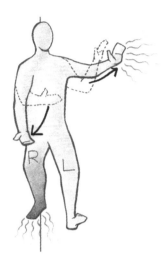

Prepare for the next three moves by moving the opposite leg back as your palm at your waist circles up near the ear, poised to push when the other hand pulls back as you shift back.

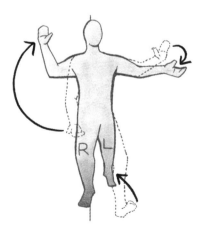

Repeat with the right hand pushing, the left hand pulling as you sink back.

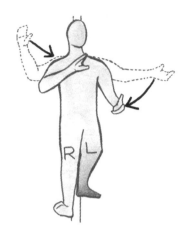

Shifting back to the left leg, Qi flows out of your relaxed torso, right shoulder, right arm, and right hand.

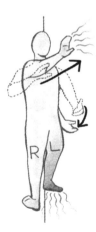

Repeat with the left hand pushing and the right hand pulling, shifting back to the right leg (see the third and forth figures of the Repulse the Monkey movement).

Repeat with the right hand pushing and the left hand pulling, shifting back to the left leg (see the sixth and seventh figures of the Repulse the Monkey movement).

Stork Covers Its Wing/ Sword in Sheath, #11

After completing the last Repulse the Monkey with the right hand pushed out and the weight back on the left, back foot, the right foot now pivots on the heel to follow the extended right arm out to point diagonally 45 degrees to left/front.

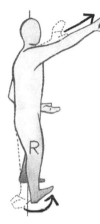

Upon completing the pivot, the weight shifts to the right foot while pivoting on the left ball and dropping the left heel in toward the right foot a bit.

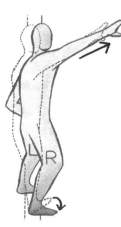

Now, as the left palm up turns into a sheath (palm turns in to face body), the weight shifts back to the left leg, and the right extended hand pulls back into the left hand's sheath between the left palm and the left hip. The right toe simultaneously pulls back to rest at the left instep.

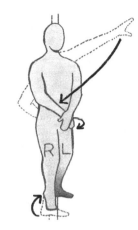

Slow Palm Slant Flying, #12

Slow Palm Slant Flying is one of the most beautiful and uplifting movements in the entire series.

The right heel goes out diagonally.

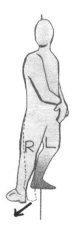

As your weight shifts to your right foot, the right palm extends slowly outward from your left hand's sheath as your left hand extends back to the opposite corner.

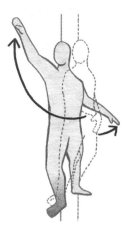

Extend your arms fully with your weight totally on your right leg; the right arm begins a great arcing circle around a bit behind your body, while the open left palm arcs up from behind until both open palms meet in front of the chest. Lift the left foot to place the left toe lightly a couple inches in front of the body below your parallel palms.

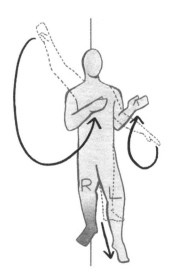

Raise Right Hand and Left: Turn and Repeat (Part I), #13

Although each movement has powerful martial applications, the goal of T'ai Chi is to "soong yi dien," to loosen the mind, heart, and body. This movement loosens the abdominal area, back, and shoulders by performing Long Qi. The palms passing one another healthfully stimulate the dan tien energy centers within the body, also relaxing the solar plexus.

Your left heel extends forward as your left arm curls around (as if hugging a tree), and your weight continues rolling up onto the left foot, as the heel of the right wrist begins to descend (a soothing Long Qi experience can be felt in the abdomen as the right palm passes the left palm as the right hand drops). Now the right hand forms a Duck's Beak and begins to lift upward.

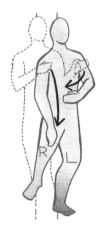

The right hand's Duck's Beak rises, as if pulling a string attached to the right foot, and pulls the back right foot up in front to touch the toe. When the Duck's Beak is above the head, the palm opens.

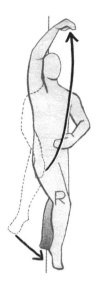

Now the right hand drops down as the right toe reaches back behind, until the right and left palms are once again parallel facing one another in front and the weight has shifted back to the right foot, with only the left heel touching.

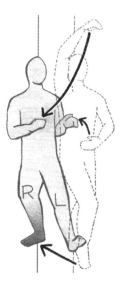

Turn to the right, pivoting on the (empty) left heel, palms arcing across in front of the chest, still parallel and facing one another.

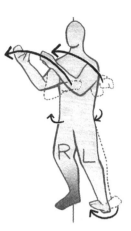

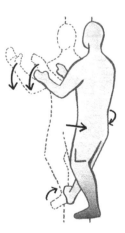

Ouch!

While moving, remember to breathe deeply into the diaphragm, but also easily and naturally. This conditions you to breathe through life's changes just as through T'ai Chi's changing postures.

As the 180-degree turn/pivot completes, the weight sinks completely back into the left leg, and the hands fall again parallel in front of the chest.

(The following sketch merely gives you a frontal view for easier viewing.)

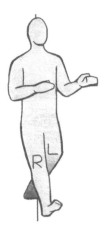

Now the left wrist begins its descent as the right arm parries as if hugging a tree and the weight begins shifting up onto the right leg.

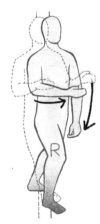

![T'ai Sci icon] **T'ai Sci**

T'ai Chi can accomplish the seemingly paradoxical goal of fostering deep relaxation *and* martial arts training simultaneously, teaching that effectiveness in all aspects of life can be effortless.

Your left hand forms the Duck's Beak, pulling the imaginary string up, bringing the left toe to touch in front as the left hand raises overhead and the weight completely shifts to the right leg.

Although this movement is very soothing to the upper body and therapeutic for the hand and arm, its martial application is powerful. As the right hand blocks a punch, the left hand lowers to block a kick. The left hand then rises to strike an opponent's face or nose as the left knee rises to kick the groin. Ouch!

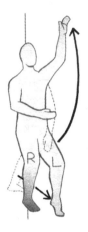

As the left hand opens and descends, the left toe reaches back, and the weight shifts back to the left foot as the palms face, parallel, in front of the chest (the right heal touching in front).

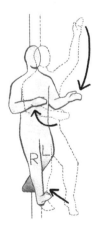

Wave Hand Over Light/ Fly Pulling Back, #14

With the palms parallel and facing each other, they rotate as if over a ball so the right palm is over the left palm.

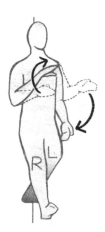

The right fingers extend straight out from chest level at your shadow opponent's throat level, as the weight shifts forward onto the right leg. The right palm curves around downward as if it has gone over and is now curving back under a sphere of light, to rest in front of the dan tien, cradled in the left palm, as the right toe pulls back to rest by the left instep.

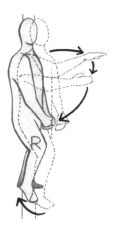

The right heel extends out front as the right palm circles, this time from "beneath the sphere of light" …

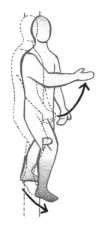

… and continuing up and over the back of the sphere of light until the back of the right hand rests in front of the chest. As the right hand is completing the circle, the left foot pulls up to rest with the toe at the right instep.

Fly Pulling Back extends your Qi forward and out in an expressive motion and then relaxes your Qi, sinking back into a retreat.

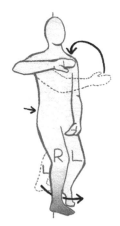

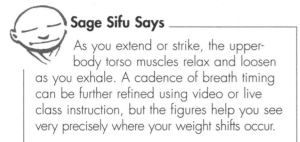

Sage Sifu Says

As you extend or strike, the upper-body torso muscles relax and loosen as you exhale. A cadence of breath timing can be further refined using video or live class instruction, but the figures help you see very precisely where your weight shifts occur.

Fan Through the Arms, #15

With the back of the right hand facing the chest and the open left palm in front of the dan tien, the left palm arcs outward to the left at shoulder height, and your weight shifts 60 percent to the left.

Your left fanning arm relaxes away from the body as the weight shifts toward the left leg. The dan tien carries the arm outward as it sinks over the left leg. Your arm moves out and up like a clock hand moving from 6 to 3 o'clock as you relax and exhale.

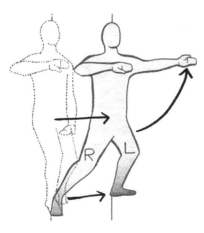

Green Dragon Rising from the Water, #16

Your weight shifts back to the right foot as the left foot pivots on the heel to point the left toe cater-corner toward the right. Your left arm follows so the entire body is turned cater-corner to the left now.

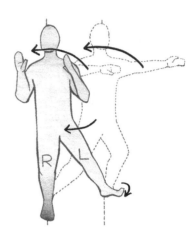

With the right and left palms falling parallel in front of the chest, weight settles back onto the left leg, and the right foot comes to the heel as your right toe comes up.

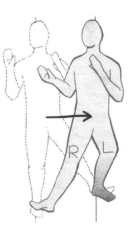

Lift your right heel slightly and replace it to extend out more cater-corner to right, then reaching open palms upward and outward while the weight shifts about 65 percent up toward the right foot.

This Green Dragon move teaches us to push and lift from your dan tien, keeping the back heel planted down, thereby reducing back pressure. This creates more power and less chance of injury while performing daily tasks.

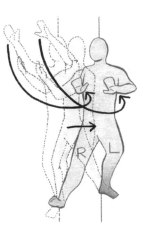

Then the right heel goes out and the hands push out from the torso.

The weight shifts on up to the right leg as you complete the push and then the hands turn to the right side, where the Duck's Beak begins for Single Whip.

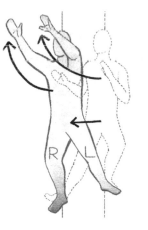

As if the hands are pulling a sphere of light back down into your heart, the weight settles back onto the left leg and the right toe pulls back to touch at the left instep.

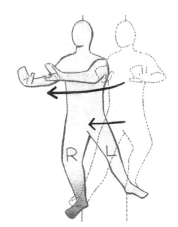

Single Whip (Part II), #17

The right hand is in a Duck's Beak (the fingers touching the right thumb), and as the left fingers stroke the inside of the right arm, the left palm pulls across the body. (Refer to the second, third, and fourth figures of the first Single Whip [Movement #3].)

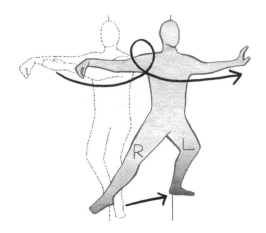

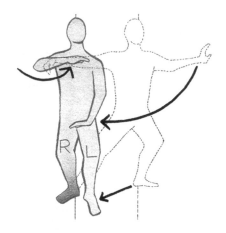

On the Duck's Beak, all the fingers on the right hand extend down to touch the right thumb. Modern carpal tunnel prevention exercises include movements like these. So among its many benefits, T'ai Chi appears to be an ergonomic carpal tunnel prevention exercise as well.

Wave Hands Like Clouds (×3), #18 (Part I, Linear Style)

T'ai Chi connects us with nature as we rise up from the water to Wave Hands Like Clouds.

As your hands draw in from Single Whip extension, turn both palms to face down. Shift the weight to the right leg, bringing the left toe out to touch in front, as the right hand comes parallel to ground at shoulder height to the center chest and the left hand comes down to arrive at the center dan tien level.

As the left toe goes straight out to the left, both hands reach straight out to the right at shoulder level.

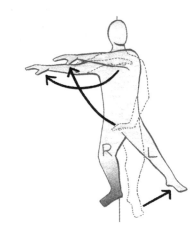

Ouch!

You'll know you are doing movements correctly if it feels good. If you feel undue strain in a knee, leg, or anywhere in the body, you're probably forcing the position. All T'ai Chi positions are designed to enable you to relax into the position. If you feel lower back pain in Wave Hands or other moves, it's usually because your lower back is overarched. Be sure as you exhale you allow the tailbone to *relax* down.

As the weight shifts back to the left leg, the right hand drops to the dan tien center, while the left hand pulls parallel to the ground across the center chest.

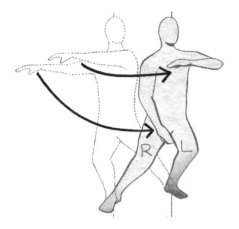

Your weight shifts to the left leg as the right leg is drawn toward the left leg and the hands reach out to the left at shoulder level.

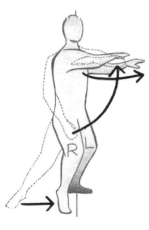

Your weight shifts to the right leg as the hands come to center (right at chest, left at dan tien).

Though obviously martial, there's also a soothing quality of imagining the hands waving like clouds. The thought unlocks an effortlessness flow throughout the mind and body.

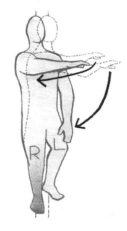

As the left toe goes straight out to the left, both hands reach straight out to the right at shoulder level.

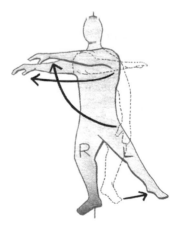

Repeat the second through sixth figures of this movement two more times (for a total of three repetitions for Wave Hands Like Clouds). However, on last repetition, leave off the action from the sixth figure of this movement, because you will be going right into a Single Whip from there. All Wave Hands Like Clouds (and there are four of them in this style) begin and end with a Single Whip.

Single Whip (Part III), #19

Refer to Movement #3's (the first Single Whip) second, third, and fourth figures, if needed, although if you are this far, you should know the Single Whip by heart by now. If not, go back and review. It's not a test, only a game. Enjoy!

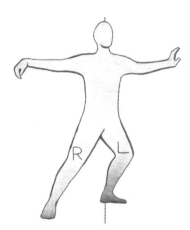

> **Sage Sifu Says**
>
> T'ai Chi is taught in three stages. First, the movements are learned. Second, the breath is incorporated into the regimen by learning an inhalation or exhalation that is connected to each movement. Third, a relaxation element or awareness of the flow of energy through the body is learned. Although the first step offers many benefits from the first day, the benefits get richer and deeper with each level you learn.

High Pat on Horse/Guarding the Temples, #20

From the Single Whip pose, the torso rotates to the right and the arms begin to curve into a horseshoe shape in front of the body. While the torso turns, you pivot on the ball of the right foot.

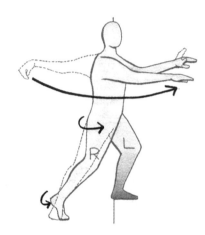

The weight now sinks back on the right leg as the left toe comes up (left heel down) and the arms settle in front of the chest.

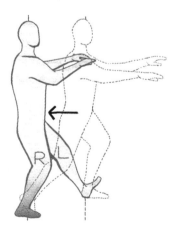

With the weight settled on the right leg, raise the left foot a bit and then touch the left toe in front, the palms patting downward a little as if patting a pony's hindquarters.

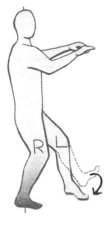

While shifting up onto the left leg, turn the palms outward, each palm arcing up to the side of the temples of the head as if protecting from a side blow, and then arcing down to form a low block by crossing the right wrist over the left in front of the dan tien. The right foot comes up to touch empty (without any weight on it) by the left instep (the left foot being filled with your weight on it).

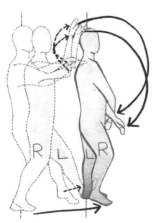

(The following sketch shows the front position of the preceding figure.)

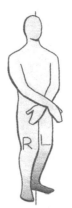

Lower Block/Upper Block, Separation of Right Foot; Lower Block/Upper Block, Separation of Left Foot, #21

With the wrists crossed at the dan tien in the preceding figure, now lift the wrists to cross them at mid-chest block (the palms still facing in toward the chest).

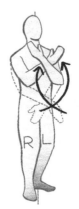

The arms continue rising as the palms turn out, causing the wrists to twist and forming an up block (with the palms facing out). It takes a

7-count to go from the low block to the up block and the kick that follows.

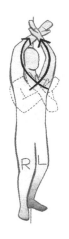

Kick the right foot up and out to the right side as the right hand chops down to meet the foot (at whatever height is comfortable—don't force it; the kicks will get higher over time). Catch the foot on its descent, and slowly settle the descending right foot down by the left foot.

Your hand may not touch the kicking foot at first. That's okay; just kick as high as is comfortable.

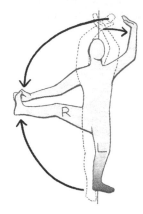

The weight shifts back into the right foot as the left wrist crosses over the right this time.

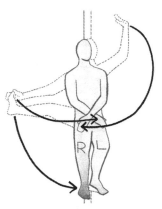

Begin the low/mid/upper block, the left leg preparing for the separation kick.

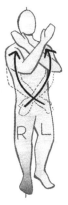

As the up block completes, the left hand begins to slip sideways to the left as the left foot prepares to kick out and up to the left.

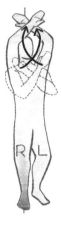

Kick the left foot out and up to the left side as the left hand chops down to meet the foot (again, kick only as high as is comfortable) and catches the left foot as it drops to slowly settle "behind" the right heel.

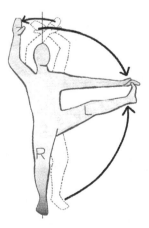

Turn and Kick with Sole, #22

As the left foot settles behind the right heel, the body turns ¼ turn to the left. The left leg fills and the right leg empties as you complete the ¼ turn.

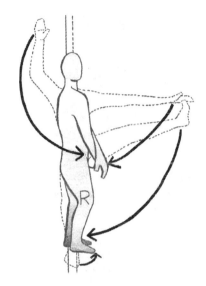

(The following sketch presents a frontal view of the pose in the preceding figure.)

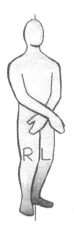

The weight shifts into the right leg as the low block rises to mid block.

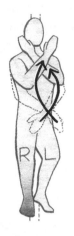

The weight sinks fully into the right leg as the mid block rises to high block as the palms twist out.

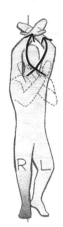

A T'ai Chi Punch Line

T'ai Chi breath is fully exhaled from the chest to the abdomen, with the tip of the tongue lightly touching the roof of your mouth so that a *full inhalation* accompanies preparations, and full *exhalations* accompany shifts, kicks, or punches.

Kick the left leg up and out to the left as the left hand swings out in front and around to the side to slap instep of the left foot (or the inside of the left leg), as the right hand chops out to the right slightly.

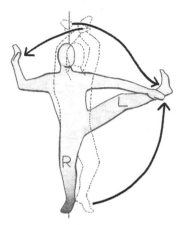

Wind Blowing Lotus Leaves (×4), #23

This is an exquisite move. It is artistically beautiful and feels fantastic because it loosens the entire torso. It also helps the body learn to push the lawn mower or perform other tasks with much less pressure on the lower back. Correct T'ai Chi movement shifts strain from the lower back to the thighs, which are much stronger and less delicate than the back's vertebrae.

After the left hand smacks the instep or the inside of the left leg, it pulls back to the head just off the right ear, and the right hand pulls behind that, as if holding a beach ball off to the right side of the head. Place the left heel down at a 45-degree angle to the left/front.

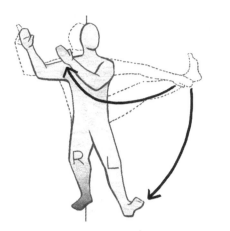

The weight shifts forward onto the left leg as the front/left arm drops down in a circular motion, blocking the groin area as the torso turns to shift over the left leg, the right hand still by the right shoulder to push as the body shifts forward. Exhale as you shift forward, relaxing.

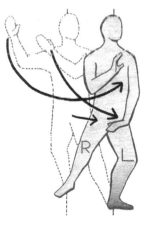

Now imagine holding the beach ball off to the left side of the head (the right hand forward of the left this time) as the right heel goes out 45 degrees to the front/right.

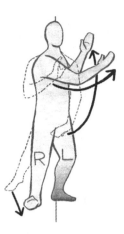

The weight shifts forward onto the right leg as the front/right arm drops down in a circular motion, blocking the groin area, with the torso turning slightly to shift over the right leg and the left hand still by the left shoulder. Exhale as you shift, relaxing.

Shift forward, as the breath seems to relax out of every cell. As your Qi sinks into the earth, its power also flows through you and out your hands. The dan tien pulls your relaxed body forward.

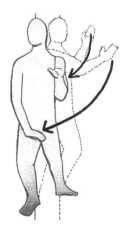

Now repeat the four figures of Wind Blowing Lotus Leaves for a total of four movements in this series, two from the right to left and two from the left to right.

Block Up/Fist Down, #24

Begin similar to the first two figures in the preceding Wind Blowing Lotus Leaves (Movement #23). However, this time, your right hand forms a fist and rises up and over to deliver a downward hammer-fist. Your left hand doesn't stop down at a groin block, but it continues circling up in front to a high block protecting your forehead, with the left palm down in a down block. As the block arcs out and up in front of the body, the palm continues to face away from the upper body even as the block is completed.

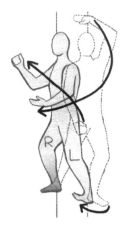

Sink back into the left leg as the pivot completes, allowing the right toe to come up pivoting on the right heel. The left open palm rests at the left hip, facing up, as the right fist swings out in front of the right shoulder.

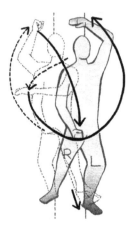

Turn and Double Kick, #25

Turn 180 degrees to prepare for the Double Kick by shifting the weight back on the right leg and pivoting on the "empty" left heel as the body turns to the right.

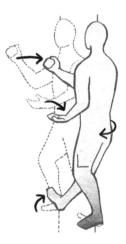

(The next sketch shows a frontal view of this last figure.)

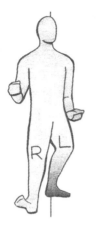

From sunken down on the right leg, shift forward and kick the left leg up and out for a left front kick.

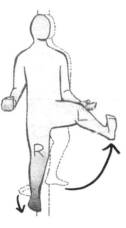

Remember that your kick does not have to be as high as illustrated.

 Sage Sifu Says

The complexity and variety of movements may seem daunting at first, but just relax and learn the move you're learning today. You'll get it, one move at a time. *A lesson for life.*

Then place the left leg out in front and shift up into the left leg …

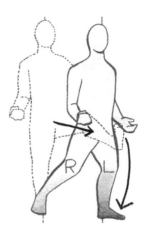

… kicking the right leg up and out front while opening the right fist and smacking the right palm down on top of the kicking right foot (or leg).

As the right leg kicks up, the right palm turns over and smacks down to slap the top of the right foot, or calf, or knee, or wherever your hand comfortably slaps without leaning forward.

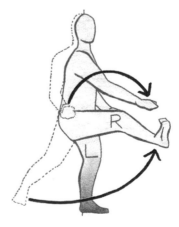

Place your right foot down in front after the kick, heel first.

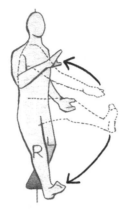

![hand icon] **Ouch!** _____
Never force or strain. Breathe easily. Let your mind and body learn to relax as you are absorbed in the silken flow of continuous movement.

Parry and Punch, #26

Step forward with the left foot while preparing the right fist near the right hip and dropping the left parry.

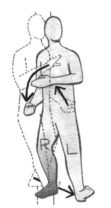

Then parry and punch as the weight shifts onto the left front foot about 60 percent forward. Again, do not lean forward as you punch. The body or vertical axis always stays stacked above the dan tien.

As the punch is thrown and Qi sinks into the forward left leg, breath is released in an easy sigh. This action is a wonderful stress release for both the hips and the upper body. Tension can be allowed to pour out the left foot into earth, and upper-body tension can be released out the punching fist.

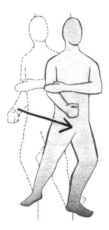

Step Back/Lower Block/ Upper Block, Kick Front, #27

Shift the weight back to the right leg, rolling up off the left heel as the hands drop out to the sides.

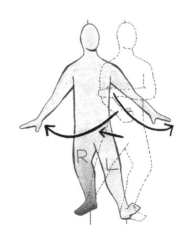

Bring the hands back down to center (the left wrist crossing on top) as the left foot comes back to touch at the right instep.

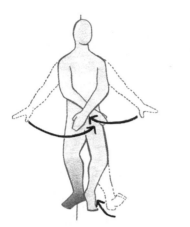

The low block rises to mid block as the left knee rises up.

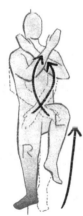

T'ai Sci

Timing on all low, mid, and upper blocks is a 7-count, but over time, the rate of your relaxed breathing will become your timer. Breath and motion become one, allowing effortless flow to fill and soothe your mind, as healing, soothing motion expands Qi and circulation through every relaxing capillary, cell, and atom of your being.

As the mid block becomes an upper block, your palms twist out and begin to strike up and out to the sides, as the left foot kicks out front.

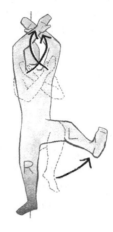

This kick is great for balance. You do not have to perform the kick as high as what's illustrated here. You may begin much lower. Go as high as is comfortable, without leaning backward out of your vertical axis. As with all movements, it is done very slowly, placing the foot out in front as you breathe. Observe your balance as you do this.

The hands slowly lower to the sides as the left foot slowly lowers to rest flat on the right side of the right foot.

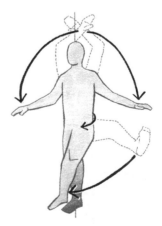

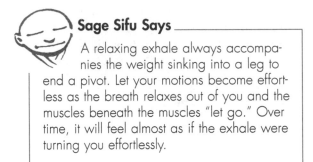

Sage Sifu Says _____

A relaxing exhale always accompanies the weight sinking into a leg to end a pivot. Let your motions become effortless as the breath relaxes out of you and the muscles beneath the muscles "let go." Over time, it will feel almost as if the exhale were turning you effortlessly.

Pivoting clockwise, shift the weight slowly to the left foot, pivoting on the right ball (you are working to achieve a ¾-turn pivot).

Shift the weight to the right foot as the ¾ turn continues to the right.

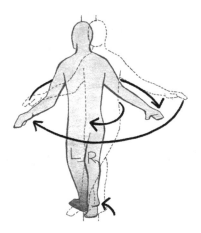

Pivot on the left ball as the ¾ pivot is completed.

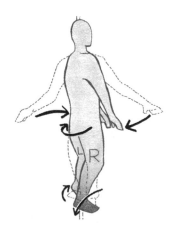

(The following figure is a frontal view of the previous figure, not more turning. See that the weight shifts back to the left foot as the right wrist crosses over the left.)

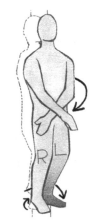

Lower Block/Upper Block Separation of Right Foot, #28

Perform a lower/mid/upper block with the right wrist crossed on top and the weight on the left foot so you can separate the right foot kick. (Refer to earlier lower/mid/upper block separation right foot kicks if you need a refresher before proceeding on to this Parry and Punch.)

Don't psyche yourself into thinking this isn't for you. It's perfect for you. If you are in a wheelchair, this movement will involve your hand arcing down. If you are paralyzed to the waist, you'll give the right-side abdominal muscles instructions to extend upward toward the arcing right hand, and this intention of motion will exercise and coordinate mind and body, relieving tension.

Parry and Punch, #29

When Separation Right Foot completes, place the right heel out to the right side and shift into it, proceeding in to a Parry and Punch. (Refer to earlier Parry and Punch instructions if you need a refresher.)

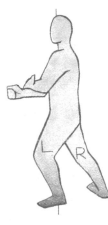

 Sage Sifu Says

When punching or pushing in T'ai Chi, remember that these martial exercises can also be about how we move through our lives: cutting the grass, washing the dishes, or putting groceries in the pantry. If we adopt good postural habits by moving from the dan tien and vertical axis while punching, pushing, or pivoting, we will likely use these habits while mowing, lifting, etc.

Chop Opponent with Fist (Pivot and Rotate Fist [×3]), #30

When turning, you must empty a leg before pivoting on it so you do not damage the knee. Once a foot is pivoted to the desired position,

the weight can be returned to it. From Parry and Punch position, your weight shifts back to the right leg as the torso pivots 180 degrees toward the right, and the "empty" left leg pivots on the heel to the right.

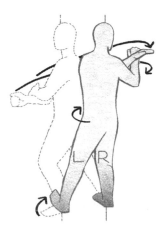

Sink back into the left leg, as the empty right leg pivots on the heel, the toes coming up, to result in a completed 180-degree turn.

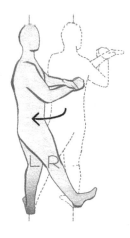

(The following figure is simply a frontal view of the preceding figure.)

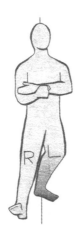

The dan tien sinks forward over the right leg, and the empty left leg comes up to place the empty left foot by the right instep.

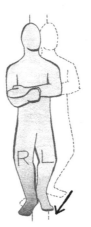

The weight now shifts onto the left leg, placing the empty right foot out, the heel first at a 45-degree angle front/right, simultaneously drawing the right elbow back to the left to prepare for the upcoming strike.

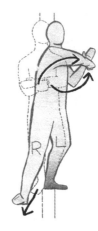

Now, shifting forward into the right leg, throw out the right elbow strike, exhaling and allowing the body to relax into the strike.

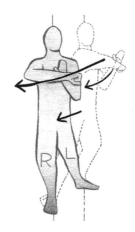

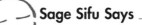

Sage Sifu Says

Allow your mind to empty as you exhale and strike. This lets the pleasure of the relaxed muscle and tissue being gently massaged by the body's motion fill your empty awareness.

The weight continues shifting onto the right foot, with the left foot placed out at a 45-degree front/left angle.

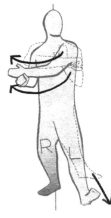

The weight shifts into the left foot as the right fist strikes a punch out to the left/front.

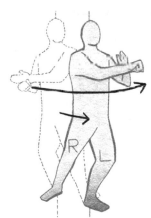

The right foot comes up to touch near the left instep and continues on out at a 45-degree angle to the front/right.

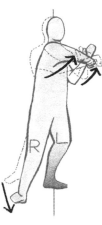

Sink the weight forward to the right foot, and throw another right-elbow elbow strike.

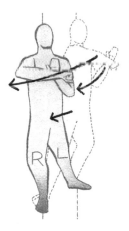

To recap, Chop Opponent involves an elbow strike stepping to the right, a punch stepping to the left, and an elbow strike stepping to the right. Over time, this movement, although martial in appearance, becomes soothing, healing, and almost dance-like in the way it lifts your mood to do it.

Sink to the Earth/Backward Elbow Strike, #31

Now drop the weight back to the left foot and throw the elbow strike out left/behind. (Don't look back; it's supposed to be a surprise.)

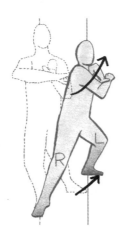

The depth of this strike is all in the bend of the left knee. If your knee feels comfortable with only a slight bend, then that is perfect for you. It will get deeper in time, and there's no rush.

Before coming up out of back stance, turn to the right and aim the right forearm to the front/right 45-degree angle.

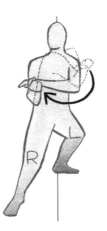

Now the right fist punches upward and the weight springs forward to settle over the right foot, the left wrist still crossed over the right fist, but then turning to follow the right hand to prepare for a Single Whip.

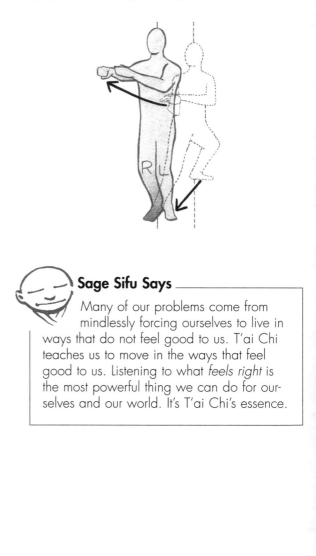

![Sage Sifu] **Sage Sifu Says**

Many of our problems come from mindlessly forcing ourselves to live in ways that do not feel good to us. T'ai Chi teaches us to move in the ways that feel good to us. Listening to what *feels right* is the most powerful thing we can do for ourselves and our world. It's T'ai Chi's essence.

Single Whip, ¾ Single Whip (Part IV), #32

This begins like normal Single Whip.

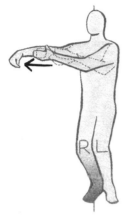

However, the left foot doesn't go all the way out to the left, but the heel touches out left/front at a 45-degree angle, and then the hand pushes out at that same left/front angle.

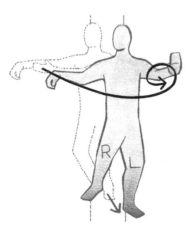

Partition of Wild Horse's Mane (×4) and Single Whip, #33

Keep the eyes looking straight ahead (ideally). The right arm/fist settles back from the Single Whip at chest level, the left hand drops down to groin level, and the left toe touches in front of the body. This is much like preparing for the Wave Hands Like Clouds position, except with fists.

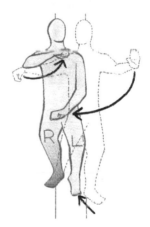

Now, as the left heel extends out front/left 45 degrees, the fists begin to roll back behind/right. The left elbow rises as the right fist lowers. Again, this is much like the hand motion you learned for Wave Hands Like Clouds, except with fists, and Wave Hands Like Clouds steps sideways, while Partition of Horse's Mane steps out at 45-degree angles forward.

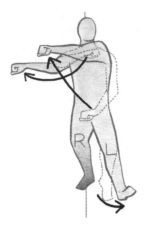

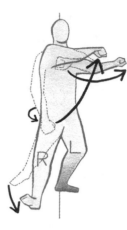

As the weight shifts up into the left leg, the left elbow strikes out.

The right elbow strikes out as the weight shifts up to fill the right leg.

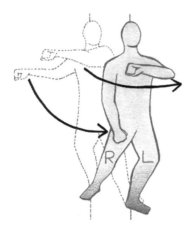

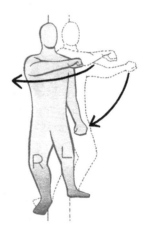

Sage Sifu Says _____

Just as in Wave Hands, in Partition of Wild Horse's Mane (and all moves, really), the dan tien actually *pulls* the relaxed body and limbs into positions effortlessly as the dan tien sinks into/over the filling leg.

Now, with the left leg full, the right leg extends out to the front/right 45 degrees, with the arms rolling back to the back/left this time.

Repeat the second through fifth figures of this movement (for a total of four Elbow Strikes, left, right, left, right strikes in Part Wild Horse's Mane). End after the last right elbow strike by stepping up to form a Single Whip.

When striking forward, the "back" heel should stay down on the floor until the vertical axis is completely over the front filling foot. Also remember never to lean into a strike, but to maintain upright posture.

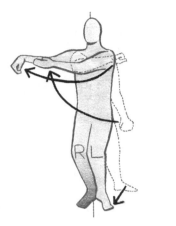

Fair Lady Works at Shuttles, #34

Fair Lady Works at Shuttles is actually a shadow-boxing routine involving blocks and punches used to spar with four opponents coming from four different directions.

From a completed Single Whip position, the right toe reaches back to behind the left heel. The left forearm points up to the sky, and the right arm comes across to rest the right open hand (palm down) just below the left elbow.

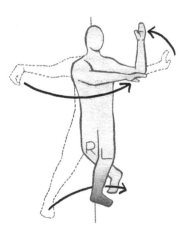

Now fill the right foot as the left pivots on the ball of the left foot. Both the body and the left foot are now pivoting toward the right for a ¼ pivot.

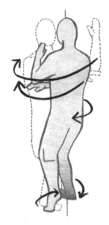

As the pivot completes, sink the weight back on the left foot pivot as the right toes come up, pivoting from the right heel. The left hand drops beside the waist to form a fist as the right hand arcs up to form an up block (palm out).

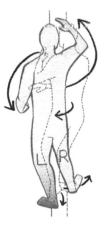

Shifting the weight forward about 60 percent into the right leg, the left hand punches out at about nose height, punching out front just beneath and beyond the blocking right forearm.

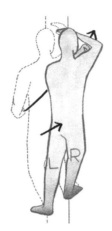

To prepare for the right-hand punch, first empty the left leg and bring it up to touch the left toe by the right instep, as the open left hand (palm down) touches under the right elbow and the right forearm points up to the sky.

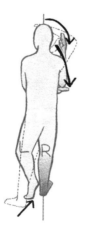

Now the left heel extends out front/left at 45 degrees, the left arm rises in an arc to up block (palm out), and the right fist drops to the right hip, preparing for a punch.

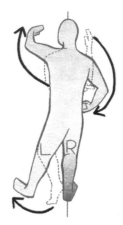

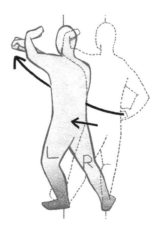

Ouch!

On all pushes, strikes, and punches, the back foot stays down until the front foot is completely full and the push or punch is complete. If you raise the back foot as you strike, the only thing behind that strike is a wobbly little ankle. However, if the back foot stays down, you have the whole planet behind it.

The weight shifts 60 percent forward into the left leg as the torso turns to the left slightly, to deliver the right-fist punch beneath the blocking left arm.

Again, note that the back foot remains down flat until the punch is complete. The body is in a state of "song" or relaxation, allowing the force of the earth to flow up through your body.

(The following figure presents a frontal view of the preceding figure.)

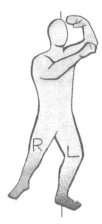

Repeat the movements shown in all these figures up to this point of Fair Lady Works the Shuttles—except, of course, beginning from this punch position, not from a completed Single Whip (as in the very first illustrated/instruction of this movement).

To proceed from the punch in the preceding figure to Grasp the Bird's Tail, continue on through the punch, stepping "forward out to left cater-corner" with your right foot reaching hands up into Grasp the Bird's Tail.

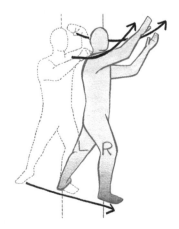

Grasp the Bird's Tail (Part II), #35

Notice this figure is simply a frontal view of the preceding figure. Refer to the earlier Grasp the Bird's Tail instructions if you need a refresher.

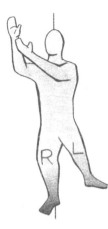

This is the same as the first Grasp the Bird's Tail, except that, to get in position, you step forward from the last punch of Fair Lady Works at Shuttles with your right foot out to Grasp the Bird's Tail.

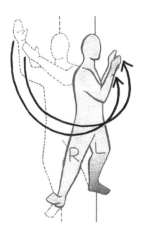

Caressing the Bird's Tail, Waving Hands Like

Clouds, and so on all can return upward cosmic experiences to the solid roots of earth—and it feels great!

Single Whip (Part V), #36

From Grasp the Bird's Tail, push out to prepare for a Single Whip, with the left leg coming forward as the push completes.

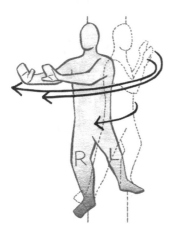

Sage Sifu Says

As you push out on Single Whip, you can enjoy a nice "cat stretch" feeling through the shoulders and back, while at other times you get more of a "deep letting go" feeling. Each time you do a movement, you can enjoy different sensations.

Refer to the first Single Whip instructions (Movement #3) if you need a refresher on Single Whip details.

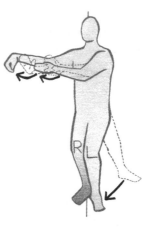

Wave Hands Like Clouds (Part II, Linear Style), #37

Refer to Wave Hands Like Clouds, Part I, if you need a refresher, but end with Single Whip "Down," as in the next figure.

Incorporate breath with each movement. This slows the movement and makes it a relaxing and centering exercise of and by itself. Be absorbed and loosened. Enjoy!

Single Whip Down, Return to the Earth (Part I), #38

Single Whip Down is performed just like regular Single Whip, except you step out left farther and on the ball of the left foot rather than the heel. Note you do not have to go as low as what's shown in the following figure. Go to your comfort level.

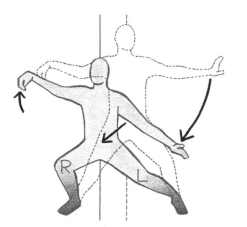

Golden Cock Stands on One Leg (×4), #39

From the Single Whip Down pose, shift the weight over to the right leg a bit more to the empty left leg completely so you can drop the left heel in slightly toward the body. Now shift the weight up into the left leg and bring the right leg/knee up while forming Duck's Beak with the right hand and sliding it down the top of the right thigh. The left hand falls palm up to the side of the left hip.

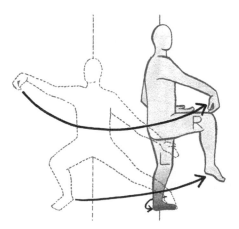

Slide the right hand Duck's Beak off the end of the right knee, up in a circular motion, and around back toward the body. The left palm up still rests next to the left hip.

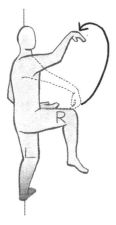

The hand completes a circle down to the chest, with the palm open and ready to push away from the body.

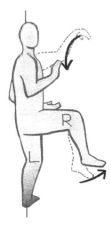

Then the right hand pushes out simultaneously as the right foot kicks straight out in front. Note you don't have to kick as high as what's shown in the figure. Just go as high as is comfortable and balanced. You'll get higher in time, so just relax and enjoy.

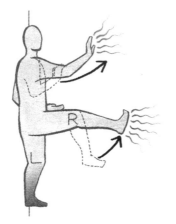

This movement may look tough if you are leafing through the book, but learning the previous movements changes your body and mind in ways that will make this movement feel easy. As always, each of us does it in our own way.

After the kick, place the right foot down slightly out in front of the body, and begin to shift the weight toward the right leg as the palm-up right hand begins dropping down to waist level and the left hand now forms Duck's Beak.

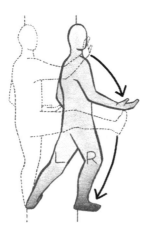

T'ai Sci

A study by Emory University found T'ai Chi to be *twice* as effective in improving balance as other therapies. By the time you get to this move, your balance is much improved!

Now shift your weight completely into the right leg, and bring the left leg/knee up while forming a Duck's Beak with the left hand, which now slides down the top of the left thigh.

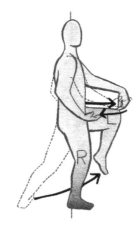

Slide the left-hand Duck's Beak off the end of the left knee, up in a circular motion, and around back toward the body.

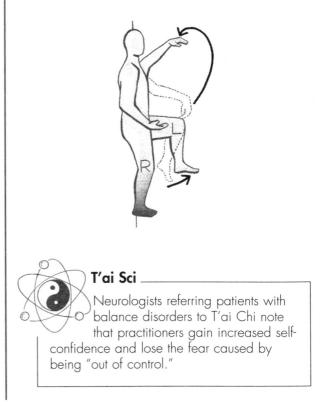

T'ai Sci

Neurologists referring patients with balance disorders to T'ai Chi note that practitioners gain increased self-confidence and lose the fear caused by being "out of control."

The left hand completes the circle down to the chest, with the palm open and ready to push away from the body.

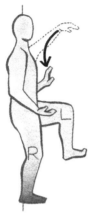

The left hand pushes out simultaneously as the left foot kicks straight out in front. Kick only as high as is comfortable and balanced; it'll get higher in time. Relax and enjoy!

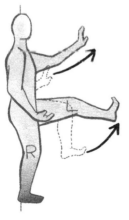

From here, repeat both right and left kicks again as in all the preceding figures for Golden Cock Stands on One Leg, but as you finish the last front kick with the left leg, put the left leg behind you and circle your right hand up from the right side to put you in position for Repulse the Monkey.

Repulse the Monkey (×3) (Part II), #40

This Repulse the Monkey series begins with the right hand pushing out, so it's only three repetitions, not four, as in the first one. Again, enjoy the soothing Long Qi as the palms pass one another, allowing a loosening of the back and shoulders.

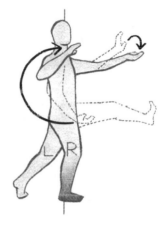

Movements #40 Through #44

The next four movements are repeats of movement series 11 through 14. *You already know them!* But go back for a refresher, if needed. The movements are as follows:

◆ Stork Covers Its Wing/Sword in Sheath (Part II), #41
◆ Slow Palm Slant Flying (Part II), #42
◆ Raise Right Hand and Left: Turn and Repeat (Part II), #43
◆ Wave Hand Over Light/Fly Pulling Back, #44

Fan Through the Arms (Backhand Slap), #45

This Fan Through the Arms doesn't come up in a rising arc to the left (as the first Fan Through the Arms [Movement #15], did); instead, it swings out front and then to the left side like a back-handed slap. As always, dan tien turning left throws slap/blow. Let the body loosen and relax the slap out from the dan tien up through the relaxed body and out through the hand.

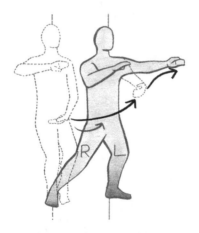

Step Push/Box Opponent's Ears/Cannon Through Sky, #46

This series, a powerful advancing attack, involves three consecutive blows and three leg lunges forward, toward the opponent.

After the Back Hand Slap, the weight shifts totally to the left leg. This movement begins with the right foot stepping forward, as the hands begin to drop, preparing you to push away in front.

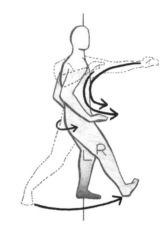

The dan tien now shifts over the front/right foot as you push out. The back heel stays down until the push is complete.

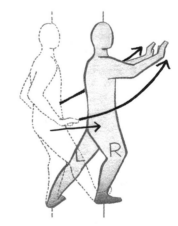

The weight completely fills the left leg so the empty right leg can come up. Now the right heel touches out front as the hands drop down and back, forming fists.

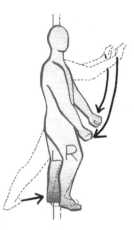

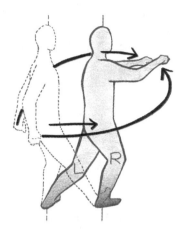

The weight shifts toward the right leg while the fists begin to fly out and forward.

Just as Fanning Through the Arm allows deep tension releases through the hips, Box Opponent's Ears can foster releases through the spine, shoulders, and head.

(The following figure is simply a frontal view of the pose in the preceding figure.)

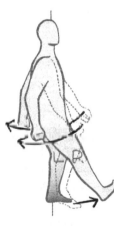

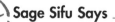

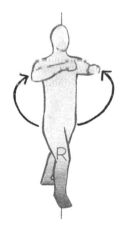

> **Sage Sifu Says**
>
> Notice that on each of these advancing attacks, the hands drop back into a preparatory position as the heel touches out front. This is like cocking a crossbow before you pull the trigger.

The fists arc around to drive into the shadow opponent's ears or temples, carried forward by the force of the dan tien shifting up completely into the right leg.

> **Sage Sifu Says**
>
> Allow the blows or strikes to flow through your relaxed body, enabling the power of the earth, beneath your back heel, to pour through your hollow frame. T'ai Chi wisely recognizes that "you" are not powerful unless you let go of the illusion of your own power and control.

The left toe comes up to touch at the right instep as the fist drops down below the waist in front (slightly to the left of the body), and the weight shifts into the left leg.

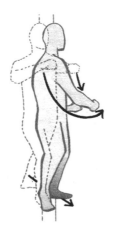

With the right heel touching out, the front fist now circles up and out to drive forward as the weight settles up into the right foot.

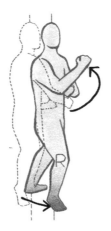

Be sure not to lean into the opponent as you box his ears, push, or strike. Remember, all punches come from shifting the dan tien forward rather than from a lunging upper body.

Single Whip (Part VI), #47

Finishing the right fist punch of Cannon Through Sky, step up with the back/left foot and turn the fist into a Duck's Beak for Single Whip, which begins the next Wave Hands Like Clouds sequence.

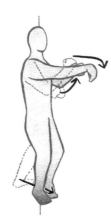

Wave Hands Like Clouds (Round Style; Part I), #48

Round Style Wave Hands is nearly identical to the original Wave Hands, except the hands are held palm up (bottom hand) and palm in (upper), as in the following figure. You already know Wave Hands, but if you need a refresher, see the figures for movements #18 and #19.

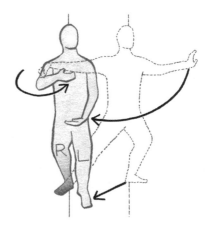

Beware of "creeping butt syndrome" as you do this exercise. Any lower-back pain is likely caused by the sacral vertebrae (or butt) creeping out behind you, causing an overarch in the lower back. As your breath relaxes out of you, allow your lower-back muscles to relax and your tailbone to drop. Don't force it—let it relax down.

Single Whip (Part VII), #49

As always, Wave Hands Like Clouds begins and ends here with a Single Whip.

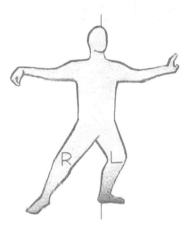

High Pat on Horse (Part II), #50

From Single Whip, the left hand stays in place as the right arm circles around. Once the right arm is around, bend both arms and relax like a horseshoe before patting the horse's behind in front. Shift your weight back to the right foot as the left toe touches out front. (If you need a detailed refresher, refer back to the first High Pat.)

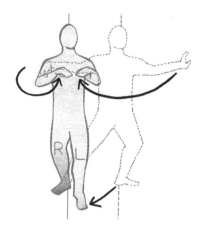

Cross Wave of Water Lily Kick (Part I), #51

From High Pat on Horse, the left heel steps out; then the weight begins to sink into it.

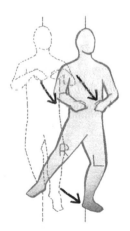

Then the right leg kicks up and out to the left side of front as the hands begin a clockwise circle up and out to the left of the body. The right leg is then pulled back across the body in an arc toward the left, where the now-descending hands circle to touch the foot or leg as it passes underneath, hearing a "pat-pat" sound as they lightly connect in passing. Note that your "pat-pat" sound may come from tapping your shin or thigh rather than your foot. That's fine; don't force it. You'll gain flexibility over time.

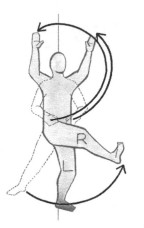

After the "pat-pat" of the hands lightly striking the foot or leg, the palms continue on out to the left as the arcing leg continues on to the right, passing by one another.

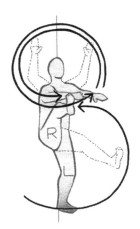

Place the right foot down in a normal Horse Stance, as the palms rise upward above the head to form a right fist and a left up block, preparing for the next movement.

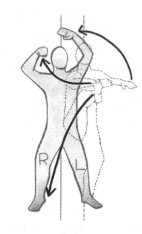

Parry Up; Downward Strike, #52

The right fist strikes down, and the left palm faces outward from the forehead. As you punch downward, try not to bend the back. Again, always maintain the vertical axis, aligning the three dan tien points vertically.

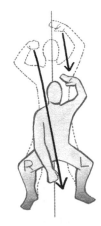

Now step forward at a 45-degree left/frontal angle to Grasp the Bird's Tail.

Movements #53 Through #56

Movements #53, #54, #55, and #56 are a repetition of movements #35, #36, #37, and #38, with one exception: this time around, Move-ment #55, Wave Hands Like Clouds, is "circular/round" rather than linear (see Movement #48 for hand placement on Round Style Wave Hands if you need a refresher). *Wave Hands is a deep loosening of torso muscles and tissue when done well, and each time you do it, your body opens more deeply to be permeated by the expanding Qi energy.*

Step Up to Form Seven Stars, #57

Form Seven Stars and the remaining movement's complexity is at first a bit mind-boggling. However, as that complexity is absorbed into our beings, we grow from it, and that growth feels great! We learn to breathe and relax through seeming chaos, which stretches the mind's capacity to comprehend, absorb, and function. This ability carries over into all aspects of our lives.

 Ouch!

Step Up to Form Seven Stars does not have to be done with your knees bent as much as what's shown in the figure. The height of stance or depth of knee bend, as always, is determined by your comfort. Many do this with only a slight bending of the knees, standing almost erect.

From Single Whip Down, shift up into the left foot, forming a fist from the Duck's Beak, and swinging it down and up into a groin punch.

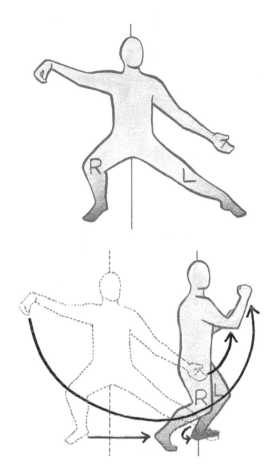

(The following figure is a frontal view of the preceding figure, to help you see the next move's details better.)

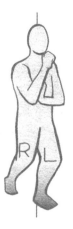

Note you can bend the knees more for a lower strike, or higher if your knees ask you to bend them less. Listen to your knees and body. That is the essence of T'ai Chi—working with your body rather than riding roughshod over it with harsh demands.

Retreat to Ride the Tiger, #58

The right foot steps back flat so the weight is about 50-50 on both feet, as the left hand swings to the left in an out block (palm out, away from body) and the right hand drops back and down to form a Duck's Beak.

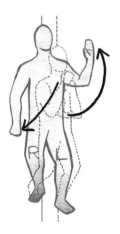

Slanting Body/Turn the Moon, #59

The weight sinks fully into the left leg so the empty right foot can pivot on the toe as the body turns to the right for a ¼ turn.

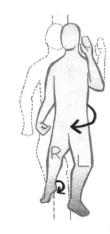

Complete the ¼ turn as the weight settles back on the right leg.

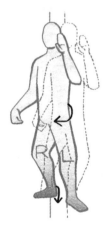

Although these blocks have very direct martial applications, they are soothing to the upper body. Breathe easily and enjoy the circular movement of the right arm blocking up and out while the left hand arcs easily down to form the Duck's Beak behind. As you memorize the movements, the silken flowing will be more and more soothing each time you perform them.

The arms exchange positions, with the right going up (palm in)/left going down (in Duck's Beak) as the left toe touches out in front.

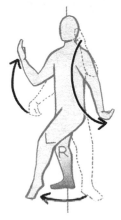

The left foot rises slightly, and as the body pivots, the left foot pivots on the empty left toe and the left heel drops in to the left (moving toward a 180-degree pivot).

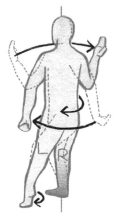

The pivot completes as the weight sinks back into the left foot and the right toe comes up, pivoting on the right heel.

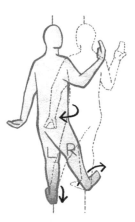

The weight shifts up into the right leg.

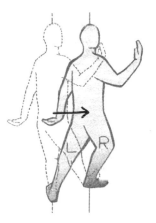

With the weight fully into the right leg, the arms again exchange places, with the left swinging up (out block, palm in facing body) and the right swinging down (side/down block) as the left foot touches the left toe out front.

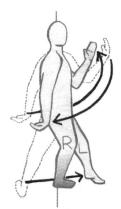

The weight sinks back up into the left leg.

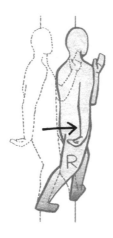

(The following figure is a frontal view of the preceding figure, to help you see the transition to the next movement.)

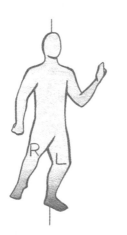

Cross Wave of Water Lily (Part II), #60

From Cross Wave Kick, keep the hands going out left for Stretch Bow to Shoot Tiger.

This movement is a repetition; see Movement #51 for details if you need a refresher.

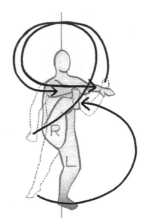

Stretch Bow to Shoot Tiger, #61

Imagine you're stretching a bow string back with the right hand, while the left hand (palm out away from the body) aims the bow out to the left at a 45-degree angle.

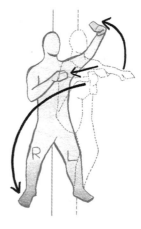

The right hand settles at the right hip.

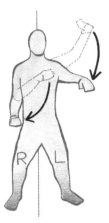

Now the right fist punches out and around to punch out directly in front of the chest.

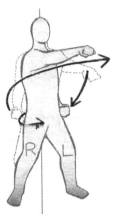

Then the left hand punches out and around while the right hand returns to the hip.

Punch three more times, right, left, right. Both hands punch and return for five punches total, beginning with the right fist and ending with the right fist.

As one hand punches, the other draws back to act as a pulley system. The hand pulling back adds power to the hand punching out. Stay loose; this is where your power is maximized.

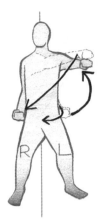

Grasp the Bird's Tail (Right Style), #62

From the last right-fisted punch, bring the fists down to the sides and the left foot over to touch by the right instep.

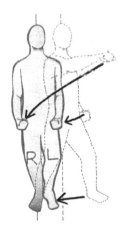

Then go into Grasp the Bird's Tail by dropping the left foot back and reaching up to the right. Complete Grasp the Bird's Tail, and if you need a refresher, go to figures for Movement #2 (the first Grasp the Bird's Tail).

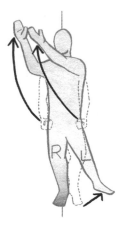

After drawing back the bird's tail, shift back to the left leg, then shift forward to the right leg, performing a movement just like Green Dragon Rises from the Water. If you need a refresher, review the second, third, and fourth figures for Movement #16 (Green Dragon Rises).

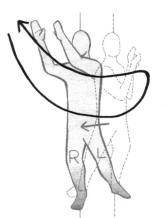

Complete the Green Dragon movement by drawing the arms back and bringing the left leg back, to now stand on both legs with fists at the sides.

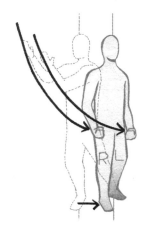

Grasp the Bird's Tail (Left Style), #63

This and the next figure mirror the Grasp the Bird's Tail and Green Dragon–like movement you did in the preceding figures, except, as you'll see, with opposite sides.

Reach up with the hands out to the left (with the left hand on top for this left-style movement and the right hand palm up underneath). The right foot goes out behind.

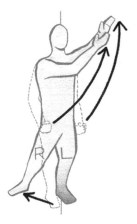

Draw the bird's tail back, then push up into the Green Dragon–type movement, this time to the left/front.

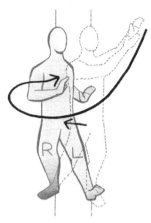

Complete the left-style motion before drawing back to the start point (as shown in the first figure for Movement #62), and now begin Grand Terminus, the very last movement.

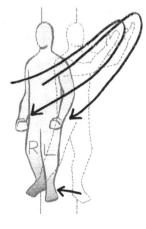

Grand Terminus; Gather Heaven to Earth, #64

Congratulations! You deserve a great, deep bow. Upon completion of learning the entire 64 posture series of the Kuang Ping Yang style form, you are now about to do the most wonderful movement of all, Grand Terminus.

This final move cleanses and reinvigorates the body, leaving you feeling about as terrific as a kid could feel, or as Dave Letterman might say, "Feeling better than people should be allowed."

 A T'ai Chi Punch Line

Grand Terminus is not only the last T'ai Chi movement, but it is also the name of that popular yin/yang symbol you see on jewelry. The white wave interacting with the black wave symbolizes a balance of all things, hard and soft, force and yielding, concentration and empty awareness. Each time you complete your T'ai Chi forms, you will have integrated all aspects of yourself. You will have centered yourself in all ways. The Grand Terminus is a completion of renewal and a gateway to greater and greater adventures. As you learn to move smoothly and effortlessly through an increasingly meaningful life, an ancient friend called T'ai Chi will always be there to console and inspire, no matter what life throws at you.

1. From Grasp the Bird's Tail Left Style/ Green Dragon movement, return to the feet-together/fist-at-sides pose to start Grand Terminus.

2. Reach the hands out and slightly back, extending the arms back and outward.

3. As you stretch up, straighten the knees for the first time throughout the entire 64 posture series.

4. Gathering the Qi from all around, the light pours over your relaxing body as the palms turn down.

5. Slowly descend the palms, invoking the cleansing light to wash through every area as the palms pass through.

6. As the hands descend back to your sides, just bask in the soothing healing of this ocean of light washing over and through. Experience effortlessness.

"Experience the light!"

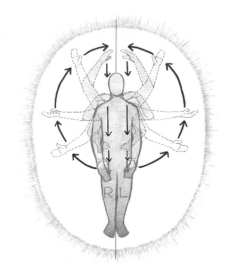

This movement is meant to gather all the light, or Qi, we have generated through the 64 movements. As the hands turn downward at the top of their arcs, allow the light to spill, washing over and through your entire being to cleanse any heavy loads or toxins. Let the feet open to release any loads right down into the earth's gentle pull. Continue to allow the light to wash over and through you throughout the day.

The Least You Need to Know

◆ Practicing movements with full, easy abdominal breaths, relax each breath out of the entire body, allowing Qi to flow into and through your limbs as the weight shifts or sinks.

◆ Allow yourself to become T'ai Chi's natural elegance, as you feel at one with the world each movement is transforming you.

◆ Push from your dan tien, not your shoulders or back. T'ai Chi's powerful self-defense moves can be soothing and can teach you to lift groceries correctly.

◆ T'ai Chi is *effortless*, showing that most battles are fought in our own minds and hearts, as we learn to let go of what's inevitable, and to positively affect what is changeable.

◆ Adjust movements to fit your mobility. No matter how expansive or limited your mobility, T'ai Chi extends it. Don't force it.

◆ Pushing and punching with your back foot planted and your body relaxed guides the force of the earth through you, as T'ai Chi connects you to both heaven and earth.

In This Part

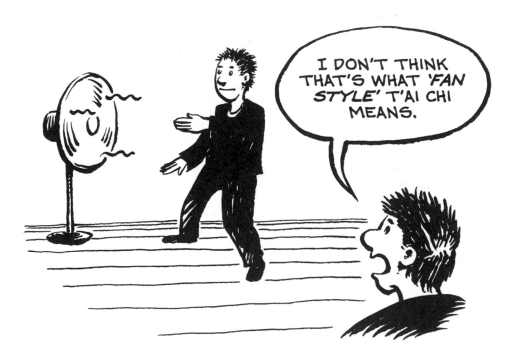

T'ai Chi's Buffet of Short, Sword, and Fan Styles

About a mere 30 years ago, almost no T'ai Chi was available to Westerners. T'ai Chi was a Chinese secret. However, today we are fortunate to live in interesting times, as the Chinese would say. In most cities today, you can find a variety of T'ai Chi styles, including not only basic forms, but the more artistic and challenging Sword and Fan Styles as well. In Part 5, feast your eyes on just a sampling of the wide variety of short forms, Sword Style, and Fan Style T'ai Chi now available to you and then choose an adventure to embark upon. On the new DVD, you'll find a noninstructional *exhibition of the entire Mulan Style Basic Short Form* and an exhibition video of the *Fan* and *Sword Mulan Styles* as well. Throughout the rest of Part 5, you are directed at various points to view the new DVD, which enhances the text explanations.

Part 5 ends with a chapter on Push Hands, explaining how this ancient aspect of T'ai Chi is not only a sparring technique, but, even more important, a way to observe our state of mind and the way we may *unconsciously* interact with the world around us.

In This Chapter

- ◆ Discovering Mulan Quan style T'ai Chi

- ◆ Learning how Mulan Quan promotes grace, beauty, and health

- ◆ Understanding what Mulan Quan can do for your heart

- ◆ On the DVD: *Exhibition of the Mulan Style Basic Short Form* and detailed video Mulan lesson excerpts

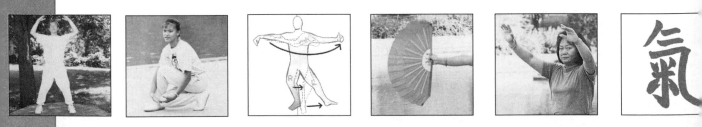

Chapter 16

Mulan Quan Basic Short Form

If Mulan Quan's main benefit could be put into one word, it would be *self-esteem*. The artistry of its forms and the mental healing of its practice expand and enhance our self-perception. Mulan's elegant promotion of grace and agility make it perfect for women, yet great for men, too.

Mulan Quan is a rather modern form of T'ai Chi, but it is derived from an ancient, nearly extinct form of Hua Chia Quan (*Hua* is "flower," *Chia* is "frame," *Quan* is "fist"; together they mean "beautiful boxing style"). The Mulan Quan T'ai Chi short form comprises 24 powerful yet delicate movements that flow one into the other. This chapter introduces the first 10 movements of the Mulan style of T'ai Chi, which are also exhibited on the DVD's *Exhibition of the Mulan Basic Short Form* (where you can view the rest of the 24 Mulan movements as well); some are also shown in the *Mulan Lesson Excerpt*.

Because T'ai Chi is constant movement, this edition of the book provides a highly useful 1½-hour DVD to give you visual support for this chapter's photo and text descriptions of the *Mulan Basic Short Form*. The DVD includes many *excerpts* of the acclaimed video programs from Mulan presenter Angela Wong-Douglas and me that, in their fully instructional format, together total more than 5 hours of content. All that obviously could not be included on the 1½-hour DVD for this book, so we've carefully chosen *valuable sections from the Mulan Basic Short Form's 80-minute program* to bring a sense of detail, timing, and flow to this chapter's general information and photo and text descriptions.

To learn the rest of this beautiful style's forms in *real-time*, classlike lessons, and to supplement the information in this chapter with fully instructional video lessons that detail all 24 of the Mulan form movements and *Mulan Moving QiGong Warm Ups* (which are the closest things to our live classes), in the comfort of your own home, please refer to the *Mulan Quan Basic Short Form* DVD or video in Appendix C.

Mulan Quan Promotes Elegance and Health

The physical elegance of *Mulan Quan* gives the practitioner a regal appearance that is mesmerizing. The practice of its forms has a wonderful impact on its practitioners' self-esteem. However, the mental healing is just the beginning because this vehicle enhances our physical beauty as well as our physical health:

> **Know Your Chinese**
>
> **Mulan Quan** translated literally is "wooden orchid fist," which means "strong, beautiful, fist." (*Mu* is "wood," *lan* is "orchid," and *quan* [ch'uan] is "fist.") This style is named after the brave young woman Mulan Fa, who selflessly took her aging father's place in the war to save his life. Her story was made famous by Disney's epic animated feature *Mulan*.

Mulan Quan is a highly effective beauty regimen for women. Its ability to simultaneously instill a sense of deep personal power and elegance in motion literally changes the practitioner's personality and outlook on life. This living embodiment of power, grace, and artistry actually transforms the practitioner. No external cosmetic can come close to the beauty treatment Mulan Quan offers. However, with a more beautiful being within, anything you adorn yourself with externally will be very effective.

Mulan Quan is recommended for many ailments and chronic diseases, including obesity, heart diseases, insomnia, and lower back problems. (Chinese T'ai Chi masters often say, "You are as young as your spine is flexible.") Reports from Chinese hospitals indicate Mulan Quan has been very useful in stroke rehabilitation treatment and as an adjunct therapy for cancer patients. The Beijing Cancer Center used Mulan as a physical therapy for patients, who then saw improved appetites, weight gain, and better overall health.

If you haven't already, begin this section by viewing the DVD's *Exhibition of the Mulan Style Basic Short Form* section to get a moving visual of the power and grace of Mulan T'ai Chi before continuing.

> **Sage Sifu Says**
>
> Refer to the DVD section titled *Mulan Lesson Excerpt (Movements 1, 2, and 3)* for a moving visual video example of the following *Step East to Lotus, Spread Wings on Lotus,* and *Floating Rainbow* movements. Note this video is provided as an exhibition, not instruction.

Step East to Lotus

This series of movements rotates both your upper and lower body joints while promoting a deep sense of tranquility. These movements improve your balance and promote an expressive attitude of elegance. The insights in this chapter go deeper than a video or live class could, due to the time limitation of classes and video. However, moving instruction offers a right-brain quality that adds a soothing and hands-free learning dimension. If you want to augment the instruction in this chapter with a video dimension, refer to the nearly 80-minute, 17-lesson, *fully instructional* video of this beautifully feminine style in Appendix C.

Step in the Eastern Direction

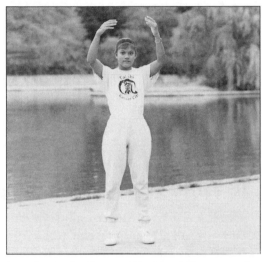

Stepping in the Eastern Direction helps you relax into your forms. This initial motion's liquid quality places the mind in a pool of tranquility as it prepares the body for what's to come.

Spread Wings on Lotus

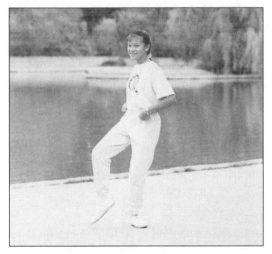

This motion fully rotates the shoulder joints, which can begin to loosen some of the daily stress that tends to accumulate there. This movement challenges and improves your ability to balance, as it carries you through a transitional move toward the next movement.

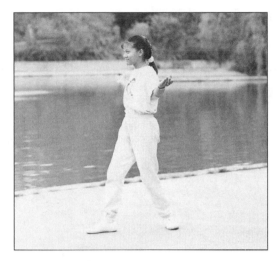

This is the preparatory movement leading to lifting the left leg.

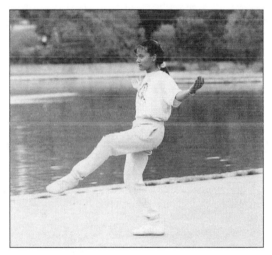

Elegance and balance are the hallmarks of this form. This movement rotates and begins to release deep tensions in the hip sockets and surrounding tissue.

Float Rainbow to Golden Lotus

This series begins with deep loosening throughout the upper body and out to the fingers. Yet it continues to open Qi's flow throughout the entire lower body as well.

Floating Rainbow

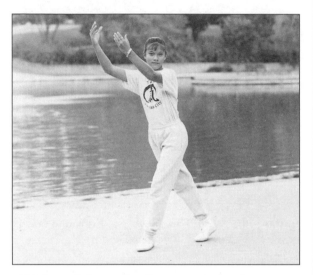

This beautiful extension lives up to its lovely name. Floating Rainbow tones the body and exercises the shoulder, elbow, wrist, and finger joints.

Sit on Golden Lotus

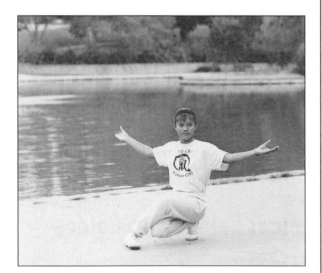

While promoting grace and balance, Sit on Golden Lotus works the thighs and legs. Some feel that the demands T'ai Chi puts on the thighs very effectively promotes circulation to the lower extremities, which allows the heart to work less hard to oxygenate the body.

Ouch!

A *Mulan Style "Ouch!"* cautionary tutorial is included in the DVD. It explains how Mulan Style T'ai Chi can be modified for those who can't see themselves, or their knees, getting into the Sit on Golden Lotus position. T'ai Chi teaches us to be flexible, so the least T'ai Chi can do is be flexible to *our* needs. *Right?*

Ride Wind to Dragon Flying

These motions promote a very subtle internal awareness of balance and movement. Every part of the body is worked and loosened in this series.

Ride With Wind and Waves

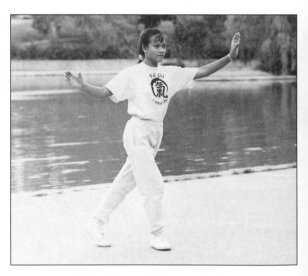

A very subtle shifting of the weight between the front and back legs exercises all the muscle groups in the lower body. The arm movements likewise loosen joints and tonify muscles throughout the upper body.

Dragon Flying Toward Wind

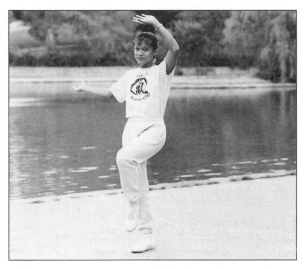

This movement is a very subtle internal motion that focuses awareness within.

Purple Swan Tilts Its Wings

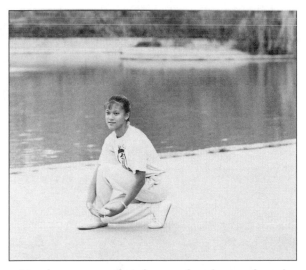

Nearly every muscle is loosened and strengthened by this move, but the abdominal muscles benefit especially. This series promotes spinal flexibility.

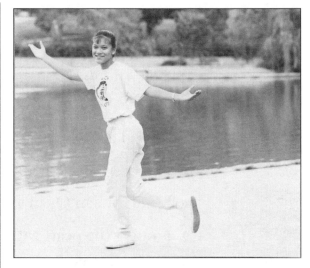

This exquisite movement is not only beautiful to the external eye, but it also promotes health, balance, and flexibility through the torso and spine.

 Sage Sifu Says

Refer to the DVD section titled *Mulan Lesson 7 Excerpt* for a moving visual video example of *Purple Swan Tilts Its Wings*. Note this video is provided as an exhibition, not instruction.

The Least You Need to Know

◆ Mulan Quan movements promote elegance and balance.

◆ Mulan Quan promotes flexibility through the spine and extremities, which may keep you feeling young.

◆ Mulan Quan can tone muscles and especially strengthen the thighs, which may be very good news for your heart.

In This Chapter

◆ Discovering the benefits of Mulan Quan

◆ Using Mulan Quan as emotional therapy

◆ Finding the pearl within you through Mulan Quan

◆ On the DVD: examples of the *Mulan Fan Style*

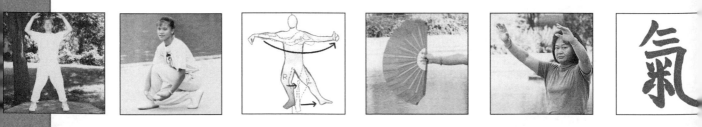

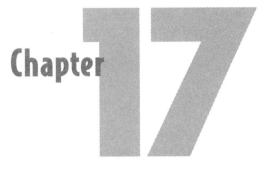

Chapter 17

Mulan Quan Fan Style

Mulan Quan is based in traditional T'ai Chi movement and *wushu* (Chinese for "martial arts"). However, it adds aspects of Chinese folk dance and gymnastics to provide a vessel of motion for the beauty of the practitioner to be poured into. Mulan Quan, therefore, reaches to the outward limits the practitioner can express, both with the wushu aspects and even as a spectacular sword form (which I introduce in Chapter 18). Yet it also explores the softest, most delicate aspects of the user, which is most beautifully expressed in the Mulan Quan Fan Style. (Note that several other T'ai Chi styles offer fan versions, in addition to the Mulan Style; by exploring via www.worldtaichiday.org and the Internet and books, you'll find much more on this.)

There are two fan styles: the single fan and the double fan. This chapter introduces you to the basic single fan style, by exposing you to how the forms look, and elaborating on how they're performed and what benefits each provides.

The motion and multidimensional quality is best learned in a live class or with video instruction. This book's DVD provides brief visual examples of the *Mulan Quan Single Fan Style*. Note this video is exhibitional and *noninstructional*. It is meant to enhance your general knowledge of Mulan Fan Style. (See Appendix C for Angela Wong-Douglas's fully instructional *Mulan "Basic" Style* video. Her instructional *Fan Style* DVD may be available soon.)

Mulan Quan styles are rapidly gaining popularity and have been involved in exhibitions and competitions from Beijing to Kansas City. Work is being done to eventually introduce Mulan Quan to Olympic competition.

Flying Bees Through Leaves

This section's movement works and stretches the entire body.

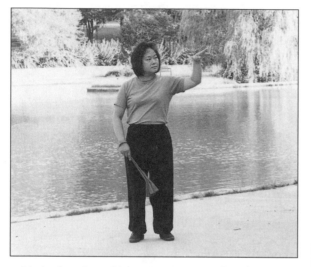

Notice here how this motion exercises the arm muscles and loosens the joints as you relax into the pose.

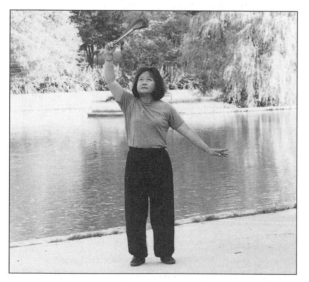

Flying Bees Through Leaves is quite graceful, but the movement is only a vessel through which to express yourself. Enjoy as you experience your own grace being poured into the vessel of your T'ai Chi. Furthermore, it tonifies the entire body from head to toe.

Stretching Cloud to Floating

Promoting equilibrium and refinement, this series is internal and subtle, yet externally strengthening to all muscles.

Stretching Left Foot

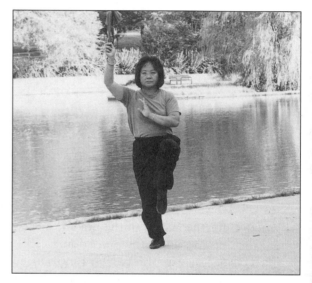

While strengthening the leg muscles, this movement fosters an internal awareness that improves your balance.

Cloud Lotus Floating

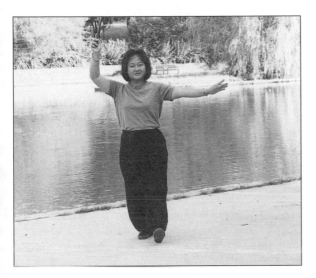

The external motion is refined by encouraging the practitioner to "feel elegant." Of course, besides that mental and spiritual benefit, it has a very practical purpose of working and loosening the arm's joints.

Miracle Touching Ocean

The beautiful names of this section are inspiring, but the movements hold even more. While creating very solid strengthening, these movements also affect the way we feel about ourselves. Mulan Quan can literally transform our self-esteem.

Miracle Dragon Lifting Head

Miracle Dragon Lifting Head is actually well named because moving in a posture of head-lifted self-esteem (which T'ai Chi requires) actually transforms the practitioner over time in ways that may seem miraculous. Mulan Quan may be a powerful adjunct therapy for the many emotionally affected conditions, such as eating disorders, facing some young people today.

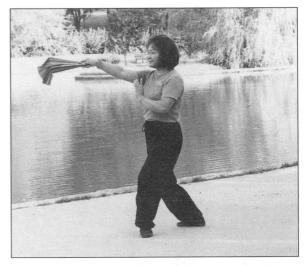

The Miracle Dragon Lifting Head encourages the practitioner to lengthen, enhancing and promoting good posture.

T'ai Sci

In Chinese folklore, the dragon represents the *yang* (expressive) aspect of power and majesty, which may be why it is commonly used in T'ai Chi imagery to help practitioners access and evoke the limitless power of their dynamic nature.

Swallow Touching Ocean

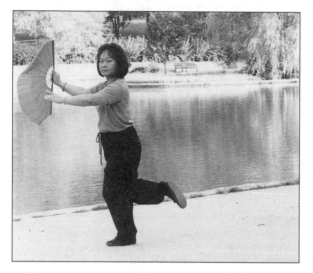

This movement powerfully strengthens the leg and back muscles while promoting release of tension through the back. (For a visual example of this movement, see it in the *Mulan Style T'ai Chi's* section on the DVD.)

Green Willow Twigs Dancing

This section offers great overall toning exercises, and its delicate footwork especially focuses on toning in the leg.

Green Willow Twigs Swaying

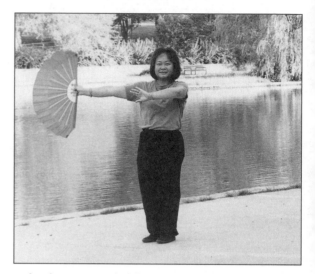

The deep rotation of the hip of Green Willow Twigs Swaying allows a subtle internal awareness of how the body shifts from its power point, or dan tien. (For a visual example of this movement, see it in the DVD's *Mulan Style T'ai Chi* section.)

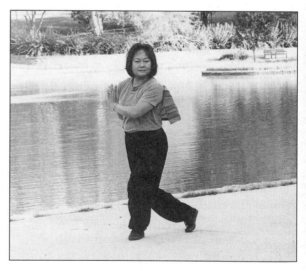

This posture works all the joints and muscles, offering great strengthening and toning throughout the entire frame.

Dancing in Wind

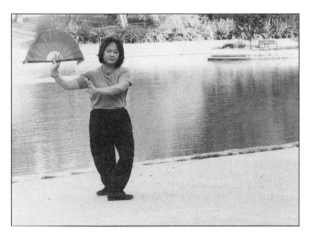

The delicate footwork of Dancing in Wind is a great toning exercise for the legs, and its subtlety offers a meditative quality as it's performed.

Dun Huang Flying Dance

While challenging the lower body to maintain balance, the upper body is rotated and flexed in a soothing, relaxed way.

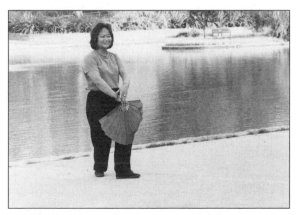

The shoulder and wrist rotations of this motion release stress and soothe your mind as you flow through its graceful ways.

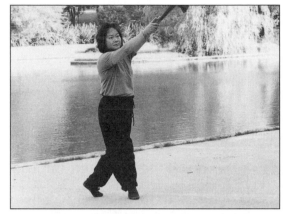

The spine and waist are flexed gently, promoting a litheness that is not only lovely but that enhances all aspects of health, according to Traditional Chinese Medicine.

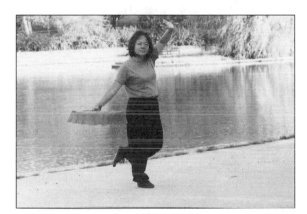

While the legs work and adjust to subtle posture changes, the upper body is gently stretched and loosened.

The Least You Need to Know

◆ Mulan Quan can change your self-image, which can positively change your physical appearance over time.

◆ Mulan Quan's self-esteem promotion may be a wonderful adjunct therapy to women facing emotional problems, as well as men.

◆ The elegance Mulan Quan offers is really within you right now! Mulan Quan only helps you to express that part of yourself.

In This Chapter

◆ Developing internal power using the sword form

◆ Promoting balance and strength through elegance

◆ Balancing raw power and subtle beauty within your mind, heart, and body

◆ On the DVD: example of Mulan Sword Style

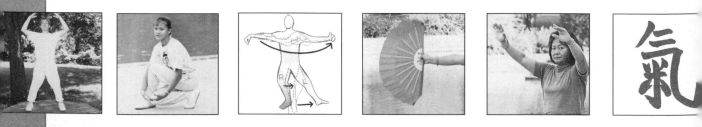

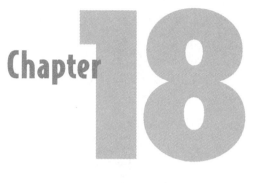

Chapter 18

Mulan Quan Sword Style

Mulan Quan is great for everyone, but women especially greatly benefit from the elegance and tender beauty it promotes. However, another profound benefit is its tremendous yet subtle power. The power of Mulan Quan is perhaps most dramatically observed in the performance of Mulan Quan Sword Style.

This chapter exposes you to some of the Mulan Sword Form postures, their benefits, and points to enrich your experience with the postures. I recommend, however, that you use this book as a supplement to live classes or video instruction. The complexity of these lovely forms can be better comprehended when you can move, follow, and hear instructions at the same time. Several styles of T'ai Chi offer sword styles as well as the Mulan. You can learn much more about various T'ai Chi sword forms from www.worldtaichiday.org, the Internet, or books.

This book's DVD provides brief exhibitional and *noninstructional* visual examples of the Mulan Quan Sword Style, meant only to enhance your *general* knowledge of Mulan Sword Style. (See Appendix C for Angela Wong-Douglas's fully instructional *Mulan "Basic" Style* video. Her instructional *Sword Style* DVD may be available soon as well.)

Preparation to Eye on Sword

This section quietly prepares the mind and body before launching into the expansive motion of the Mulan Quan Sword Style.

Preparation Stance

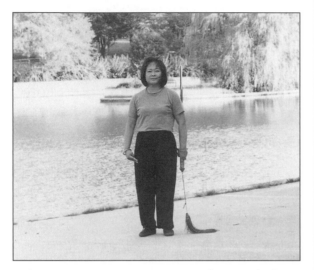

The Preparation Stance is meant to focus and relax the mind, body, and heart.

Left Foot Half-Step with Eyes on Sword

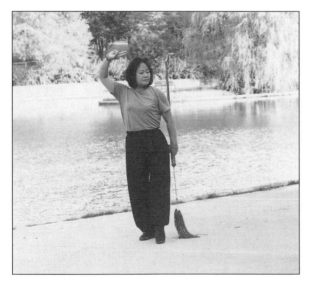

Here is a full rotation of the shoulder and arm as the sword arm goes into a clockwise rotation. (For a visual example of this Mulan Sword Style movement, see the *Mulan Style T'ai Chi* section on the DVD.)

Forward Step to Low Jab

This series works the entire body, loosening and lengthening it from head to toe.

Forward Step, Holding Sword Under Elbow

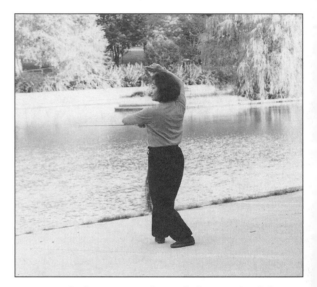

Your right foot steps right, with the weight shifting forward. Bring your sword-wielding arm straight out to the side and then around to the front, bent elbow. This movement helps to loosen the entire body as you breathe and allow your Qi to flow through all your limbs, as well as through the sword hand. (For a visual example of this Mulan Sword Style movement, see the *Mulan Style T'ai Chi* section on the DVD.)

Sword Exchange, Turn Body, and Low Jab

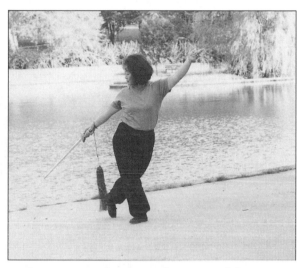

This movement fosters an elongation of the entire frame as the hips are rotated and the body loosens. (For a visual example of this Mulan Sword Style movement, see the *Mulan Style T'ai Chi* section on the DVD.)

Sword Upright to Balance Body

In these motions, your entire body is strengthened with very desirable and select muscle toning.

Body Return, Step with Sword Upright

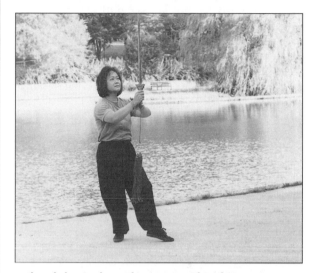

The abdominal muscles are toned in this movement as the back and legs are worked as well. (For a visual example of this Mulan Sword Style movement, see the *Mulan Style T'ai Chi* section on the DVD.)

Vertical Sword and Balance Body

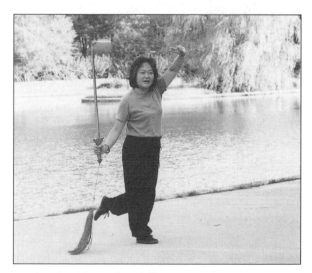

The shoulder and wrist joints are exercised here, which helps the practitioner avoid calcium deposit buildup in joints that might negatively affect flexibility. Mulan Quan enables you to age while maintaining fluid, elegant flexibility.

Turn Around to Up-Jab

Balance, posture, and leg strength are found in this set of movements.

Turn Around, Lower to Sitting Position, Sword Upright

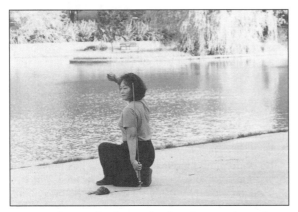

Leg muscles are both stretched and strengthened as you breathe and lengthen through this movement.

Step Up, Lower to Sitting Position, Sword Up-Jab

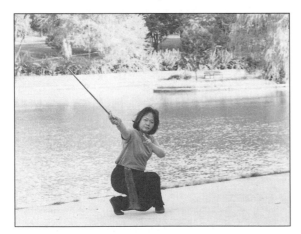

Practicing this movement with an attitude of "elegance and style" will have a wonderful impact on both your balance and your posture. (For a visual example of this Mulan Sword Style movement, see the *Mulan Style T'ai Chi* section on the DVD.)

Level Sword to Lift Leg

The following set of postures tonifies and beautifies your body in many ways.

Level Sword, Turn Body, and Lift Knee

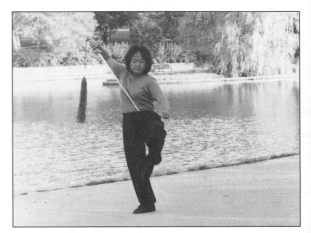

While improving your balance, Level Sword, Turn Body, and Lift Knee also tones and strengthens.

Lift Leg, Side Step, Side Chop with Sword

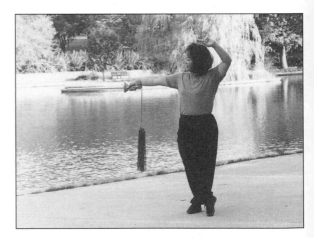

This may be the most beautiful of all Mulan Quan movements, yet it also works to loosen the body's muscles and joints.

The Least You Need to Know

◆ The sword form promotes a sense of gentle power.

◆ Remember to make the forms fit your body.

◆ Let the thought of elegance elongate your form through the practice of these movements.

In This Chapter

- ◆ Learning the art of Push Hands
- ◆ Using Push Hands to learn about yourself
- ◆ Discovering how masters resist many opponents effortlessly
- ◆ On the DVD: T'ai Chi does not overextend

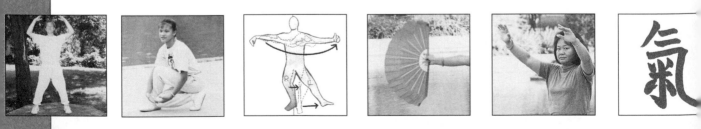

Getting Gently Pushy with Push Hands

Push Hands is a paradox. It is a sparring technique in a way, but it is also a quiet tool of self-awareness. The way you see Push Hands says as much about you as it does about Push Hands. To one person it may look like a delicate dance, while another may see a physical contest not unlike a sumo-wrestling match. Actually, it can be a tiny bit of both.

By moving your dan tien in toward your opponent, your weight shifts toward your front foot and your Qi flows through the body, exerting a very relaxed force (like the unbendable arm). So as your hand pushes toward your opponent, if your opponent is stiff, this will likely uproot his stance, causing him to lose his balance. If he is supple and yielding, he will absorb your attack and respond in kind.

The goal, however, is not necessarily to forcefully uproot your opponent. Rather, the purpose of Push Hands is to become accustomed to the ebb and flow of physical energy expressed in motion and how *you* respond to it. If your opponent is pushy and abrupt, he will likely overextend himself as he attacks. This attack isn't violent; it's just his arm extending into your chest or heart area. When he overextends, he will come in off-balance if you yield. When he retreats to try to catch his balance, he is vulnerable. A slight push can send a larger, more powerful opponent reeling when he is out of center. The *T'ai Chi Long Form* and *Mulan Basic Short Form Exhibitions* on the DVD illustrate how the practitioner does not overextend when pushing or receding, but maintains postural alignment while flowing through the changing positions.

When pushing hands, you seek to maintain a delicate contact with your opponent while remaining flexible and calmly aware of yourself. Push Hands is mainly about observing and responding with the most power and least effort. The expanded awareness and practice of experiencing different aspects of self that Push Hands promotes makes us more fluid and better able to become whatever is required and most useful at any given moment. Push Hands is training in being all things.

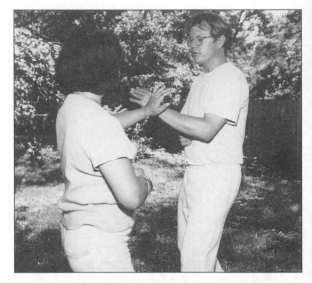

The goal of Push Hands is not to resist, but to yield and deflect incoming power.

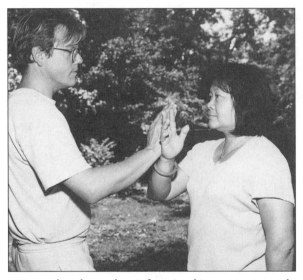

Notice that the pusher is focusing his energy toward the other by facing his palm toward the opponent as he pushes. The energy center, Lao Gong, on the Pericardium energy meridian is in the center of the palm of the hand. This is a highly sensitive point and also projects energy outward.

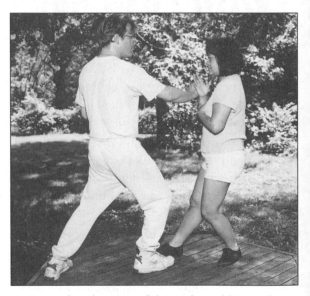

Remember the story of the snake yielding to the white crane's attacks.

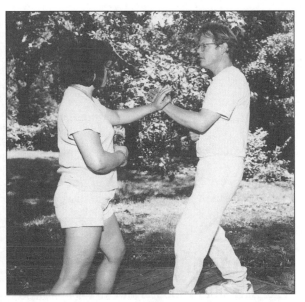

Think of a butterfly resting between the exchanging hands or wrists as you push or retreat from your opponent. Try to be sensitive enough to anticipate motions so your advancing opponent does not crush the butterfly as you lithely retreat.

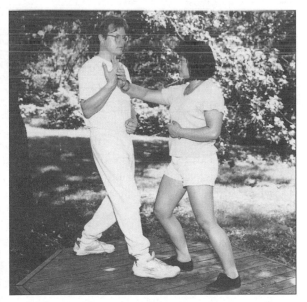

Realize that, just as with all T'ai Chi, Push Hands is not physical force as we usually think of it.

Sage Sifu Says

When pushing hands, envision a butterfly poised between your wrist and the wrist of your opponent. Try to have just enough pressure between them so the butterfly doesn't fly away, yet not so much that you crush it. Your goal is to maintain subtle contact, yielding when attacked and advancing when your opponent yields.

Push Hands is done with the same effortless power as the Unbendable Arm presented in Chapter 4. Also notice that, in this exercise, the unused hand is a fist held at the ready near the chest. In T'ai Chi, as in all martial arts, nothing is done without reason. The resting hand is ever ready to spring into action. Don't think in fear, but in relaxed alertness.

The Psychology of Push Hands

Push Hands is about observing. As with all T'ai Chi, it is all-encompassing and has as much to teach us about our mind and heart as it does about our physical balance and dexterity.

If I am pushy and overpowering in life, this will show up in my Push Hands technique. I will often find myself overextending or over-emphasizing the attack, with little thought of staying centered. Likewise, if I am too timid, the dancing exchange of Push Hands will seem limp and lifeless—not much fun. The goal, as always, is to strike a balance between the raging bull and the shrinking violet that reside within. Both aspects of self are perfect and absolutely necessary to making us a whole being, just as nature is perfect because it contains these extremes and everything between.

Practicing Push Hands can raise the raging bull from the shrinking violet and bloom delicate petals from the raging bull. As T'ai Chi expands your beingness, Push Hands can help by illustrating in an external social element the internal tendencies you may not have noticed about yourself or others.

Eventually, Push Hands may become a powerful business or marriage-counseling tool because it helps illuminate how people interact. It's not about labeling one person's technique as good or bad, but rather about becoming aware of people's tendencies so we can interact more effectively, no matter where they're coming from.

Different Forms of Push Hands

There are several different forms of Push Hands. Some incorporate very directly applicable martial techniques that involve deflecting blows and tripping your opponent as he loses his balance. These are fun but not necessary for most T'ai Chi training. If you're curious about these techniques, shop around for an instructor well versed in Push Hands. If your instructor does not do Push Hands, you may find weekend workshops that teach the techniques, or video instructionals, or perhaps there may be someone who knows at T'ai Chi club gatherings. Contacting the T'ai Chi organizations listed in Appendix A or at www.worldtaichiday.org may help lead you to teachers or events that specialize in Push Hands.

> **Ouch!**
>
> For people in a more frail physical condition using T'ai Chi as therapy, more martial Push Hands techniques are not advised and really not necessary. You can play a basic Push Hands routine with a partner you can trust to be gentle enough. Or you can skip Push Hands altogether. These tools are toys to play with. We play only with toys we enjoy and that make us feel good, which is the point of toys in the first place.

Legends of the Masters

There are stories about T'ai Chi masters who exhibit almost superhuman strength when being pushed or when pushing others. Bill Moyers' documentary on the healing mind showed an old Chinese master who could withstand the onslaught of a half-dozen pushing students without being budged and seemingly without really exerting himself. This same master also sent those students flying off across the lawn with hardly any indication of movement on his part.

There is an area of T'ai Chi that focuses on energy projection, called *fa-jing*, and it is claimed that some masters (like the one Bill Moyers met) can use the force of their Qi to withstand attacks and send opponents flying. However, there may be a physical element to this ability as well.

If the human body is a structure like a building, engineering principles may explain some of this. If just the right structuring of materials in just the right way can build buildings that resist massive pressure in weight-bearing demands, can't the body likewise do so? If a T'ai Chi master were very attuned to how his body aligned bones and muscles with the support of the earth beneath, he may be able to resist great external force by using internal engineering principles. Also, as in Push Hands, if one was so self-aware of these principles, one could be subtly attuned to when this opponent offered the slightest break in solidity. Then the master would be able to uproot the opponent with the least bit of force. This would seem magical to the untrained eye, just as a remote control would seem magical to a caveman. However, it may really be just a matter of subtle awareness.

The Least You Need to Know

- Push Hands helps you become self-aware.
- Push Hands improves your balance and power.
- For those rehabilitating from injuries or with balance problems, Push Hands may best be avoided.
- Masters' feats may seem magical, but at their root are part of a high human science evolved in China.

In This Part

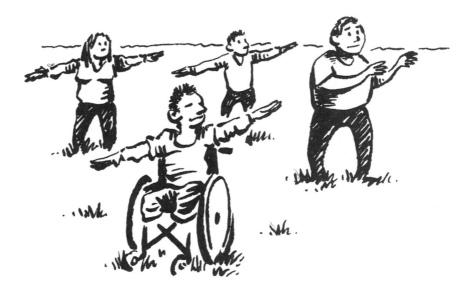

Part **6**

Life Applications

Part 6 demonstrates how T'ai Chi can change your life and our world. T'ai Chi becomes a gateway to looking at life and health in a completely different way. By seeing our world and ourselves in a proactively empowered way, we can literally change the course of our lives and make our world a much better place.

Part 6 details illnesses T'ai Chi can help treat. It also explains how corporations can support their employees' development of healthy lifestyles while maximizing profits by increasing productivity. You'll also learn how, in addition to business savings, society may save big on avoided social problems by incorporating T'ai Chi at all levels of society, beginning with elementary public education.

Last but not least, you discover how T'ai Chi and QiGong can help literally change our world by enabling all of us to maximize our ability to be a healing force in this world.

In This Chapter

- ◆ Kids, seniors, women, and men—everyone can benefit from T'ai Chi

- ◆ T'ai Chi and sports: a winning combination

- ◆ T'ai Chi as a health therapy

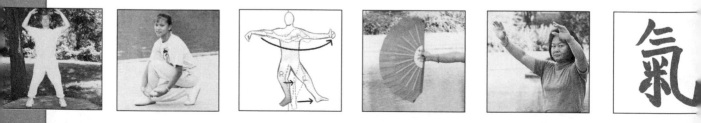

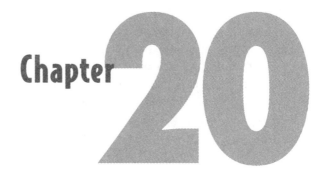

Chapter

20

T'ai Chi as Therapy for Young and Old

T'ai Chi is for everyone, and this chapter provides details on how T'ai Chi benefits specific people, their health conditions, and their athletic activities—with even more information in this third edition. In fact, anyone, but especially health professionals and T'ai Chi/QiGong teachers, will find the last part of this chapter a powerful reference, with maladies listed in alphabetical order and details on how T'ai Chi or QiGong may help.

If you are treating a specific condition, you will find here an introduction to how T'ai Chi may assist your ongoing therapy. Seniors will find out why T'ai Chi is the very best thing they can do for themselves. Specific reasons why children, men, and women should practice T'ai Chi are provided as well.

This chapter will also assist parents and T'ai Chi teachers who want to start a T'ai Chi class for kids. Kids are taught differently from adults, and this chapter gives teachers or parents some great insights into helping their kids make the most of T'ai Chi—and have fun doing it. With specific information on new research regarding T'ai Chi's benefit to young people with attention-deficit and hyperactivity disorder (ADHD).

T'ai Chi for Kids

Kids are the embodiment of change, and change can be very stressful. Their minds and bodies grow at phenomenal rates, so they are constantly having to work with new and different bodies, making coordination and balance a big issue. T'ai Chi, with its emphasis on balance, is well suited to address these challenges.

Preparing for Athletics and Life

T'ai Chi works to integrate the mind and body, skeletal and muscular systems, and left brain and right brain. In physical terms, this centering is built around an awareness of moving with good posture and from a low center of gravity, or the vertical axis and the dan tien.

Some people, such as gifted athletes, are naturals at this kind of self-awareness and movement. Because most of our kids are not naturals, T'ai Chi can be a most effective way to help them prepare for athletics and simply be comfortable in their rapidly changing bodies.

Treating Attention Deficit Disorder

Attention deficit disorder (ADD) is a growing problem not only with children, but with adults as well. T'ai Chi is a wonderful adjunct therapy for treating ADD because it augments many of the mood-management techniques recommended for ADD sufferers. A University of Miami School of Medicine study shows T'ai Chi is a powerful therapy for ADHD. The children participating in the study saw a drop in ADD symptoms and an enhanced ability to focus, concentrate, and perform tasks.

Edward M. Hallowell, M.D., and John J. Ratey, M.D., experts on the management of ADD, wrote, "Exercise is positively one of the best treatments for ADD. It helps work off excess energy and aggression in a positive way, it allows for noise-reduction within the mind, it stimulates the hormonal and neurochemical systems in a most therapeutic way, and it soothes and calms the body."

T'ai Chi's slow, mindful movements have much to offer people who suffer from ADD. The following table explains why T'ai Chi may be a perfect ADD therapy.

T'ai Chi and ADD

What Experts Suggest	What T'ai Chi Offers
Set aside time for recharging batteries, something calm and restful, like meditation.	T'ai Chi is a mini-vacation.
Daily exercise that is readily available and needs little preparation can help with the blahs that occur and with overall outlook.	T'ai Chi is easy, requires no preparation, and is a daily mood-elevator.
Observe mood swings; learn to accept them by realizing they will pass. Learn strategies that might help bad moods pass sooner.	T'ai Chi is a tool for self-observation of feelings and for letting those feelings go.
Use "time-outs" when you are upset or over-stimulated. Take a time-out; go away, and calm down.	T'ai Chi can be performed in the bathroom at school or work, giving you a break from the stress.
Let go of the urgency to always finish things quickly by learning to enjoy the process.	T'ai Chi's slow, flowing routine is about letting go of the outcome and learning to love the process.
ADD usually includes a tendency to over-focus or hyperfocus at times, to obsess or ruminate over some imagined problem without being able to let it go.	T'ai Chi teaches the practice of letting go on a mental, emotional, and physical level with each exhale.

Ouch! _____

Check with your child's therapist or physician before beginning T'ai Chi. Also find an effective, understanding T'ai Chi instructor who has experience teaching children.

Teaching T'ai Chi to Kids

All kids—not just kids with ADD—usually have difficulty with the slowness of T'ai Chi. Therefore, you simply speed it up when teaching children. But do teach each child at his or her own pace; some can go slower than others.

Sage Sifu Says _____

T'ai Chi for kids with ADD will not look like T'ai Chi for adults. It will be faster.

Give kids constant recognition for their T'ai Chi accomplishments. Ask each kid to demonstrate his or her new movements for the class at the end, and have everyone applaud. If a kid forgets a move, jump in and do it with them. Over the weeks, they will look forward to the recognition and will practice more.

T'ai Chi is a loose thing, not a rigid thing. It can work for everybody and can be taught in many fun ways. Keep a kid's T'ai Chi class moving, and include stretching exercises from yoga or aggressive calisthenics to use up excess energy. Then, as the kids get more tired, ease them into slower movement.

Kids can do QiGong meditations, too. It isn't anything like adult meditations; more and different images work. Try the children's meditation tape offered in Appendix C for examples.

T'ai Chi for Seniors

Seniors can find no better exercise in the world than T'ai Chi. *Prevention* magazine has reported that "T'ai Chi may be the best exercise for people over the age of 60 … providing cardio fitness, muscle strength, and flexibility all in one simple workout that is easy on the joints." According to some studies, T'ai Chi may help build bone mass and connective tissue, with zero joint damage. Other studies show T'ai Chi is twice as good as any other balance exercise in the world. Because complications from falling injuries are the sixth-largest cause of death among seniors, this is a very big deal. For seniors with chronic conditions, T'ai Chi can help treat many maladies. (For details, see the section "The Therapeutic Powers of T'ai Chi and QiGong" at the end of this chapter.)

If your mobility is limited in some way, even if you're in a wheelchair, that's no problem. There is a T'ai Chi class for you, and if you are persistent, you'll find a teacher and a class perfect for you.

Ouch! _____

Each condition is different, so discuss with your physician T'ai Chi's potential benefits to your case. T'ai Chi is extremely gentle and should not be confused with the harder martial arts, but consult your doctor before beginning the class.

T'ai Chi for Women

T'ai Chi is the ultimate exercise for women, in part because of its ability to cultivate both elegance and power. In today's working environment, where women are competing with men and trying to break through the glass ceiling, T'ai Chi's ability to cultivate an inner sense of confident power can be very helpful. However, T'ai Chi can be helpful to women for many biological reasons as well.

Halting Bone Loss

Bone loss is a big problem with many women. Studies indicate that stress may be a major factor contributing to the loss of bone mass in even relatively young women. The daily stress relief T'ai Chi promotes provides a powerful preventive therapy to help ensure a long, active life for women.

Studies have shown that QiGong practice raises estrogen levels in women, including those over 45. This is highly desirable because reduced estrogen levels after menopause cause a loss of calcium from the bones and increase the risk of osteoporosis and heart disease.

Treating Eating Disorders

Women suffer from eating disorders 10 times more often than men do. Although often thought of as an adult problem, anorexia and bulimia most often start in the teenage years, while the sufferer is still living at home. Although I am unaware of any studies on the effectiveness of T'ai Chi as therapy for anorexia or bulimia, the underlying issues and symptomology seem to suggest that T'ai Chi practice embodies much of the treatment criteria for eating disorders.

For example, it is recommended that anorexia and bulimia sufferers strengthen their inner core of self and self-worth. The self-esteem T'ai Chi practice builds and encourages can be a highly effective way to discover the power within one's self. The need for a restoration of biochemical and hormonal balance may be facilitated with T'ai Chi's ability to create a homeostatic effect throughout the body, not only physically, but also mentally and emotionally. T'ai Chi addresses the need to balance internal rhythms and needs with life's demands

by those who practice it so they can become quietly mindful of subtle feelings and needs before they suffer from a crisis born of acute stress or panic.

> **Ouch!**
>
> Do not attempt to self-treat any disorder, including an eating disorder. Suggest T'ai Chi and QiGong to your physician or therapist as an adjunct therapy. It may be a powerful addition to your ongoing treatment, but discuss it with your doctor.

Mood swings and depression are a part of bulimic bingeing, and feelings of lack of personal control are a part of many teenagers' anorexia or bulimia. Food, or denying ourselves food, provides us with a feeling of self-control over an out-of-control world. T'ai Chi's regular practice is designed to help us realize that we have a great deal of control over how we are impacted by the world. This centering enables us to feel more accepting of the fact that much of the world is beyond our control.

Preparing for Childbirth

T'ai Chi has much to offer a pregnant woman, if practiced very gently and with care. Most pregnant women can practice its slow and gentle movements. Its gentleness and relaxed motion promote the circulation of energy and blood throughout the body, while its smooth abdominal breathing fully oxygenates the bodies of both mother and child. However, *only practice when it feels good*, and *never strain yourself*. Rest whenever you need to, and modify or forgo any movement or exercise that doesn't feel right.

T'ai Chi breathing is a wonderful way to prepare for delivery. The famous Lamaze breathing technique is based on QiGong breathing techniques and pain-management tools. This aspect of T'ai Chi makes it perhaps the most effective exercise to prepare you for a safe, natural childbirth. Remember to breathe.

 Sage Sifu Says

Although T'ai Chi is very gentle, some postures may be too low or somewhat strenuous for pregnant women. Do not practice these postures, or adjust them so they are less strenuous for you. As your pregnancy progresses, change your T'ai Chi to make it less strenuous with each passing month. Always go slow and listen to your body. Do not do anything that doesn't feel good. Be sure your physician approves of T'ai Chi before beginning classes.

T'ai Chi for Men

Just as T'ai Chi can help women develop their powerful dynamic side, T'ai Chi helps men develop their passive or receptive side as well, thereby helping men become better homemakers and parents.

T'ai Chi's goal is to strike a balance between our dynamic (male/yang) side and our receptive (female/yin) side. Men and women have both qualities, and T'ai Chi helps balance them.

T'ai Chi helps us let go of old self-concepts and prejudices, just as it teaches us to let go of tensions and fears. As our physical bodies relax and become more fluid, we become more flexible mentally and emotionally.

However, T'ai Chi can help you be that big, strapping stud of an athlete as well. In fact, maybe it can help you keep up with the women who are advancing in every sport today.

T'ai Chi and Sports

T'ai Chi is the ultimate sports training tool because its goal is to cultivate balance, calm, and power—the basis for excelling in any physical activity. T'ai Chi can enhance any athletic performance. T'ai Chi's cultivation of awareness of the dan tien, or center of gravity, can be especially helpful for surfing, skateboarding, snowboarding, and skiing. In fact, T'ai Chi instructor Chris Luth conducts "T'ai Chi Skiing Workshops."

However, the self-awareness, or biofeedback, element of T'ai Chi and QiGong can bring out the giant in any athlete. Several blind golfers are very accomplished. Yes, you read right—*blind* golfers. When asked, they explain that golf is more of a game of "feeling" than sight (as are most sports at their core). They explain that the sighted golfer is handicapped in a way because of their obsession with *outcome* rather than *process*, or *feeling*. T'ai Chi takes the awareness of the athlete internal to the *n*th degree, maximizing the power of any athlete in any sport, blind or sighted.

Weight Training

Gil Messenger, a student of Master Kuo Lienying, was a sports trainer as well as a T'ai Chi instructor. He often taught a form of QiGong meditation to weight trainers, who were surprised to discover that they could then lift more weight. We think when we are pumped and straining we are more powerful, but these weight lifters discovered that by allowing the body to let go, to fill with light, and to move from a calm center, they increased their physical power.

Golf

At an American QiGong Association conference in San Francisco, I had the pleasure to meet a golf coach who had worked with Tiger

Woods and had written a book about Tiger's incredible, almost superhuman golf swing. His book theorized that the reason for Tiger's immense power was that as a young child he had practiced QiGong exercises with his dad. This introduced him to "feeling" his swing in a heightened way and also taught him to swing from the dan tien at a very young age. You see the results, as Tiger has dominated professional golf for many years of his career. That's yet another reason all children should be learning T'ai Chi and QiGong from kindergarten through university!

In golf, instructors encourage you to "swing with the belly button." This is another way of saying to swing with the dan tien. Many golfers discover that they can drive the ball much farther after practicing T'ai Chi for only a few months.

> **Ouch!**
>
> The concept of swinging from the dan tien may also help reduce "golfer's back" problems. By thinking of swinging from below the navel (or dan tien) rather than from the navel, your lower back twists less.

Also, T'ai Chi's relaxed motion allows the limbs to be swung by the dan tien's motion with no muscle resistance. This, in turn, allows the entire force of the dan tien's turning to be projected outward through the hands and club into the ball.

Tennis and Racquetball

The same force used in golf is brought to bear in tennis and racquetball. If you play either of these racquet sports, you will also find an increased sense of control. Sometimes tennis players describe a sense of slowing down, as if T'ai Chi practice made the game seem a bit slower than before.

Tennis players also often discover less pressure in the knees after practicing T'ai Chi. Consciously moving from the dan tien can bring less pressure to bear on the knees when coming to an abrupt halt because when the head or upper body leads the movement, the knees must work harder to stop your momentum. T'ai Chi can also give you an off-day exercise that is soothing to the joints but still keeps the mind and body working together at a fine edge. You may be able to have fewer days on the court while still improving your game, which may save your knees as well.

Baseball

The concept of swinging with the dan tien is exemplified in baseball's batting motion. Many batting coaches speak of "squashing the bug," which is another way of saying swing with the dan tien or body: as the body pulls the bat around and the back foot pivots, an imaginary bug beneath the back foot is squashed. When performed correctly, the most powerful swings appear almost effortless. The mental calming and focus T'ai Chi promotes can also improve the hit-to-strike ratio, as well as improving defensive reactions when fielding.

T'ai Chi's ability to improve balance is excellent for infielders, who must move on a dime and reach outward to make plays. However, pitchers are probably the greatest beneficiaries of T'ai Chi training. Just before going into a pitch, pitchers must hold their balance on one leg for a moment. This moment of balance is the most crucial point in a pitcher's windup and can determine both force and accuracy. Therefore, the amazing balance improvement T'ai Chi provides can be the most powerful weapon in a pitcher's arsenal.

The "Hard" Martial Arts

In the 1970s, the world was surprised to see a 19-year-old Canadian win the World Karate Championship. His secret? T'ai Chi. The centering, balance, looseness, and focus T'ai Chi promotes greatly enhance the power and speed of any boxer or martial artist. More than any other exercise, T'ai Chi promotes increased reaction speed because it is therapy not just for external muscular performance, but for the mental and neural processes as well.

T'ai Chi as Therapy

The following sections provide an introduction to how and why T'ai Chi and/or QiGong may be an effective therapy for your condition. If you or your doctor are interested in more in-depth explanations, refer to the end of this chapter for an alphabetical listing of maladies found to benefit from T'ai Chi or QiGong therapy. Master Ken Cohen's book *The Way of Qigong: The Art and Science of Chinese Energy Healing* may be very helpful as well (see Appendix B). The QiGong Institute's QiGong Computerized Database, at www.qigonginstitute.org, is also a great resource, as is www.worldtaichiday.org's medical research library.

Cancer Treatment

In Chinese hospitals, T'ai Chi and QiGong are often used in conjunction with chemo or radiation therapies. QiGong and T'ai Chi therapies can lessen the side effects of radiation treatments, but T'ai Chi has many other benefits to offer. For example, a sense of hopelessness or helplessness can diminish the effectiveness of standard treatments. T'ai Chi, however, engages the patients in the healing process, giving them a sense of empowerment.

In China, QiGong may be a primary therapy for advanced, inoperable, and medically untreatable cancer. It can slow the progression of the disease while maintaining appetite and helping with pain management. Beyond that, the emotional and mental clarifying aspects of T'ai Chi and QiGong can help a patient prepare for life transition in a more meaningful and spiritual way. By helping them become more at peace in their lives, they may find the transition to death a less fearful event, thereby enabling them to make the most of their remaining days.

Cardiac Rehab and Prevention

Many cardiologists prescribe T'ai Chi as an adjunct therapy for treatment of heart problems or as preventive therapy. T'ai Chi provides a gentle exercise that promotes circulation, but its meditative quality may offer even more benefits. T'ai Chi's stress-reduction qualities foster a feeling of self-acceptance and safety in the world, allowing practitioners to let go of the control issues that can make life seem like an endless state of panic.

 Sage Sifu Says

When you release a deep breath, think of the muscles letting go of the bones. On the next exhale, think of the brain, the mind, and the cranial muscles letting go of thoughts and worries. On the next release of breath, think of letting the heart and the muscles around it relax. Each release of breath becomes a deep cleansing and letting go on many different levels: physical, emotional, mental, and other levels you're not conscious of.

T'ai Chi gives us a daily dosage of homeostatic feelings of well-being. As we become familiar with this feeling of optimum health, we get more attuned with what foods, drinks, or activities promote or detract from that wonderful feeling. This biofeedback feature can be instrumental in helping people make lifestyle changes that may extend their lives by many years.

Stroke Recovery

Doctors often recommend T'ai Chi for stroke recovery because T'ai Chi's soothing demands of left brain/right brain interaction and mind/body interaction can epitomize a physical therapy for stroke victims. T'ai Chi challenges patients to coordinate movement, but at the same time helps them feel at ease in the face of the frustration this challenge might cause. If balance is a severe problem, a spouse or friend can spot you to help maintain balance.

In Kansas City, we are pioneering a new approach to T'ai Chi for stroke victims with balance problems. By securing a mountain-climbing harness to the ceiling by a hook, a patient may perform T'ai Chi without fear of falling. One of the main balance benefits all T'ai Chi practitioners get comes from constantly testing the limits of their balance. As one drifts in and out of balance, the mind and body exchange data that effortlessly improves the balance, which often continues to improve for life. The following figure shows the harness approach. Note that the harness pictured is only illustrative and is not sufficient to prevent falls; *a full-body harness, including a shoulder harness that secures in front of the upper chest, is required to prevent falling.*

Hospitals all over the world eventually will provide rooms filled with hooks for climbing harnesses so stroke rehab or other balance-challenged patients can come and practice T'ai Chi without fear of falling. These same patients may want to have a qualified contractor install harnesses in their homes. Contact your hospital and show them this section of the book. Physical therapists can consult with

mountain-climbing supply stores to find the optimum full-body harnesses.

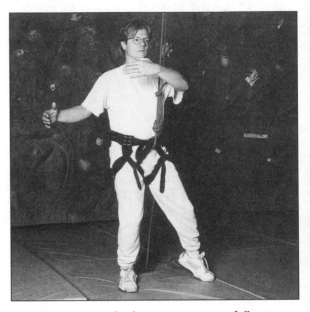

Do not use this harness to prevent falls.

Ouch!

If you have a balance disorder and want to use a climbing harness to prevent falls, discuss the exact purpose of the harness with a climbing expert so he or she can ensure that the harness you use is appropriate to keep you from falling. This security will help you relax more, allowing you to get more benefit from T'ai Chi. Ask the expert about a full-body harness, often used in caving as well as climbing.

Addictions

T'ai Chi, as well as acupuncture, is being successfully used to help people break addictive patterns. A research program working with heroin addicts revealed that withdrawal symptoms decreased much more rapidly than in non-QiGong control groups. Furthermore, breaking an addiction, whether it's to cigarettes or heroin, is a very stressful endeavor. The body and mind crave and yearn constantly. This study also showed that the QiGong group had much lower anxiety and was able to find restful sleep five times faster than non-QiGong-practicing addicts in recovery. The reason QiGong is so powerful lies in the essence of what an addict, or any of us stuck in unhealthful behaviors, craves.

What is it that they crave? Ultimately, it is life energy. When a smoker gets a cigarette or an addict gets a fix, the first thing this person does is sit back, enjoy the moment, and relax into the pleasure of the cigarette or fix. This moment of relaxed, focused awareness opens the mind and body to an increased flow of Qi or energy. This is why a raging drunk can have so much energy, even when filled with alcohol. The problem is, the cigarettes or drugs are destroying the body to open up to Qi; when the drug wears off, the body clamps down, squeezing off the flow even more. So learning to open to Qi in a healthful, expansive way is one means of healing an addiction.

Note the pattern of addiction:

1. A prospective user is looking for access to Qi, or life energy, whether he or she realizes it or not. When Qi is flowing through us, we feel good, at peace, and capable.

2. When cigarettes, drugs, or alcohol are first used, the ritual of using them and/or the chemical they put in the body causes the user to relax and open to Qi flow. But this is a false and unhealthful way to open to it.

3. Because this is an artificial way to open up to the flow of Qi, the mind and body do not learn how to keep the flow open.

4. In fact, when the drug, whether it's nicotine or heroin, is gone, the body and mind tighten up even more than before. The chemicals and their reactions in the body are unhealthful and cause the mind and body to get tighter, squeezing off more Qi than ever before.

5. The user is then required to use more of the drug or to use it more and more often because now it takes a more forceful dose to open the mind and body's gates to allow the Qi to flow through.

6. Eventually, the user's dosages, no matter how large, do not open the user to increased Qi flow or a feeling of "highness." Eventually, even the largest dosages give the user only a lower-than-normal flow of Qi.

7. People who are heavily hooked on cigarettes or alcohol (even more so with harder drugs) have a look of lacking life. They are becoming void of Qi. Their mind and body have become tight.

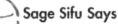 **Sage Sifu Says**

The more we can tap into ways to fill our bodies with life energy using tools such as T'ai Chi, the less we will have to look outside ourselves for satisfaction. Our consumption level drops as our needs diminish. Therefore, T'ai Chi can also help the environment because less consumption means less trash.

T'ai Chi and QiGong provide us with a healthful pattern of access to life energy, or Qi. This is what we all want. When we hug a loved one, we feel their Qi mingling with ours. When we pet our dog or cat, they revel in feeling our loving intention in our Qi flowing from our hand to their body. T'ai Chi and QiGong are tools to fill us with life, and they can be very effective tools for helping addicts find their way out of the maze they have stumbled into, finding a way back to being truly alive.

The best drug program is preventive. T'ai Chi and QiGong will eventually be taught in schools worldwide. By teaching the mind/body awareness and powerful stress-management tools these health sciences offer, many future drug, alcohol, or other addicts will avoid the desire for mood-altering drugs or addictive behaviors or substances. Educating every student from kindergarten through university in mind/body internal awareness and health development techniques like T'ai Chi and QiGong as a matter of standard education makes perfect sense.

The Therapeutic Powers of T'ai Chi and QiGong

Although T'ai Chi and QiGong can play a positive role in many existing conditions, each condition is different, and you must discuss T'ai Chi or QiGong as an adjunct therapy with your physician.

The following list contains some conditions T'ai Chi and/or QiGong may help. Realize that some of the research mentioned is sourced from research being done worldwide, with varying qualities of scientific method, sometimes involving QiGong medical treatment by professional QiGong doctors or therapists using "emitted Qi." (Refer to the "Chi, I'm a Healer?" section in Chapter 10 to give you some idea of what emitted Qi is, but not necessarily fully reflecting the treatment used in the study.) The following section is meant to encourage a more expansive dialogue of treatment options between you and your physician, and is not meant to replace your standard care.

Many of the following listings are based on information provided by the QiGong Institute's Computerized QiGong Database, which contains 3,500 research abstracts. You, your teacher, your doctor, or anyone else can obtain this excellent research tool at www.qigonginstitute.org. This QiGong Database is a must for every health professional/health reporter in the world today. You should recommend this database to your doctor or health center. Other research came from the resource library at www.worldtaichiday.org. You can visit the worldtaichiday.org library to obtain article references for some of the T'ai Chi research referred to in the following list and to keep abreast of new research on T'ai Chi and QiGong as it emerges from research centers worldwide. Also, visit the Headline News section of www.worldtaichiday.org for the latest breaking health news on T'ai Chi and QiGong.

ADD and ADHD. Research at the University of Miami School of Medicine has shown that adolescents with ADHD displayed less anxiety, daydreaming behaviors, inappropriate emotions, and hyperactivity and showed greater improved conduct after a T'ai Chi class 2 days per week over 5 weeks. T'ai Chi meets many of the criteria for mood-management techniques recommended for ADD (see the "Treating Attention Deficit Disorder" section earlier in this chapter).

Aging, slowing the aging process. Research at Baylor Medical School has found that some cells from the bodies of long-term QiGong practitioners live *five times longer* than the same cells from non-QiGong-practicing test subjects.

Other research from The Shanghai Institute of Hypertension looked at several aspects of aging. They determined that QiGong is an effective measure in preventing and treating geriatric diseases and delaying the aging process.

AIDS. Studies indicate regular T'ai Chi practice may boost one's T-cell count while improving outlook and providing a soothing gentle exercise. The relaxed forms effectively oxygenate the body while moving blood and lymph throughout.

Allergies and asthma. The stress-reduction benefits of T'ai Chi and QiGong help the body maintain elevated DHEA levels. Low DHEA levels have been directly linked to allergies. High stress levels are linked to the frequency and intensity of asthmatic reactions as well.

Angina. Biofeedback aspects of T'ai Chi and QiGong can help students learn to regulate blood flow by awareness of warmth in hands and feet. Evidence suggests this skill may alleviate some forms of angina.

Anorexia/bulimia. See the "Treating Eating Disorders" section earlier in this chapter.

Anxiety, chronic. The relaxed abdominal breathing T'ai Chi and QiGong promote can be a beneficial adjunct to therapy.

Arthritis. T'ai Chi's low impact causes no joint damage (unlike other higher-impact exercises), while its weight-bearing aspect may encourage development of bone mass and connective tissue. *Note:* Those with arthritic knees may want to do modified T'ai Chi forms, sharing weight on both legs rather than fully centering the weight over one knee.

Back pain. *Prevention* magazine reported a study in which, after 1 year of T'ai Chi classes, a group of men and women ages 58 to 70 found increased strength and flexibility in their back, helping to reduce the odds of back pain.

Balance disorders. T'ai Chi practitioners fall only half as much as those practicing other balance training, as reported by an Emory University study, among others.

Baldness, premature. QiGong and T'ai Chi promote stress management and blood circulation. Some QiGong exercises, such as Carry the Moon, specifically promote circulation in the scalp.

Behcet's Disease. Behcet's Disease is a chronic, recurring disease. Neijing Central Hospital (China) of Management claims to have cured five patients of Behcet's Disease. It believes this was due to QiGong's ability to build up immunological function and increase blood flow volume, and by promoting saliva flow and increased oxygen intake.

Brittle bones/bone loss in women. Research from the National Institute of Mental Health reports that the stress hormones found in depressed women caused bone loss that gave them bones of women nearly twice their age. T'ai Chi and QiGong are known to reduce depression and anxiety, and provide weight-bearing exercises to encourage building bone mass and connective tissue.

Bronchitis/emphysema, chronic. Over time, Sitting QiGong and/or T'ai Chi may show positive results in appetite, sleep, and energy levels, but also rather dramatically and healthfully in decreasing breaths per minute.

Burns, healing of. Researchers at the Navy General Hospital of Beijing, China, studied emitted Qi on burned rats. They noted that the QiGong treatment in some ways expedited the healing ability of burned rats.

Cancer. Several clinical studies reported that a combination therapy of drugs with personal practice of QiGong provided a better outcome than drug therapy alone.

Carcinoma. The Guangzhou College of Traditional Chinese Medicine, Guangzhou, China, researched the effects of emitted Qi on carcinoma. It reported, "The emitted Qi may promote normal function of human immune cells while killing the tumor cells, suggesting that QiGong is a feasible means to the treatment of carcinoma."

Cardiovascular benefit. Research has shown that the extremely gentle and low-impact T'ai Chi exercise can provide the same cardiovascular benefit as moderate-impact aerobic exercise. The *Harvard Women's Health Watch* reported, "Studies support T'ai Chi [use] for heart-attack and cardiac-bypass patients, to improve cardiorespiratory function and reduce blood pressure."

Chronic Fatigue Syndrome (CFS). Research in the *British Medical Journal* (February 2001) showed 84 percent of CFS patients adding exercise to their CFS standard care got "very much" or "much" better, as opposed to only 12 percent of patients receiving only standard care. CFS's chronic pain limitation may make T'ai Chi and QiGong's gentle motions and deep breathing (with its pain-management benefits) an optimum exercise for CFS sufferers.

Chronic Fatigue and Immune Dysfunction Syndrome (CFIDS). The Chronic Fatigue and Immune Dysfunction publication the *CFIDS Chronicle* (Summer 1999 edition) contained comments from a CFIDS sufferer on success using T'ai Chi as therapy. (For more information, contact the CFIDS Association of America at 1-800-442-3437, or visit www.cfids.org online.)

Chronic pain. Students often find anything between mild pain relief and complete alleviation of chronic pain by using T'ai Chi and/or QiGong. In some cases, patients find complete relief from long-term chronic pain conditions.

Circulation and nervous system disorders. T'ai Chi promotes circulation and can have a very integrating effect on the mind and body.

Compulsive, obsessive disorders. T'ai Chi and QiGong's mindful awareness of self and constant reassurance that we can breathe through and relax into any situation may be a helpful adjunct to therapy for OCD, which gently exposes patients to their fears. Again, introduce T'ai Chi and QiGong only with your therapist's approval.

Concentration/QiGong uses in education. Although researchers in a study in Xinjiang, China, admit limitations in their research, they find encouraging signs that QiGong exercises could greatly enhance the educational experience for primary school children and beyond.

Coronary disease. Ganshu College of TCM in China claimed to have found strong evidence that QiGong exercises may help with coronary disease.

Depression and mood disturbance. Regular (daily) T'ai Chi practitioners usually find less incidence of depression and overall mood disturbance.

Diabetes. T'ai Chi's stress-management and increased circulation qualities make it ideal for diabetes. A Beijing University of Chinese Medicine and Pharmacology study found that blood sugar could be lowered successfully by doing QiGong exercises. In the study, 42.9 percent of patients were able to take less medicine while having more staple foods. Nanjing University's study found that T'ai Chi exercise helped regulate metabolic disorder of type 2 diabetes mellitus with geriatric obesity by regulating the nervous-endocrine system in the body.

Digestion, improving. T'ai Chi's gentle massage of internal organs and stimulation of blood circulation and Qi promote healthy digestion.

Drug uptake. The QiGong Institute reviewed voluminous studies done worldwide and concluded that QiGong and drug therapies are superior to drug therapy alone. The reason for this is believed to be found in QiGong's ability to enhance Qi and blood circulation to that area so nutrients may more efficiently be delivered to the affected cells. Also, waste products in the stressed tissue can be removed more readily.

Fibromyalgia. Fibromyalgia is a modern epidemic, a chronic pain condition affecting 6 to 8 percent of the U.S. population. Some health professionals have recommended T'ai Chi as a very desirable adjunct therapy for sufferers. In 2000, the University of Maryland School of Medicine, Baltimore, conducted a study of a nonpharmacologic intervention in fibromyalgia. Twenty of 28 subjects completed at least 5 of the 8 sessions of a QiGong program. Significant improvement was seen in the Fibromyalgia Impact Questionnaire and a range of other outcome measures, including tender points and pain threshold. Improvement was sustained 4 months after the end of the intervention.

Flexibility enhancement. *Harvard Women's Health Watch* reported an Emory University study showing that T'ai Chi may possibly improve elasticity in ligaments and tendons, create stronger knee flexors and extensors, and create better posture.

Gallstones. The Navy General Hospital, Beijing, China, did a study using emitted Qi to determine whether a particular emitted Qi therapy could help people pass gallstones. It found a positive treatment rate of 93.33 percent.

Gastritis. Chronic atrophic gastritis (CAG) is a common yet difficult illness, according to researchers at the Institute for Industry Health in Xian, China. Studying the effect of a combination of QiGong exercise with Tuina (Chinese therapeutic massage), researchers found that 97.1 percent of patients gained some benefit.

Gastrointestinal malignant tumors. The Department of Chinese Medicine, Second Affiliate Hospital with Jiangxi Medical College found that a group of patients using QiGong exercises with their standard chemotherapy, radiotherapy, and Chinese medicine had a significantly higher survival rate than those getting only standard medical therapy with no QiGong exercises.

Geriatric fitness. *Prevention* magazine reported, "T'ai Chi may be the best exercise for people over the age of 60 … providing cardio fitness, muscle strength, and flexibility all in one simple workout that is easy on the joints." Other studies show that T'ai Chi is by far the best balance conditioner. Research finding that T'ai Chi may also lessen tissue brittleness further adds to the case that T'ai Chi is the best possible exercise for seniors.

Heart disease. At the Institute of Psychology, Academia Sinica, a research study found that T'ai Chi and QiGong practice can positively affect the states of mind of subjects to lessen the incidence of Type-A behavior patterns, believed to increase the risk of heart disease.

Hemorrhoids. Some QiGong breathing involves the sphincter muscles, which may directly alleviate hemorrhoid symptoms. T'ai Chi's ability to reduce constipation lessens the aggravation of hemorrhoid symptoms.

High blood pressure. T'ai Chi can significantly lower high blood pressure in many cases.

Infections. Regular T'ai Chi practice is believed to increase the T-cell count. T-cells are thought to consume viruses, bacteria, and even tumor cells.

Insomnia. Insomnia is a growing problem in our rushed and digitized world. T'ai Chi and QiGong students often remark of improved sleep and reduced insomnia after a few weeks of regular T'ai Chi and QiGong practice. Researchers at the QiGong Department of Ningbo Hospital of TCM, in China, gave 78 patients suffering from insomnia treatments involving QiGong Meditation (Sitting QiGong), coupled with QiGong self-massage of several acupressure points, including in the wrists. After 1 course of treatment, 35 cases were cured (good sleep for more than 6 hours a day, no concomitant symptoms anymore), 22 cases showed obvious effect (sleeping for 4 to 6 hours per day, with other concomitant symptoms ameliorated obviously), 9 cases showed some effect (better sleep than before, with other concomitant symptoms ameliorated a little), and only 2 cases showed no effect (just like before). So *76 out of 78 found relief from insomnia using QiGong without the need for drugs.*

Knee strengthening. Knee problems are common as we age. The University of Illinois at Urbana-Champaign conducted a study on older adults using 20 weeks of T'ai Chi training. The overall findings suggest that T'ai Chi training improves knee extensor strength and force control in older adults.

Leukemia. The Immunology Research Center, Beijing, China, studied the effects of externally emitted Qi to see how it affects leukemia cells in mice. It found the mice treated with Qi emission had reduced numbers of L1210 cells (malignant tumor cells). However, researchers cautioned that the mechanism and the way emitted Qi does this need to be further investigated.

Liver disease, hepatitis B, and the like. Researchers at Lixin County Hospital of TCM in Anhui province, China, found that 10 kinds of liver diseases, especially B type hepatitis, could be cured with the combination of drugs and QiGong.

Lou Gehrig's disease. Many support groups of neuromuscular diseases recommend T'ai Chi. Check with your doctor to discuss introducing T'ai Chi as an adjunct to your therapy.

Low blood pressure. At Lixin County Hospital of TCM, researchers believe QiGong combined with standard drug therapy to be good for low blood pressure.

Menopausal therapy. The QiGong Institute reviewed voluminous studies done worldwide and concluded that QiGong combined with drug therapy is superior to drug therapy alone, including in the case of menopausal treatments. This mechanism of enhanced drug delivery suggests that QiGong could make possible smaller doses of drugs, which would cause less adverse side effects. For example, QiGong is reported to restore estradiol levels in hypertensive menopausal women, leading to the possibility that estrogen-replacement therapy might not be necessary or might be used at reduced levels.

Menstrual disorders. Researchers at PLA General Hospital in Beijing, China, used acupressure, massage, and emitted Qi to treat 76 cases of various gynepathic diseases. The results were that 52 cases (68.42 percent) were nearly cured, 14 (18.42 percent) were markedly effective, and 10 (13.16 percent) found the treatment to be effective.

Mental health. The Institute of Psychology, Chinese Academy of Sciences, Beijing, China, conducted studies to see how QiGong practice would affect mental health. The result: a group that had practiced QiGong for more than 2 years had a curative rate on symptoms of psychosomatic disorders about *twice* as high as that of a QiGong group practicing less than 2 years.

Migraine. Biofeedback aspects of T'ai Chi and QiGong can help students learn to regulate blood flow by increasing awareness of warmth in hands and feet. Evidence suggests this skill may alleviate some forms of migraines.

Multiple sclerosis. MS support groups recommend T'ai Chi.

Muscle wasting (and other tissue deterioration). Studies indicate that T'ai Chi may be an ideal exercise to help older people suffering muscle wasting.

Neurotransmitters, QiGong's effect on them, and how that impacts health. Researchers at Anhui College of TCM assert that their research indicates that QiGong practice affects neurotransmitters in such a way to help regulate the function of the neuralgic system to prevent and help cure diseases.

Ovarian cysts. Researchers at PLA General Hospital, Beijing, China, found a high success rate using a combination of acupressure, massage, and emitted Qi in curing or positively affecting the majority of cases of various gynepathic diseases, including ovarian cysts.

Paralysis. Researchers at the PLA General Hospital of Beijing, China, studied the effect of emitted Qi combined with QiGong exercises in treating paralysis. The effect of the treatment judged by the indexes of rehabilitation commonly used was "excellent" in 23.25 percent of cases, "good" in 46.5 percent, "fine" in 23.25 percent, and "bad" in 6.99 percent of cases, with an overall effective rate of 93.01 percent.

Parkinson's disease/improving motor-skill control. Parkinson's support groups recommend T'ai Chi, and many students claim significant reduction in tremors with T'ai Chi practice.

Posture problems. T'ai Chi's gentle, mindful awareness of postural adjustment makes it a wonderful therapy for posture problems and for alleviating the pain or chronic tension associated with them.

Psychotherapy. A German researcher points out that QiGong is gradually gaining prominence as a therapeutic tool in Germany and pointed to positive effects of QiGong exercises for those dealing with neurosis, depression, anxiety, psychosomatic disorder, and psychosis. The researcher cautions that a wrong practice of the exercises, as pertains to specially sick people, can have bad effects, and these subjects require competent guidance and assistance.

Rehabilitation and immunity strengthening. The Institute of Medical Science at Wonkwang University, Korea, found that of those patients who used QiGong, 84 percent of respondents reported improvement in recovery time, 66.6 percent reported reduced inflammation after QiGong, and 50.3 percent reported no scarring as compared to before. In addition, 59.9 percent of respondents reported an increase in resistance to the common cold after 4 months of QiGong.

Respiratory diseases, chronic. A collaborative study with the Research Institute of TCM, Tainjin College of TCM, and Tianjin Thorax Surgery Hospital was done on patients suffering from chronic bronchitis, asthma, pulmonary emphysema, and cor pulmonale. A group treated with QiGong exercise and drugs fared better than the one treated only with drugs.

Rheumatism. *OT Week* magazine reported, "Areas where T'ai Chi has proven effective include rheumatism; weight management; treatment of back problems; management of high blood pressure; and stress reduction … and may speed recovery in postoperative patients …."

Sexual performance. T'ai Chi's stress reduction and promotion of circulation can make it a very healthful way to improve sexual performance.

Stomach carcinoma. The General Navy Hospital in Beijing studied the effects of emitted Qi on NK cells, which they believe play a role in cancer. They found a statistically remarkable effect of emitted Qi killing both adenocarcinoma cells of the stomach and the NK cells.

Strength enhancement. After 1 year of T'ai Chi classes, a group of men and women ages 58 to 70 found increased strength.

Tears, cleansing mechanisms, and QiGong. *Psychology Today* reported that the Tear Research Center has discovered crying may cleanse chemicals from the body that build up during emotional stress, including ACTH, a hormone that is considered the body's most reliable indicator of stress. Sitting QiGong's progressive relaxation therapy often leaves practitioners wiping away tears, perhaps explaining why we feel clearer and lighter after practice.

Thrombosis. At the Department of Pathology, Weifang Medical College in Shandong, China, researchers claimed their research indicates that "QiGong exercise could reduce thrombosis, RBC aggregability and blood viscosity, and could prevent and treat cardiovascular and cerebrovascular diseases."

Ulcers. QiGong relaxation therapy coupled with reductions in external stress factors has shown substantial success, even with long-term ulcer problems.

Weight loss. *OT Week* magazine reports that T'ai Chi has been proven effective with weight loss. T'ai Chi promotes healthful weight loss in many ways; it burns calories but also helps reduce stress levels. This stress reduction helps reduce nervous snacking. Furthermore, T'ai Chi's slow, quiet mindfulness helps us get in touch with our *homeostatic* or healthful potential and what that feels like. That steers us away from foods or activities that do not promote health and toward those that do.

Know Your Chinese

Modern psychologists refer to a state of mental and emotional well-being as **homeostasis**, or a **homeostatic state**. T'ai Chi promotes this by smoothing our Qi, the life blood of our mental, emotional, and physical being. T'ai Chi is the epitome of a homeostatic exercise.

Hopefully, this book will be shared with physicians throughout the world to encourage more worldwide research on these health tools. The Department of Physical Medicine and Rehabilitation at the Medical College of Ohio aptly stated that "research into the efficacy of T'ai Chi, QiGong, and Yoga clearly is in the beginning stages. What little has been conducted thus far is promising. These methods may serve to add valuable contributions to the continuity of care of ambulatory and non-ambulatory patients." The National Center for Complementary and Alternative Medicine (NCCAM) in Bethesda, Maryland, was established in 1998 by the United States Congress to conduct and support basic and applied research and research training, and disseminate information with respect to identifying, investigating, and validating *complementary and alternative therapies.* Current NCCAM projects are investigating T'ai Chi, QiGong, meditation, and other natural therapies. It is likely that in coming years, the world will be ever more stunned by the profound benefits T'ai Chi and QiGong offer all of us.

The Least You Need to Know

- T'ai Chi helps kids with physical development and focus.
- Teach kids faster T'ai Chi, and spice it up with harder exercises.
- T'ai Chi is perfect for all ages—and athletes, too.
- If your physician or therapist is unfamiliar with T'ai Chi and QiGong, show him or her this book!
- No matter what ailment you have, T'ai Chi and/or QiGong can probably help.

In This Chapter

◆ Understanding the benefits of starting a T'ai Chi program at work

◆ Learning why T'ai Chi is a natural for the office

◆ On the DVD: exhibitions to show how T'ai Chi fits in at the office

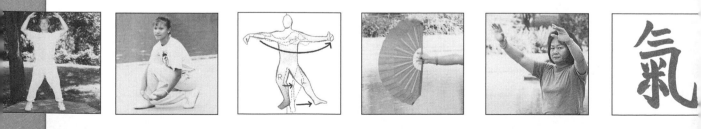

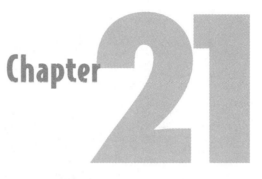

Chapter

21

"Tie" Chi: Corporate T'ai Chi

Corporations all over America are integrating the powerful health and personal growth tools of T'ai Chi into the fabric of the workplace. Why? Because T'ai Chi can save companies big money, is very applicable to the office, and can lessen workplace injury, reduce stress, and boost performance.

This chapter details how T'ai Chi accomplishes these goals so you can speak with authority to your company's wellness director about incorporating T'ai Chi into your workplace. Many companies will pay for a T'ai Chi program, making it well worth your time to suggest it to your wellness director.

The Bottom Line on Stress Costs to Business

You can help your company understand how sponsoring T'ai Chi classes is in its best interest as well as yours. One of corporate America's highest unnecessary production costs is in lost productivity due to *employee stress*. U.S. businesses are losing $300 billion per year due to stress (that's more than $7,500 per employee, per year), which may be why the Occupational Safety and Hazard Administration (OSHA) has declared stress a workplace hazard.

Using T'ai Chi as Stress and Pain Relief

Companies and corporations are increasingly turning to T'ai Chi as a solution to stress. Companies that have offered T'ai Chi to either their employees, clients, or executive staffs include Sprint; Hallmark, Inc.; Black and Veatch Corp.; Associated Wholesale Grocers; BMA (Financial); and Columbia Hospitals, to name a few.

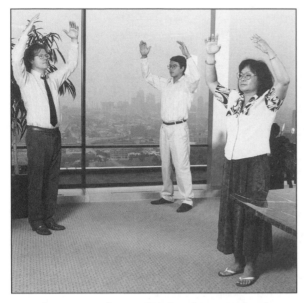

Penthouse T'ai Chi at BMA's headquarters has been a popular wellness program. Approximately 100 employees attended the introductory stress-management workshop.

A community college near Kansas City provides T'ai Chi classes as a wellness program to its staff, and many participants are finding alleviation of chronic pain conditions, less stress, and fewer sick days. T'ai Chi is rapidly becoming the most popular wellness program for many companies. Isn't it great that companies are realizing that what is good for the employee is good for the company's profits as well?

Investing in Creative Potential

If T'ai Chi can help employees recover from illnesses and thereby reduce absenteeism, that can also mean major savings. But what about creativity? T'ai Chi's meditative quality enables practitioners to become more creative as they let go of being locked into old patterns.

A popular corporate expression is to "think outside the box," or look beyond the established way of doing things to try to find new and innovative approaches, capitalizing on constantly changing tools and technology. It's a useful concept, but how do you really think outside the box? You have to release the old ways of doing things. Again, T'ai Chi is about letting go of everything—mentally, emotionally, and physically. That requires releasing prejudices and preconceptions, making you clearer and more open to new possibilities and potential. If T'ai Chi can help employees think outside the box, this will open them to fresh, innovative approaches and may boost profits more than anything you could begin to measure.

> **Sage Sifu Says**
>
> Albert Einstein said, "Imagination is more important than knowledge." When T'ai Chi and QiGong help us let go of physical, emotional, and mental tension, our "imagination muscle" literally expands. As we let go of old patterns, we open to new and exciting concepts that our old, tense bodies and minds couldn't comprehend. We also learn more easily and are more creative in using what we learn.

Helping with Lower Back Problems and Carpal Tunnel

A large part of costly, unscheduled absenteeism is due to employees' lower back problems. T'ai Chi is very effective at helping with chronic lower back pain, as well as other chronic pain problems.

Because T'ai Chi is the very best balance training in the world, causing participants to be half as likely to suffer falling injuries as other exercises, T'ai Chi can reduce workplace injuries dramatically. Tell your company's safety director to look into Emory University's T'ai Chi study on balance. It will get his or her attention.

Some T'ai Chi exercises are very similar to exercises designed to prevent repetitive stress injury, such as carpal tunnel syndrome. You may be hitting several birds with your well-thrown T'ai Chi stone.

T'ai Chi Is a Natural for the Office

One thing that makes T'ai Chi uniquely ideal for the workplace is that it requires no special clothing or equipment. If you have 15 minutes and a quiet room, you are all set to experience some amazing stress reduction and energy boosting.

Because T'ai Chi is so slow and gentle, you often need not work up a sweat when taking a T'ai Chi break. By simply loosening your tie or kicking off your heels, you are ready to play. (See the *T'ai Chi Long Form* and *Mulan Basic Short Form Exhibitions* on the DVD to see how T'ai Chi can be done anywhere, in little space, and with no special wardrobe needs.) In fact, Sitting QiGong or simple Moving QiGong can be done right at your desk. As employees become more adept at these tools of breath and relaxation, they'll use them throughout the day to reduce stress and boost performance.

A T'ai Chi Punch Line

British dominance of the seas in the 1700s can, in part, be linked to the simple discovery that citrus fruits cure scurvy. Feeding British sailors limes, therefore, made it possible for British ships to stay at sea for much longer missions than enemy ships. Today's captains of industry who realize that stress is the greatest threat to their crews and who give their people tools such as T'ai Chi to avoid illness and burnout will dominate in business.

The Least You Need to Know

◆ "Tie" Chi can save companies big money.

◆ T'ai Chi can be done in work clothes in an office. Just loosen your tie or kick off your heels, and you're ready to go.

◆ T'ai Chi can help employees get along.

◆ Show this book to your wellness director, and you might get free T'ai Chi classes at work.

◆ Companies can increase productivity by offering T'ai Chi classes to their employees.

In This Chapter

◆ Eating a T'ai Chi diet plan

◆ Discovering herbs and teas as medicine

◆ Increasing health and prosperity by using Feng Shui

◆ Learning about yourself with the *I Ching*

◆ Using T'ai Chi to really enjoy life

◆ On the DVD: 64 flowing, changing T'ai Chi Long Forms physically symbolize the 64 *I Ching* life change symbols

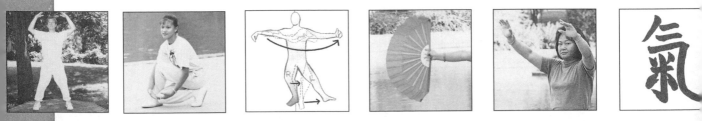

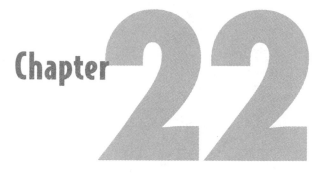

Chapter 22

T'ai Chi's Philosophy of Balance and Flow

T'ai Chi is not an end in itself. T'ai Chi is a passageway to a more healthful lifestyle. Dietary changes, the inclusion of regular massage therapy, acupuncture tune-ups, and the power of positive thinking can all catapult you forward into even greater rewards T'ai Chi offers. This chapter exposes you to many interesting and wonderful tools to further your life adventure in self-awareness and limitless growth.

The Yin Yang of Diet

T'ai Chi's movements are a blend of hard and soft, exertion and relaxation, force and yielding. In fact, the T'ai Chi symbol is the yin/yang symbol—the symbol of balance. Just as T'ai Chi and QiGong are built upon the concepts of balance, so is every other aspect of healthful living.

Chinese cooking adheres to these same principles. In Chinese cooking, a good cook balances the use of yin foods and yang foods to create a meal that is not only delicious, but also provides optimum health benefits. In a way, a good Chinese chef is almost like a pharmacist, blending nutrients, herbs, and Qi into a prescription that treats the eyes, palate, and health.

Green vegetables are yin food. They are cool and easily digested, and helpful for certain parts and functions of the body. Meat is a yang food. Yang is power and provides great energy to the body, but it is less easily digested. Chinese herbs are divided into cool and hot, dry and wet, each of which is good for certain conditions. Your food becomes not only a culinary treat, but also a prescription for optimum health.

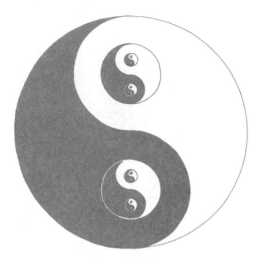

This ancient yin/yang symbol is actually called "T'ai Chi." It represents two things: that everything in the universe exists within each individual thing (even you), and that we should seek balance in all things.

Sage Sifu Says

Many nutritionists see the Chinese diet as optimum, encompassing approximately 50 percent grain (rice), 30 percent vegetables, and 20 percent meat. Each person is unique, and our needs vary depending on our current health and activities. Ask your physician or a qualified dietician to discover your optimum diet.

Be aware that just eating Chinese food does not mean a healthful diet, however. There are healthful and unhealthful Chinese foods as well. Stick to stir-fried rather than batter-fried meats and vegetables. Steamed fish is excellent, too. Use your own good judgment.

Chinese Herbs and Teas for Health Conditions

Ginseng tea is made from ginseng root, which resembles a person's head and body. Ginseng has yang qualities. If a person's condition is overly yin, or cool and damp, an herbalist may suggest herbs promoting the yang qualities of dry and hot. For example, fresh ginger tea may be good to treat some early cold symptoms. Bitter melon soup, a yin food, may be used to treat an overactive yang condition such as nosebleeds. Consult a qualified herbalist for more detailed information. Be sure your physician is aware of any herbal therapy you may engage in.

Ouch!

The Chinese health philosophy frowns on iced drinks because they introduce too much yin into the body too quickly. This shocks the body and upsets the balance. Hot or tepid drinks are preferred because the body is naturally warm.

Feng Shui: Architectural T'ai Chi

The Chinese believe that Qi, or life energy, flows not only through living things, but through *all* things. According to this belief, we move in a great ocean of invisible energy that affects and interacts with energy from other beings, nature, and even buildings. In fact, the Chinese have developed an architectural style to affect the way energy flows through your home or business to maximize health, happiness, and prosperity. *Feng Shui* (pronounced *fung shway*) is like architectural T'ai Chi, or T'ai Chi for your house.

Know Your Chinese

Feng Shui means "wind" and "water." Wind represents universal forces, while water represents Earth forces. Balancing the two creates optimum health and prosperity.

Have you ever noticed how almost all Chinese restaurants have aquariums, many near the front door? This arrangement is based on Feng Shui because running water is very good for the room's Qi.

Western architecture often uses running water for decorative purposes. However, science is now suggesting that the use of water in architecture is also functional. Many homes and geographical areas are bombarded by positive ions in the air. This can aggravate allergies or cause other physiological or mental discomforts. Some of this positive ion overload is because of modern electricity, but some is a natural phenomenon. Running water produces negative ions, which can balance the ions in a room, home, or business, making it more pleasant and more healthful. If a restaurant makes you feel more at ease, you will likely come back there more often, making the restaurant more prosperous. So Feng Shui works on principles based on a subatomic understanding of the energy dynamics in a room, which, in the end, can lead to a happier, more prosperous existence.

The *I Ching*

There are many ways to use the *I Ching*, and there is some debate about how or what it really does. Some think it is a fortune-telling device, while others see it as a tool for self-analysis or self-contemplation. There are 64 possible hexagram combinations, which represent all the possible ways life can transform.

Some modern analysts compare the *I Ching*'s hexagram system to the Rorschach test, where the person reading the hexagrams is really defined by how she sees them. To read your *I Ching*, you throw out the hexagrams or shake yarrow sticks from a cup, and the way they fall tells you what to look up in books that list the hexagrams meanings. The meanings are often just vague enough so you must interpret for yourself the detailed meaning for your life.

Therefore, when we use this method of divination, we are compelled to introspection, to understand who we are, what we want, and where we want to go in life. Seen in this light, the *I Ching* can be a very healthful and potentially invaluable tool. Some bookstores will have books, or even kits, so you can practice using the *I Ching* system yourself.

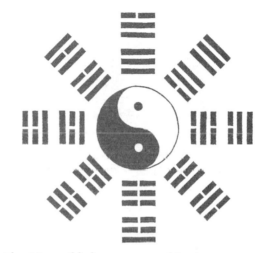

The 64 possible hexagram combinations represent all the possible forms of life's changes, just as styles of T'ai Chi, like the one with 64 movements, represent all possible physical changes we go through. (See Chapter 15 and the *T'ai Chi Long Form Exhibition* on the DVD to view the flowing changes.)

Rest and Rejuvenation

T'ai Chi's yin and yang symbol reminds us that we must balance our natures in our bodies and in the world around us. In our modern, fast-paced lives, we are too reliant on busyness and constant noise. We consider television a form of relaxation. While a small amount can be, the number of hours most Americans watch television is actually unhealthful. In fact, the American Medical Association has stated that more than 2 hours per day is unhealthful.

A T'ai Chi Punch Line

One day my wife and I went to a temple in Hong Kong, and while there, we had our fortunes forecast by a priest using the *I Ching*. After divining our fortune, the priest told my wife, "You are pregnant." We laughed because we knew we had been careful. Two days later, my wife got dizzy, so we rushed her to a clinic, where the doctor did blood tests. The doctor came back and announced, "You are pregnant."

Just as activity is important to our health, so is absolute rest. Most of us probably find it difficult just to sit, to simply be and serenely enjoy the absence of stimulation. At first, the slowness and quiet quality of T'ai Chi and QiGong drive many people a little nuts.

Sage Sifu Says

A famous Vietnamese monk once said that we are like glasses of dirty water. Each day the dirt gets shook up, and we become cloudy and unclear. If we take time to sit still, our stress settles down, and we again can see clearly.

This is a cleansing process. The more anxiety we feel, breathe through, and let go of, the more we settle into a clarity and calmness that we eventually learn to enjoy. By sitting still, we become aware of anxieties and tensions we may have buried in our subconscious mind. These repressed feelings can manifest as muscle tension, asthma attacks, volatile emotions, and so on, unless we become aware of them, feel them, and begin to breathe through them by physically letting the muscles let go and the mind relax. The cleansing pleasure of that "empty awareness" is perhaps the most healthful thing we can do for ourselves. It gives our mind a chance to

rest, heal, and recharge. This also gives our spiritual nature an opportunity to come forth. We can get a new perspective on life just by sitting. Just as a drug addict must go through a period of anxiety to let go of the craving for drugs, those of us who are addicted to "busyness" and constant stimulation (TV or whatever) must go through that same anxiety period. But eventually we tap into the bliss of stillness of mind. As always, remembering to *breathe* makes the transition more tolerable.

T'ai Chi Teaches Mindful Living

T'ai Chi's slow process and seemingly endless progression from one movement to the next teaches us to let go of the outcome and be in the moment. In the West, this is called "stopping to smell the roses." With T'ai Chi, we don't just think about stopping to smell the roses; we simply must do it. You cannot stand to perform a 20-minute slow-motion exercise like T'ai Chi and stay in a rush-rush-hurry-hurry mentality. It is impossible. Therefore, T'ai Chi is like a magic formula that actually changes who you are. Its methodology forces us to love the act of living, just as we must love the feel, the sensation, *the breath*, and the motion of each T'ai Chi movement so we don't anxiously wait for it to be over. Life becomes a sacrament, every moment and every person we touch becomes sacred and a miracle. As T'ai Chi's slow mindfulness causes us to subtly attune to the miracle of our own existence, we see the world as miraculous. On a physical level, as we daily immerse ourselves in Qi, or life's energy, we connect with that quality in all living things.

The mindful living T'ai Chi teaches spills out into every aspect of our lives. To help bring forth T'ai Chi mindfulness, practice the following exercises:

◆ **Savor the smell and taste of liquids.** When you take a sip of water with a lime twist or hot tea, really smell the rich aroma as you drink. Let the fragrance fill your awareness. As you swallow it, feel the heat or cold go down your throat. Experience its descent all the way into your stomach.

◆ **When you hold a hot cup of tea, watch the steam rise.** Get your face right up next to it. The steam is agitated atoms that burst free of the surface and scream outward into space, just like the huge bursts that erupt from the surface of the sun. Enjoy this fabulous display of erupting atoms.

◆ **Simplify your diet.** Drink more water with a lime twist and less soda or beer. Take the time to really taste and smell the lime. Lime is an exquisite gift we've been given. Usually we drink very sweet, over-flavored things because we don't slow down enough to really taste them. So we need the shock value of 13 sugar cubes and the other sticky stuff that comes in most cans of soda.

◆ **Eat more fruits and vegetables.** Really stop and chew them. Feel their texture, sense their temperature, and savor their subtle flavor and smell.

◆ **When you cook, feel the food as you cut it up.** Listen to the sizzling as it cooks, and really smell the richness of its aroma. Pretend for a moment that this was your last day on Earth and you would never be able to smell these smells, hear these sounds, or taste these tastes again.

◆ **Sit and watch nature.** Nature cannot be analyzed or fixed. Nature simply washes over you. Watch the clouds move, the trees sway, and the weather unfold. This world is a miracle placed here for your enjoyment. Don't take its beauty for granted.

◆ **Just listen** when your spouse (or children or friends) talks to you. Observe their faces and the excitement in their voices. Let the images of their day wash over your mind. Do not worry about how you are "supposed" to respond. Enjoy their presence.

Sage Sifu Says

The T'ai Chi symbol, or yin/yang symbol, literally means the supreme ultimate point in the universe. When you follow the suggestions to allow T'ai Chi to weave its mindfulness into your life, you begin to feel more and more as though you are in the center of the universe.

◆ **Observe people; experience them.** Imagine for a moment that you were the only person on Earth and there was never ever going to be anyone else but you. You probably would be filled with desire to speak to others, to enjoy their existence. Here they are, now. Enjoy.

◆ **Let life wash over you.** Do what needs to be done, whether it's washing dishes or paying bills, with a sense of unhurried pleasure, like the way T'ai Chi movements are done. If we don't run from what we must do, it can be pleasant, and all things simply work out, as if we did nothing at all.

The Least You Need to Know

◆ Balance your diet; balance your life.

◆ Drink "fresh" ginger tea at the first sign of a cold.

◆ According to Feng Shui, an open, flowing interior design does much more than just look good.

◆ The *I Ching* may help you understand yourself better.

◆ T'ai Chi teaches savoring life and smelling the roses.

In This Chapter

- ◆ Lowering unemployment and health-care costs

- ◆ Helping schools

- ◆ Reducing crime and violence

- ◆ Cleaning up the environment and healing our world

- ◆ On the DVD: *Long* and *Basic Short Form Exhibitions* show a physical model of *effortless adaptability*

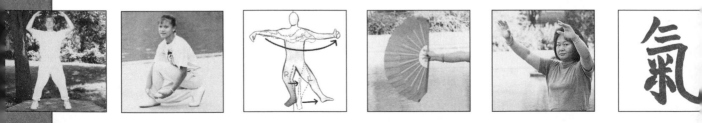

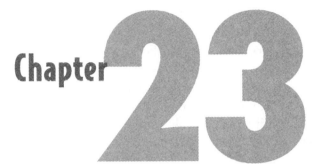

Chapter 23

Do T'ai Chi and Change the World

T'ai Chi is widely misunderstood. Is it an exercise, a martial art, or a meditation *technique?* Actually, T'ai Chi is all those things, but it also offers so much more. T'ai Chi can be a key to discovering our personal empowerment. As we find that we can take control over our body's circulation, our blood pressure, and our stress responses, we are empowered. This empowerment begins to resonate out to every aspect of our lives—work, relationships, and society.

As we feel empowered and T'ai Chi works its clarifying magic, we find learning easier and more exciting. We become drawn to learning as the world becomes fresher and more magical because of our new attitude of well-being. T'ai Chi cultivates and supports our childlikeness, curiosity, and zest for life. When we treasure each moment of our lives, we are much less likely to engage in acts that endanger our health or our freedom. When we feel at peace within ourselves, we are much less likely to hurt others. Much violence is the act of someone in personal pain who externalizes that pain on others. T'ai Chi can help heal that pain, thereby reducing much violence.

T'ai Chi and Unemployment

Because people who grew up in high-stress households have higher unemployment rates, T'ai Chi may help both parents and children change that pattern. Furthermore, because the modern economy forces many people to change careers several times, T'ai Chi's promotion of letting go of the past and relaxing into change can be helpful to adults in today's job market.

England's Royal Academy of Pediatrics College released a study that concluded that "stressful" households caused problems for children that could last a lifetime. One thing it discovered was that children from such households endured higher unemployment levels than kids from more peaceful households. We know stress limits our creativity and can affect our self-esteem. T'ai Chi's ability to provide children with a tool that can help them find a calm place within, even when home is less than calm, can be of powerful help to them.

It is estimated that most of us will change, not jobs, but careers more than five times in our lifetime. For people who find change difficult, this can be excruciatingly stressful and even life-threatening over time. In a world of constant and relentless change, T'ai Chi's ability to help us mentally, emotionally, and physically let go can be a great help.

> **Sage Sifu Says** _____
>
> Change in and of itself is an essential and wonderful part of life. Our unhealthful responses to change are the problem. T'ai Chi is a tool to lubricate our way into the challenging and exciting future that awaits those who rise to the occasion.

By being able to let go of past employment and being open to new information and self-definitions, we can be ready to flow into our next occupation. This flowing can happen not only less stressfully, but with an adventurous anticipation, just like when we were kids. This is what T'ai Chi can help us do as individuals and as a society. View the *Exhibition of the T'ai Chi Long Form* and *Exhibition of the Mulan Basic Short Form* sections on the DVD to see how the physical model of flow and release can provide a daily example of how we can begin to flow with less resistance through all aspects of life.

When you catch yourself considering worst-case scenarios while engaged in a task or project, take a deep breath and let your entire body release thoughts, tensions, and fears. Then make a list or flow chart of what is required for your

success. This will let you realistically decide whether to proceed rather than resist change because of irrational fears. T'ai Chi promotes a sense of being in the moment, of dealing with the tasks at hand, and of letting go of fear-based projections of the future.

T'ai Chi and the Health-Care Crisis

Approximately 80 percent of the illnesses that send us to the doctor are due to stress. The six leading causes of death are stress related. Today's health-care crisis is literally due to stress. Stress can be managed, and perhaps no more effective stress-management tool exists than daily T'ai Chi and QiGong meditations.

Hospitals and insurance carriers are incorporating T'ai Chi and QiGong into what they offer clients. Physicians, neurologists, cardiac and hypertension specialists, and mental health providers are prescribing T'ai Chi for a host of physical, emotional, and mental conditions. Medical university nursing programs are also introducing T'ai Chi to their students as part of their training. Other schools are considering offering it to all medical students.

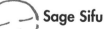

> **Sage Sifu Says** _____
>
> To get the maximum benefits from T'ai Chi and QiGong, make time to practice every day. After a while, it won't be a chore at all. You will relish and savor your T'ai Chi moments, looking forward to them like a schoolkid looks forward to the weekend.

T'ai Chi begins to show us that we have a health-care crisis simply because we choose to have a health-care crisis. Each of us has it within our own power to dramatically lower our dependence on general health care, pharmacology, and surgery. The fastest-growing investment industry in the United States today is pharmaceuticals. The three top-selling medications are ulcer, high blood pressure, and mood-altering medications. T'ai Chi and/or QiGong can have significantly positive effects on all three of these conditions, in some cases.

> **Sage Sifu Says**
>
> When going to the doctor, think less of expecting the doctor to "heal you." Rather, think in terms of you and the doctor in partnership. Ask the doctor what healthful habits or activities you can engage in to facilitate your healing. Your question should be, "How can I heal me?"

T'ai Chi and QiGong are not at odds with modern Western health care. They can be partners with it. You don't decide between medication or surgery and T'ai Chi. If you need medication or surgery, then use it. However, medication and surgery should not be the first line of defense. If we practice T'ai Chi, we might never develop the need for certain medications or for much heart surgery. If we daily water our "T'ai Tree" roots with the soothing balm of life energy, we will be less likely to ever need that medication or surgery, saving ourselves pain and money, while saving society a great financial burden.

We cannot afford to ignore our body's signals and our health until we are in a crisis situation and then expect society to lavish money upon us for expensive surgery or medication. This isn't just about Medicare alone; *all* our health insurance premiums are skyrocketing due to a national need to become mindful of our health. T'ai Chi can save us all big money and help us feel good while doing it.

T'ai Chi in Education

Studies show that change, even change for the better, is stressful. A good example is when you upgrade your computer. The newer program gives you new tools to make your work faster and more efficient, but letting go of the old ways and learning the new is often stressful.

In many ways, each day our children are learning new ways to do everything, both at home and at school. Kids today are under tremendous stress because the world is changing very fast, and they will see changes we never dreamed of in our lives. Therefore, the best tool we can give them to launch out upon the world with confidence and health is, you guessed it, T'ai Chi.

Helping Students Stay Current in a Fast Current!

T'ai Chi brings you back to the calm center, no matter how fast life's carousel is spinning. In today's rapidly changing world, this is a very important tool to give our children. No matter how much math, science, and economic facts we give them, they will be lost if they don't know how to thrive healthfully in a world of change. Why? Because our understanding of math, science, and economics is changing on an almost daily basis. Of all the discoveries made since the inception of man, nearly all have been made in our lifetimes, and the world is only getting faster with the explosion of the information age. Therefore, children with mind/body training that can help them adapt to new ways more easily and more healthfully will have a distinct advantage over kids *who learn only* the current ways things are done or the current textbook facts.

Chronic stress can even inhibit our thinking processes, literally shrinking parts of the brain. So by teaching children T'ai Chi, we help them be calm and provide them a physical model to relax through changes, which thereby can improve their mental function.

> **A T'ai Chi Punch Line**
>
> If you look at many long-term T'ai Chi practitioners, Chinese or Western, you will find very vibrant people, often at the pinnacles of their professions. T'ai Chi practitioners do not fear and run from change, but find it essential to a full life.

Studying Health from the Inside Out

Hopefully, every school will eventually provide T'ai Chi instruction through all levels of education and to teachers as well. T'ai Chi is a cross between physical education and health science, and may eventually become a staple of health science. What better way for kids to learn about their bodies and health than by paying attention to the laboratory they walk around in every day, their own miraculous minds and bodies, through practicing T'ai Chi's mindful exercises?

Although most of the high school T'ai Chi classes I've taught have been in health science, instructors in physical education, art, and drama are considering T'ai Chi as an adjunct to their classes.

Helping Students Avoid Drugs

Some schools are already providing T'ai Chi to students. I have taught T'ai Chi and QiGong relaxation therapy to students in elementary, junior high, high school, and university levels through health science, college-preparatory programs, and drug-abuse-prevention programs,

as well as for developmentally disabled students. Health science teachers have told me that students claim the main reason they begin smoking or using drugs and alcohol is to alleviate stress. Of course, those of us with more life experience know that, in the end, drug abuse creates more stress, but it is not enough to simply tell kids to "just say no." We must take the next step and provide them with tools to manage the enormous stress they face in an increasingly complex world.

T'ai Chi and Crime and Law Enforcement

T'ai Chi is now being taught in prisons, as well as in court-sponsored rehabilitation programs. T'ai Chi's ability to build self-esteem, heal childhood trauma, and manage potentially violent stress makes it an incredible coping tool for anyone trying to change. If we want to reduce crime, finding ways people can become productive parts of society is a cost-effective and just plain effective way to do it. It costs twice as much to send a child to prison as it does to send that child to Harvard. Per capita, the United States has incarcerated more of its children than any nation in the world. It is time to find creative solutions such as T'ai Chi and mind/body fitness training to heal the very roots of crime—*the potential criminals.* Doing this before the crime occurs will save us all much pain and vast amounts of money.

> **A T'ai Chi Punch Line**
>
> Many people using T'ai Chi to rehabilitate from drug-abuse problems like the fact that T'ai Chi gives them something to replace the old habits with. Rather than just denying themselves the high they loved, they are growing toward a new life as T'ai Chi helps them improve each and every day.

Law enforcement officers work in constant danger and often see only the worst sides of people. This can be very stressful. Historically, law enforcement officials have suffered from stress-related maladies such as alcoholism, drug abuse, coronary heart disease, diabetes, and suicide, according to *Police Chief Magazine* and the U.S. Public Health Service. T'ai Chi may be an effective, multipurpose way to help law enforcement officers deal with job-related stress. T'ai Chi's martial applications are an added bonus to officers learning T'ai Chi's soothing stress-management tools.

T'ai Chi can help in several ways. First, it can help officers dump job stress after work. Then if they do go out for a drink after T'ai Chi class, they will be doing it for pleasure rather than for stress reduction. This can mean the difference between a couple social drinks and a mind-numbing binge.

Second, if officers are less stressed on duty, they will likely see more options in any given situation. Problems can be defused more easily when in a calmer, clearer state. Even in difficult situations, T'ai Chi's calming effects can resonate, especially if it helps the officers sleep better, which T'ai Chi is known to do. T'ai Chi's calming aspects can help defuse potentially dangerous situations, which leaves the officer with less stress to take with them off duty. Less stress begets less stress, and so on and so on.

Hopefully, departments will eventually provide officers with 7-hour shifts and use the last hour for T'ai Chi decompression time. This will make business sense for all the reasons listed in Chapter 21 on corporate T'ai Chi, but these benefits are magnified because law enforcement officials' stress can be even higher.

T'ai Chi and Violence

Most domestic violence is a very ineffective form of stress management. Domestic violence is a way a very unhappy person takes out personal stress on his or her loved ones. It's ineffective because as we tear down those around us, that eventually tears us down. We create a sanctuary of pain rather than a loving home.

T'ai Chi can change that from many angles. If children begin to use T'ai Chi's mind/body fitness stress-management tools to self-heal in school, the cycle of pain at home will be changed and diminished in some ways. Then if parents are encouraged to learn these tools through community services, they can change the cycle even more effectively. There is a great spider web of connection in a community that will be affected as well. If one parent breaks a cycle of abuse and pain, his or her children will not spread that pain by being mean to the children around them at school or by growing up and passing it down to their kids by being violent to them.

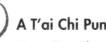 **A T'ai Chi Punch Line**

Many T'ai Chi practitioners hear others tell them they have "changed," "are calmer," or "are easier to be around" before they even notice the changes in themselves. Even when you are feeling stress, others may see you as "mellow" in comparison to the rest of the world.

Alcohol and other substance abuses aggravate much domestic violence. (The benefits of T'ai Chi for drug rehabilitation are discussed in Chapter 20.) Substance abuse and domestic violence all set a destructive dynamic in motion that reaches far beyond the home. A famous "kick the cat" story shows how a community is affected by one person's calm or rage:

An executive gets a traffic ticket on the way to work and then fumes at his administrative assistant. She, in turn, snaps at the other executives and employees she deals with. They get ticked off and snap at their co-workers, who are testy with people in the other companies they deal with on the phone, and so on. Eventually, thousands of people who have had a lousy day hit the freeway and begin to give the one-fingered salute to other motorists. And so it goes.

Finally, all these seething people get home and yell at their spouses, who yell at the kids, who walk upstairs and kick the cat.

T'ai Chi can inverse this process, and thousands of family cats can get a loving caress by kids growing up in a more loving world, nurtured by parents who work at companies that provide health tools to them like T'ai Chi. Sound far-fetched? Not really. Stress is the source of much of our communal pain, and stress management such as T'ai Chi can act as a balm and dramatically heal it.

 A T'ai Chi Punch Line

Once you learn T'ai Chi, you'll begin to notice people practicing everywhere you go, in any country in the world. T'ai Chi is an international language. My students have done T'ai Chi with people in England, France, Japan, Vietnam, Mexico, China, El Salvador, and Cuba, to name a few. As you travel, T'ai Chi will give you a pleasant vehicle to interact with and meet other people, even if you don't speak their language.

A study done by the Transcendental Meditation Foundation (which teaches an excellent form of stress management called Transcendental Meditation, or TM) found that when a small percentage of the population of a community, school, or organization practiced TM, it had a positive impact on that entire social body. Therefore, even though many people

will never practice T'ai Chi, those who do may change the entire community in positive ways.

T'ai Chi and the Environment

At first, it may not seem like T'ai Chi has anything to do with our world's environment, but it does. The words *T'ai Chi* mean "the Supreme Ultimate Point in the Universe." Every single part of the entire world exists within each and every thing, even you and me. Modern physics demonstrates this by explaining that all things are made of energy—*the same energy*. You, I, the sun and moon, and Earth's oceans and mountains are all made of the same energy. We are connected. This is brought home even more as science explains that you and I and everyone on this planet have breathed an oxygen atom breathed by Jesus, Buddha, and Mohammed. The world gets smaller.

Sage Sifu Says

Each time you walk outside, look up at the sky and at the trees or grass. Let the full breadth of nature's beauty wash over you. Think of opening your body to the universal energy as if you were an open, airy sponge that could fill with the life around you, and likewise you can expand out to merge with it. If you make this a habit and take 30 or 60 seconds to do this each time you walk in or out of your home, it will change your life.

When you practice T'ai Chi and especially Sitting QiGong, you often feel at peace, somehow connected to the world around you, as if you were the center of the universe. This experience leaves you feeling as though you matter, yet it also leaves you feeling as though every other person and every other thing in this world are of vast and profound importance as well.

T'ai Chi and QiGong remind us that we are energy by immersing our mind and body in the experience of it each day. This constant immersion reminds us how closely we are linked to all things. This isn't an illusion. The illusion is that we think we are separate from the world. The rainforest and ocean are the earth's lungs and thermostats. Without them, we perish. To feel "connected" to the world is to become real. T'ai Chi and QiGong help us become more and more real.

Our decisions about how to live in our world will be healthfully influenced by the "realness" T'ai Chi cultivates. This will be a powerful asset to building a cleaner, healthier world. As with all things, the world's environmental health begins with our own state of health. Your heart beats to supply oxygen to your entire body. However, the first thing the heart feeds is itself because if it is healthier, stronger, and clearer, it is more useful to its world (your body). By feeding yourself the healing force of life energy every day, you enable yourself to be a healing force as you flow through the world *around you.*

The Least You Need to Know

- T'ai Chi helps heal our society, our world, and us.
- T'ai Chi saves money in health care and may lower crime and unemployment rates.
- T'ai Chi helps us all "just get along."
- T'ai Chi influences our environment in a positive way.

In This Chapter

◆ Unleashing your power to change the world

◆ Connecting to T'ai Chi and QiGong world events, teachers, and resources with one source: www.worldtaichiday.org

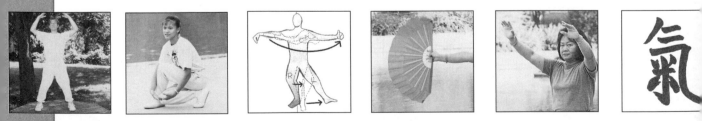

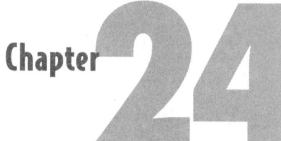

Chapter 24

Celebrating World T'ai Chi and QiGong Day

> If we want to make something truly spectacular of our world, there is nothing whatsoever that can stop us.
>
> —Rainer Maria Rilke

Not only are *you* truly profound and unique, but you are holding a truly profound and unique book: the first edition of this book actually *launched a world event, changing the world in a healing way*. World T'ai Chi and QiGong Day, through coverage by *CNN*, *The New York Times*, *The South China Morning Post, and media worldwide*, has educated millions about T'ai Chi and QiGong. Therefore, this book doesn't just "talk the talk"—it *walks the walk* of T'ai Chi's expansive personal power.

Too often in our lives we underestimate and undervalue our power as human beings. The practice of T'ai Chi and QiGong is designed to unblock the rigid limitations we hold so the greatest potential within us can flow up and out through our relaxed mind and body.

It's actually very unhealthy for human beings to settle for less than their greatest potential, for *repression of enthusiasm and hope can diminish our health*. Studies reveal that when people give of themselves to make the world a better place, it improves their physical and mental health—kind of an "instant karma," if you will (kudos to John Lennon). And T'ai Chi and QiGong help energize and motivate us for "right action," as T'ai Chi philosophy extols us to aspire to.

Participating in World T'ai Chi and QiGong Day is a way you can expand your T'ai Chi and QiGong journey to include joining with hundreds of thousands of like-minded people worldwide each year to be part of a fun and beneficial global health and healing event known as World T'ai Chi and QiGong Day.

Unleash the World-Altering Power Within You!

As we practice T'ai Chi, we realize it changes our lives by showing us that most of what holds us back is not "out there" in the world as much as it is *in our own mental and emotional limitations* in the form of rigidity we've constrained ourselves with unconsciously. As earlier chapters explained, this mental constraint actually affects circulation and health functions over time. But it also holds back our lives. My T'ai Chi and QiGong practice enabled me to open to large, expansive ideas, such as, for example, creating World T'ai Chi and QiGong Day, first by announcing it in the first edition of this book. Then these powerful tools gave me the stress-management techniques needed to endure the stress of actually fulfilling that dream.

Ouch!

When you catch your mind revolving around the negatives of "I can't do this" or "I can't change that," practice the QiGong breathing/energy exercise taught in Part 3. Let your mind and body *let go of everything*. Releasing negatives fills you with hope as you fill with light.

The same T'ai Chi and QiGong energy empowered teachers and organizers in cities worldwide to envision and create massive (and smaller) World T'ai Chi and QiGong Day events locally in 60 nations that make this global event the historic annual reality it has become. This event has since been recognized by the United Nations World Health Organization, governors, mayors, and senators worldwide.

The purpose of World T'ai Chi and Qigong Day is twofold: to educate millions worldwide of the profound health and healing benefits of T'ai Chi and QiGong and how they can heal society and save hundreds of billions of dollars annually; also, by bringing humanity together across racial, economic, and geopolitical boundaries each year to wrap the earth in a healing wave of energy, we create a vision of what is possible for the world when we focus on health and healing.

We are entering an extraordinary time in human history with access to modern *and ancient wonders* to make life better and better. We are learning that by healing ourselves, we heal the world, and vice versa. And today we have access to the best of both modern and ancient sciences. By marrying the dynamic power of our modern Western technological world's information age with the inner peace and clarity that ancient Eastern wisdom has cultivated and refined for us over the last 2,000 years, we may be at the beginning of a wondrous human renaissance where health and clarity merge with limitless potential to *create the world of our dreams.*

Bookmark www.worldtaichiday.org and enjoy the free resources there, and get involved in this global movement for health and healing. Encourage friends and family to utilize the many free resources there as well.

The Least You Need to Know

◆ You have the seeds for wondrous change *in you*.

◆ Fear limits our ability to expand our mind and world to open to hopeful visions.

◆ T'ai Chi and QiGong can help you breathe and relax, open to limitless possibility.

◆ Joining in World T'ai Chi and QiGong Day can help change the world by lessening stress and fear, and expanding health and hope.

◆ Your world and our world become limitless as we practice life tools enabling us to relax into the future.

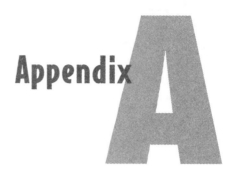

Appendix A

The T'ai Chi and QiGong Yellow Pages

Although two chapters in this book relate to particular T'ai Chi styles (Chapters 14 and 15), the majority of this book is a valuable resource for anyone exploring any style of T'ai Chi or QiGong. In fact, this book is used as a student primer and textbook by many teachers of many different styles worldwide. With that in mind, I created this appendix to expose readers to the many styles and schools in their communities.

For those who find it difficult to attend local live classes, the 4-hour instructional DVD listed in Appendix C can be a godsend. Its classlike format is similar to attending classes *in the comfort of your own home.* The video details the illustrated instructions in Chapter 15. You may also find that after learning at home, it's easier to learn in live classes, even if the styles are different.

In this appendix, you'll find an extensive listing of T'ai Chi and QiGong organizations, schools, and teachers in the United States, Australia, New Zealand, Canada, South Africa, and the United Kingdom. For continually updated telephone numbers, e-mail addresses, or websites for your local school/teacher listings below visit www.worldtaichiday.org, and click on Beginner Resources. (If you're not Internet-equipped, go to your local library, show this to the librarian, and ask for help.) You will also find contacts there for more than 50 other countries. Due to the volume of listings, the authenticity of each listing cannot be verified; rather, this listing is a clearinghouse of information to assist in your search for a school near you, not an endorsement. You are your best judge of what school or teacher is right for you. Always use discretion when contacting and choosing a school or teacher.

The following listings are arranged by city, school, and country. *Note:* For purposes of this directory, all "Tai Chi," "Taiji," or "T'ai Chi" references will be abbreviated as "TC." All "QiGong" (or Chi Kung) references will be abbreviated as "QG." All "Martial Arts" will be seen as "MA." "Kung Fu" or "Gung Fu" is "KF."

Visit www.worldtaichiday.org to find phone numbers, e-mail addresses, and website links and continually updated information for all the following listings, as well as listings worldwide.

National T'ai Chi and QiGong Organizations and Schools

National Registries

World T'ai Chi & Qigong Day Assn.
www.worldtaichiday.org

International Tai Chi Association (ITCCA) Italia
www.itcca.it

National QG Assn.—Nationwide and Int'l.
www.nqa.org

Canadian Taijiquan Federation
www.canadiantaijiquanfederation.ca

Tai Chi Union for Great Britain
www.taichiunion.com

British Council for Chinese Martial Arts
www.bccma.com

Taijiquan and Qigong Federation for Europe (TCFE)
www.tcfe.org

Registries by State

Alabama

Birmingham, AL
New Forest Way

Daphne, AL
Shaolin TC Inst. @ YMCA

Dothan, AL
School of TC
Frederic Lecut

Fairhope, AL
TC for All
Ron Driesbach

Florence, AL
North Alabama Tang Soo Do

Mobile, AL
The Mary Abbie Berg Ctr.

Mobile, AL
Liu Inst. Int'l. Shaolin TC

Alaska

Anchorage, AK
Dao Dancing TC

Anchorage, AK
Jade Lady Meditation TC/QG

Anchorage, AK
N. Dragon Taoist Arts

Anchorage, AK
The Oriental Healing Arts Ctr.
Inst. of Med. QG/MQ/QH/TC

Anchorage, AK
Shifting Wind TC/QG

Anchorage, AK
Sifu Ray's Studios

Anchorage, AK
Touch of Tao

Ketchikan, AK
Chi-Lel QG

Soldotna, AK
Kenai Peninsula College

Arizona

Chandler, AZ
Yang's TC of Arizona

Fountain Hills, AZ
Body in Harmony

Mesa, AZ
g.e.t.i.t. intgrtv. arts TC/QG

Mesa, AZ
House of Karate

Mesa, AZ
Spalding's World Class Karate, TC/MA

Phoenix, AZ
Deanne Hodgson

Phoenix, AZ
Garden Paradise TC

Phoenix, AZ
TC/QG/Feng Shui
Don Fiore

Phoenix, AZ
Two Fishes Swimming

Phoenix, AZ
World MAs

Prescott, AZ
Shen Yi Healing Arts of AZ

Sierra Vista, AZ
Acdmy. of Fitness

Surprise, AZ
Sher Dano

Tempe, AZ
World TC

Tucson, AZ
American Wu style TCquan Assn.

Tucson, AZ
Chi Works AZ

Tucson, AZ
Great Harmony TC Chuan

Tucson, AZ
Inst. for Conscious Change

Tucson, AZ
Wu Style TCC Inst. of Tucson

Arkansas

Little Rock, AR
Four Winds TC

California

Albany, CA
The Possible Scty. QG/AquaChi

Alhambra, CA
Tai Ji Club
Sun Anuang

Arcadia, CA
Draco Arts
Marvin Quon

Arcata, CA
TC for Life
Glenda Hesseltine

Atascadero, CA
Energetic Arts Ctr.

Bakersfield, CA
TC Institute
Sabrina Kusek

Benicia, CA
Daoist MA

Berkeley, CA
Ashkenaz Dance/Cmty. Ctr. QG

Berkeley, CA
Bay TC with HeartLove!

Berkeley, CA
Bodymind Healing Ctr.

Berkeley, CA
Brkly. YMCA AquaChi

Berkeley, CA
Cal. TC
William Dere

Berkeley, CA
Chi Nei Tsang Inst.

Berkeley, CA
Inner Communications

Berkeley/San Francisco, CA
Shaolin One Finger QG
Arleen Kwan

Berkeley/Kensington, CA
White Magnolia TC/QG

Beverly Hills/L.A., CA
Pat Akers TC

Burbank, CA
Jian Mei Int'l., MA Assn.
M. Wen Mei Yu

Cardiff by the Sea, CA
Enhancing Tech. Unltd.

Carlsbad, CA
San Diego QG
Fay McGrew

Carlsbad, CA
Shadow Dragon MAs

Carlsbad, CA
The Yoga Ctr.

Carmel Valley, CA
Jing Chi Shen

Cerritos, CA
Cerritos College Cmty. Ed.

Chula Vista, CA
Bonita Tai Chi

Claremont, CA
Shaolin Wei Tuo QG

Concord, CA
TC for Arthritis/QG
Robin Malby

Corona, CA
Ron Sahli/Corona Parks

Costa Mesa, CA
QG in the Park

Duarte, CA
Dan Lee Acdmy. of TC

El Cerrito, CA
Wen Wu School of MA

El Segundo, CA
AEA TC Club

Escondido, CA
Nina Sugawara

Eureka, CA
TC for Life
Glenda Hesseltine

Fair Oaks, CA
Sacramento Chen TC

Fairfax, CA
Energy Arts
Bruce Kumar Frantzis

Fort Bragg, CA
Neighborhood TC Assn.

Fullerton, CA
Yang and Tung
Tom Walters

Glendale/L.A., CA
TaiChiME4Health
Arnell Bertumen

Hayward, CA
TC Chih
Athene Mantle

Idyllwild, CA
Peaceful Dragon TC

Imperial Beach, CA
Golden School of TC

Imperial Beach, CA
T'ai Chi by the Sea

Irvine, CA
Anthony Ho's Wu TC
Lee Scheele

Irvine, CA
JoAnna Gee Schoon
TC, QG

Laguna Beach, CA
Kuang Ping TC

Laguna Niguel, CA
Flowering Hands TC

Laguna Niguel, CA
Michael Mohoric QG

Lakewood, CA
King's KF and TC Assn.

La Mesa, CA
Hsing-I MA Inst.

Lodi, CA
TC for Hlth.
Brenda Norris

Loma Linda, CA
L. L. Univ./Drayson Ctr.
TC
Sifu Kurland

Lomita, CA
Shaolin
Manuel Marquez

Los Angeles, CA
Hsing Chen Internal Arts

Los Angeles/Malibu, CA
Nat'l. TC Ch'uan
Assn./J.M.I.M.A.
Doria Cook-Nelson

Los Angeles, CA
Nat'l TC Chuan Assn.
Dan Paik

Los Angeles, CA
Universal Tao of Los
Angeles

Los Angeles, CA
Zhao Bao Wu Dan TC

L.A./Beverly Hills/Santa
Monica, CA
Tim O'Connor's
Acdmy./TC Chuan

L.A./Irvine, CA
Red Road School TC
Samuel Barnes

L.A./Santa Monica/
Idyllwild, CA
Peaceful Way TC

L.A./Ventura, CA
Tai Xing yi Bagua

Malibu/Studio City, CA
Doria Cook-Nelson

Marina del Rey, CA
Therapeutic Bodywork/QG

Menifee, CA
Mt. San Jacinto College

Menlo Park, CA
The QG Institute

Mill Valley, CA
TC for Seniors
Mark Johnson

Mission Viejo, CA
Saddleback College

Modesto, CA
Kung Fu Inst.
Sifu Neil Thomas

Monterey, CA
Cynthia Fels

Monterey, CA
Monterey Bay Healing Tao

Moraga, CA
Into Being
Wendy Helms, Ph.D.

Newport Beach, CA
Chi Arts Assn.

Oakland, CA
Bay Area Healing Tao (QG)

Oakland, CA
Creation Spirituality
University QG

Oakland, CA
Dayan QG: Gentle Path to
Health/Fitness

Oakland, CA
TC Chih QG

Oakland, CA
Way of Joy QG/Vicki

Oakland, CA
Women's QG Alliance

Ojai, CA
Embracing Your Chi

Orinda, CA
Bodymind Healing Ctr.

Palm Desert, CA
TC/Bagua/QG
Bernard Shannon

Palm Springs, CA
Scott Cole's TC/QG

Palm Springs, CA
Sun TC/Medical QG
Rob Haberkorn

Palo Alto, CA
TC Chih with Dona
Marriott

Palm Springs, CA
TC Education and Research
Inst.

Palo Alto, CA
TC/QG
Cindy Mason, CMT, Ph.D.

Pico Rivera, CA
TC for Seniors
Bill Ferrel

Poway, CA
Poway Kenpo Karate

Rancho Cucamonga, CA
Chaffey College PE Dept.

Redlands, CA
Grace TC Ctr.

Richmond, CA
Richmond Senior Ctr. QG

Riverside, CA
NWTCCA/Myra Allen

Riverside, CA
SoCal NWTC Chuan Assn.
Sifu Ruth Villalobos

Riverside, CA
UCR/Sifu Harvey Kurland

Riverside, CA
UCR Student Rec. Ctr. TC

Riverside/Corona/
Norco/Moreno Valley, CA
Young at Heart TC
Villalobos/Kurland

Running Springs, CA
Tension Masters and
QG/TC

Sacramento, CA
Jan Polin

Sacramento, CA
Judy Tretheway

Sacramento, CA
Tara Stiles

Sacramento, CA
TC and QG

Sacramento, CA
TC for Beauty

San Bernardino, CA
Ctr. for Spirit Enrichment

San Diego, CA
Chi Healing Ctr.

San Diego, CA
Flowing Waters TC

San Diego, CA
Golden Leopard Kempo

San Diego, CA
Golden School TC
Gene Golden

San Diego, CA
Hsing I MA Inst.

San Diego, CA
KF Acdmy.

San Diego, CA
Natural Healing Specialties

San Diego, CA
S.D. TC and QG Assn.

San Diego, CA
TC Chih

San Diego, CA
TC Chih/18 Forms QG

San Diego, CA
TC/QG Healthways

San Diego, CA
TC Wellness Ctr.

San Diego, CA
Wisdom Healing QG

San Francisco, CA
American QG Assn.

San Francisco, CA
Authentic Breathing QG

San Francisco, Bay Area, CA
Donald/Cheryl Lynne Rubbo

San Francisco, CA
East/West Acdmy. Hlg. Arts
Effie Chow

San Francisco, CA
Int'l Tibetan QG Assn.

San Francisco, CA
Michael S. Isaacs

San Francisco, CA
Shaolin One Finger QG
Angela Lee, L.Ac.

San Francisco East Bay Area,
CA
TC Chih/QG School

San Francisco, CA
Waving Clouds

San Francisco, CA
World QG Fed.

San Francisco/Bay Area, CA
American Chen TC Society

San Francisco/S. Bay, CA
Bay Area Chen TC

San Jacinto, CA
Mt. San Jacinto Clg.

San Jose, CA
Arnold Tayam, D.M.Q.

San Jose, CA
Morning Crane
Chris Shelton

San Jose, CA
Quang Ping TC

San Leandro, CA
Java Gym Holistic Exercise
Studio

San Leandro, CA TC, SL
Adult School
Rosalind L. Braga and Mary
Ellen Waite

Santa Barbara, CA
Inst. of Integral QG/TC
Roger Jahnke, O.M.D.

Santa Barbara, CA
SB Clg. of Oriental Med.

Santa Cruz, CA
Santa Cruz TC

Santa Cruz, CA
TC Natural Health Club

Santa Cruz/Aptos, CA
Shaolin One Finger QG
Teresa Halliburton

Santa Monica, CA
Emperor's College/Trad'l.
Oriental Med.

Santa Monica, CA
SMTC Chuan/QG
Joe Lopez

Santa Monica, CA
Tao West Arts

Santa Monica/L.A., CA
Peaceful Way TC Chuan

Santa Rosa, CA
Redwood Empire TC
Kevin V. Powers

Santa Rosa/Occidental, CA
Jane Golden's TC/QG

Sausalito, CA
Shaolin MAs KF/TC

Sebastopol, CA
Integrative Body Works

Sebastopol, CA
Taoist Med. QG Ctr.

South Pasadena, CA
South Pasadena TC Club

Stockton, CA
Stuart Alve Olson/Valley
TC/QG

Sunnyvale, CA
TC and CK for Health

Valley Springs, CA
Sheng Chi KF

Ventura, CA
Dr. of Oriental Medicine
Fred Siciliano, O.M.D.,
L.A.C., M.H.

Walnut Creek, CA
TC Chih/QG

Watsonville, CA
Cass Redmon

Westminster, CA
Bone Marrow QG

West L.A., CA
UCLA Extension

Whittier, CA
TC 4 Kids/Adults/Seniors
Deborah Moen

Colorado

Boulder, CO
Human Performance Assn.

Boulder, CO
Transformations/QG
Groups

Boulder, CO
Trinity QG
Carolyn Eberle

Colorado Springs, CO
4 Branches Healing Arts

Colorado Springs, CO
Adam Sewell Fitness

Colorado Springs, CO
Mvmt. for Well-Being
JudyAnne Light

Colorado Springs/Wdlnd.
Pk., CO
Daoist Practices Ctr.

Denver, CO
Ancient Harmony TC
Mearl Thompson

Denver, CO
The Gift of Qi
Steve Bradley

Denver, CO
Home for Int'l. Arts
Mary C. Ryan

Denver, CO
Jewish Community Ctr./TC

Denver, CO
TC Chih
Anna Pergola

Denver, CO
TC Project: Joe Brady
Jacqui Shumway

Greeley, CO
Jade Mountain TC

Lakewood, CO
Green Mtn. Rec. Ctr.

Nederland, CO
QG Research/Practice Ctr.

Pagosa Springs, CO
Pagosa Springs TC/QG

Paonia/Hotchkiss/Cedaredg
e/Basalt, CO
Robert Cook School of TC,
QG, and KF

Parker, CO
Omega MA/American
Acdmy. of MAs

Pueblo, CO
Gaia Inst. Wellness Ctr.

Thornton, CO
CO Budo Ctr. Karate
Schools

Woodland Park, CO
4 Branches Healing Arts

Connecticut

Branford/West Haven, CT
Silent Dragon Schools

Chaplin, CT
Starfarm TC

Coventry, CT
Silver Dragon TC

Danbury, CT
Grand Master T. K. Shih

East Haddam, CT
Peaceful Wolf TCC/QG
David Shaver

Elmwood, CT
White Lotus MA

Gales Ferry, CT
South Shaolin KF School

Glastonbury/Crmwl., CT
Daoist Practices Ctr.

Greenwich, CT
Greenwich Hospital

Manchester, CT
Ju Nan Shin MA Acdmy.

Manchester, CT
Malee's School of TC/KF

Meriden, CT
Central CT TC

Middletown, CT
Eagle's Quest TC
David Chandler

Mystic, CT
Gary Donovan TC/QG

New Haven, CT
Silent Dragon KF/TC

Newington, CT
Dragonfly TC

North Westchester, NY
(also in CT)
Red Lion TC
Linda Schneiderman

Norwalk, CT
Brian Buturla QG

Norwalk, CT
Waterwheel TC

South Windsor, CT
Shaolin Wushu Ctr.

Waterford, CT
C. C. Chen's Yang Style TC

West Hartford, CT
White Lotus MA/Reiki Ctr.

West Haven, CT
Silent Dragon TC/KF

Woodbury, CT
USA MA

Delaware

Camden-Wyoming, DE
Traditional Chinese TC
School

Georgetown, DE
TCC

Newark, DE
Chinese MA and TC Inst.

Newark, DE
Ming Tao TC Ch'uan
Studio

Wilmington/Newark, DE
Sun KF School

Wilmington, DE
TC for Life

Florida

Boca Raton, FL
Equisol Oriental Med. Ctr.

Boca Raton, FL
KF Conservatory

Bradenton, FL
Tang MAs Ctr.

Clearwater, FL
Chinese MAs Ctr.

Deerfield Beach, FL
Theosophical Society

Deland, FL
BlueSky Yoga and TC Ctr.

Deland, FL
Warrior MAs Ctr.

Dunedin, FL
Chinese MA Ctr.

Ft. Lauderdale, FL
Supreme Science QG Ctr.

Highlands County, FL
YMCA and SFCC Classes

Hollywood, FL
Chungs's TC/KF

Hollywood, FL
Healing Tao of S. FL.

Jacksonville, FL
Ctr. for Ntr'l. Health

Lantana, FL
MAs Acdmy.

Longwood, FL
White Dragon KF/TC

Miami, FL
Natural Motion Systems

Miami, FL
Wing Lung KF/TC Assn.

Miami, FL
WITHIN Wellness Ctr.

Miami Shores, FL
TC with Todd Plager

Naples, FL
Maria Baum

Naples/Bonita, FL
Dragon's Gate

Neptune Beach, FL
Cobalt Moon Hlg. Ctr.

New Smyrna Beach, FL
TC by the Sea

Orlando, FL
Life-Align

Orlando, FL
Wah Lum KF/TC of USA

Pompano Beach, FL
Harmony Ctr.

Pompano Beach, FL
Pen and Sword TC

Pompano Beach, FL
QG Care

Sarasota, FL
3 Treasures School

Sebastian, FL
City of Sebastian Cmty. Ctr

Sebring, FL
Private class: 863-385-1234
SFCC and YMCA classes

Siesta Key/Sarasota, FL
Tantra TC/TC Chih

Stuart, FL
Internal Arts Institute

Tamara, FL
White Crane Healing Arts

Tampa, FL
Hwa Yu TC Ch'uan
Mark McGee

Tampa, FL
Univ. of S. Florida's TC

Tarpon Springs, FL
Bob Messinger

Tarpon Springs, FL
Soho Studio

Titusville, FL
MAs Unlimited

Vero Beach, FL
Vero Beach TC/KF Club

Vero Beach, FL
Vero Beach QG Society

West Palm Beach, FL
TC of Palm Beach

Winter Haven, FL
TC and MA
Michael Smith

Winter Haven, FL
QC
William J. Neff, Dipl. Ac.

Georgia

Atlanta, GA
Chinese Shaolin Ctr.

Atlanta, GA
Sifu Christopher Gresov,
Ph.D.

Atlanta, GA
TC Ch'uan Atlanta

Atlanta, GA
TC Chuan

Carrollton, GA
Tallapoosa Ctr.

College Park, GA
TC Health Society

Columbus, GA
Hughston Wellness Ctr.
Penny Pennington

Columbus, GA
TC for Health/Stress
Philip Chan, M.D.

Decatur, GA
Tai-Chi Assn., Inc.

Lawrenceville, GA
TC at UUCG

Marietta, GA
Chinese Shaolin Ctr.

Norcross, GA
Chinese Shaolin Ctr.

St. Simons Island, GA
TC/QG
Damian G. Fedorko

Hawaii

Big Island, HI
TC Assn.
Sifu Howard James

Hilo, HI
Peter Tam Hoy's Scl. of TC

Honolulu, HI
Cheng Man Kang Seow TC

Honolulu, HI
Dong's Int'l. TC/QG Assn.

Honolulu, HI
TC Chih

Honolulu, HI
Tse QG Ctr.

Honolulu, HI
Wu's TC Chuan Acdmy,
Hawaii

Kailua-Kona, Big Island of
HI
Nei Wai Kung MAs Acdmy.

Kapaa, Kauai, HI
QG Kahuna Valley
Francesco
Daisy Garripoli

Kaua'i, HI
Kaua'I School of TC

Lihue, HI (Kauai)
dba Ke ala T'ai Chi
Nii and Bailey, LLC

Makawao, Maui, HI
HI TC Ch'uan Assn.

Idaho

Boise, ID
Dancing Bear TC/QG
School

Illinois

Alma, IL
TC for Healthy Living
Jenni Balis

Arlington Heights, IL
Forest View Ed. Ctr.

Aurora, IL
Quiet Dragons TC

Belleville, IL
TC for Wellness
Jan VanLeuven

Brookfield, IL
Phoenix TC and QG

Charleston, IL
Jazzercise/TC Fitness Ctr.

Chicago, IL
Chinese KF Institute

Chicago, IL
The Human Process/TC
Chicago

Chicago, IL
Hyde Park TC

Chicago, IL
PowR Healing

Chicago, IL
Wai Lun Choi's Chinese
MA

Effingham, IL
Champions MAs

Effingham, IL
Private TC, QG, and BZ
Trng.

Effingham, IL
Restorative TC\QG
Shar Marvel

Effingham, IL
TC for Arthritis
Marvel/Purcell

Evanston, IL
Heartwood Ctr.

Evanston, IL
The Human Process/TC

Joliet, IL
TC and Massage
Jeff Lindstrom

Kankakee, IL
KVPD Cmty. Wellness Ctr.

Lake Zurich, IL
LZ Park District

Mascoutah, IL
Dolores Gordon

Mattoon, IL
East-West Fitness/Self-Def.

Mattoon, IL
Internal Boxing
Rusty Hays

Oak Park, IL
TC and QG classes/Oak
Park

Peoria, IL
TC for Life

Rockford, IL
TC with Sue Michaelsen

Salem, IL
TC for Healthy Living
Jenni Balis

Skokie, IL
San He QG Ctr.

Springfield, IL
Wellness Institute

St. Charles, IL
Gentle Path TC Assn.

St. Charles, IL
TC Shaolin Chuan Assn.

Villa Park, IL
White Tiger TC Chuan
Acdmy.

Waukegan, IL
Juhua Shan Yangsheng
Gong
S. E. Alleyne

Winfield, IL
Lightheart Ctr.

Indiana

Bloomington, IN
The Arana Ctr.

Bloomington, IN
New School TC

Highland, IN
Krucek QG Acdmy.

Indianapolis, IN
TC of Indianapolis

Indianapolis, IN
Tigerlily TC/Aikido
Gary Mohr

Michigan City, IN
Mssg. Therapy/Wellness
Ctr./QG

Milan, IN
Kissell Shaolindo

Seymour, IN
Middle Way TC

Terre Haute, IN
Terre Haute TC Club

Whiting, IN
Arts of Wisdom KF/TC

Iowa

Ames, IA
Dragon Arts Life Arts and
MAs

Des Moines, IA
Aurora TC Circle

Des Moines, IA
Chinese MA Acdmy.

Guttenberg, IA
Guttenberg Karate and TC
Inst.

Waterloo, IA
Covenant Wellness Ctr.
TC/QG

Waterloo, IA
Zhu's TC Healing and
Fitness

Kansas

Augusta, KS
Augusta MAs
Michael Huddleston

Dodge City, KS
Nats Yoga and Dance

Overland Park, KS
Mulan with Angela Wong-
Douglas

Overland Park, KS
TC/QG with Bill Douglas

Overland Park, KS
Yang Tai Chi/OP Cmty. Ctr.

Shawnee, KS
TC/QG with Bill Douglas

Topeka, KS
TC/QG w/Peggy Wheeler

Wichita, KS
Chi Lin TC Group
David Larsen

Kentucky

Louisville, KY
KY TC Ctr.

Madisonville, KY
Scott Vander Ploeg TC

Murray, KY
TC Assn. of Murray

Salyersville, KY
Wayne Hall TC/Chi QG

Versailles, KY
KY TC Ctr.

Louisiana

Metairie, LA
Liu Inst. Int'l Shaolin and
TC

New Orleans, LA
Acdmy. of MAs

New Orleans, LA
Heiping Pai TC Chuan Fa

New Orleans, LA
Shaolin and TC QG Inst.

Shreveport, LA
Lee's KF/TC Ctr.

Slidell, LA
TC Journey

Maine

Bethel, ME
TC/QG for All

Brunswick, ME
N. Chi MA Ctr.

Houlton, ME
Laughing Dragon TC

Portland, ME
Full Circle Synergy TC

South Freeport, ME
Maine Coast TC

Turner, ME
Yeung Style TC

Wiscasset, ME
Wiscasset Rec. Ctr.

Maryland

Annapolis, MD
TC with Jan Graves

Annapolis, MD
TC on the Bay

Annapolis, MD
QG with Kimberly

Arnold, MD
Jing Ying Inst.

Baltimore, MD
Communications
Health/Network

Baltimore, MD
Elementary TCC Study
Group

Baltimore, MD
New Circle TC

Baltimore, MD
TC in Baltimore

Bethesda, MD
Cloud Hands TC

Camp Springs, MD
Skyvalley Tai Ji

Chestertown, MD
Chesapeake TC/QG
Wayne McGuire

Chevy Chase, MD
Tai Chi Center

Columbia, MD
Moving in Stillness
Karl Ardo

Eldersburg, MD
Wednesday Evening
TC/QG

Ellicott City, MD
Ohashiatsu

Finksburg, MD
Three Treasures Health

Frederick, MD
Scott Acdmy. of MA

Gaithersburg/Wash. DC,
MD
Dancing Mtn. TC Quan

Hollywood, MD
Theory In Motion, TC and
QG

Laurel, MD
School of TC of MD, Inc.

Owings Mills, MD
USKA

Rockville, MD
www.davidchentaichi.com

Salisbury, MD
A Peaceable Place

Silver Spring, MD
MD Dance of Phoenix QG

Takoma Park, MD
Wu Shen Tao Hlth./MA
Ctr.

Massachusetts

Boston, MA
Bow Sim Mark TC

Boston, MA
Gin Soon TC Chuan
Federation

Boston, MA
Nam Pai Acdmy.

Boston, MA
Yang's MA Assn.

Brookline, MA
Mindfulbody TC Chuan

Cohasset, MA
KF/TC w/Jade Forest

Dedham, MA
Dedham Cmty. House

East Bridgewater, MA
Wu Li Acdmy.

Greenfield, MA
J. R. Roy MAs Studio

Holliston, MA
New England School of TC

Leominster, MA
Trdtnl. Arts Inst. TC/QG
Jeff Cote

Marblehead, MA
United MAs Ctr.

Martha's Vineyard, MA
Chilmark QG

Mattapoisett, MA
Watercourse Ctr. for
Healing Arts

Millbury, MA
Wah Lum KF and TC Inst.

Northampton, MA
Deer Mountain TC Acdmy.

North Andover, MA
Yang's MAs

Norwood, MA
Guang Ping Yang TC Assn.

Norwood, MA
In the Moment Wllns. Ctr.

Peabody, MA
Tao for All Seasons

Plymouth, MA
Dragon Gate Internal Arts

Shrewsbury, MA
TC Arts Assn.

Sutton, MA
TC Arts Assn.

Watertown/Brighton, MA
Pooled Resources
Judith Poole

Wayland, MA
Longfellow Club, QG

Westford, MA
NCM TC School

Woburn, MA
8 MAs for Health

Yarmouthport, MA
MA Guang Ping Yang TC
Assn. Hdqtrs.

Michigan

Alpena, MI
Alan LaCross MAs Ctr.

Ann Arbor, MI
Peaceful Dragon TC and
QG

Ann Arbor, MI
Wu's TC Chuan Acdmy.
Ann Arbor

Bloomfield Hills, MI
Taoist TC Society of MI

Dearborn, MI
Celestial Crane TCquan
and QG

Detroit, MI
Wu's TC Chuan Acdmy.—
Detroit

Grand Haven, MI
W. Michigan Yangjia
Michuan TC

Harbor Springs, MI
Smooth Moves

Kalamazoo, MI
Kehoe's TC

Lansing, MI
8 Willows KF Rsrch. Grp.

Lansing, MI
Moving Stillness

Livonia, MI
Taoist TC Society of MI

Livonia, MI
Traditional Arts—Orient

Mendon, MI
Rouhe Daoquan

Monroe, MI
Pierce MAs Institute

Muskegon, MI
City Ctrs.

Sterling Heights, MI
Energetic Arts of MI

Stevensville, MI
Lakeshore TC

Traverse City, MI
Simply TC
Barbara Jones Smith

Troy, MI
Michigan TC Ctr.

Minnesota

Bloomington, MN
Normandale TC
Quan/Internal Arts

Cannon Falls, MN
Roaming Dragons TC
Chuan

Duluth, MN
Christal Ctr.
Richard Tosseland

Duluth, MN
Healing Tao
Kate Pearson

Ely, MN
Chickadee TC

Ely, MN
Dao of Well-Being

Ely, MN
Int'l Qigong Alliance

Minneapolis, MN
World Inst. for Self-Hlg.

Minneapolis/St. Paul, MN
Dragon Door QG
John Du Cane

Plymouth, MN
TC Ch'uan and Internal
Strength

St. Cloud, MN
St. Cloud Karate/TC Inst.

Mississippi

Long Beach, MS
Gulfcoast Wing Chun and
TC

Missouri

Branson, MO
Branson TC Assn.
Sifu Ken Kersh

Columbia, MO
Chajonshim MAs

Jefferson City, MO
Synature TC/QG

Joplin, MO
School of TC

Kansas City, MO
Sifu Scott Winokur

KC Metro, MO
Stress Mgmt. TC/QG

KC Metro, MO
TC with Linda Bowers

Milan, MO
Shin Tai Dojo TC
Dale Green

Mineral Point, MO
Black Dragon KF Hlg. Arts
Ike Bear

Raytown, MO
Kansas City TC/KF

Springfield, MO
Cox Fitness Ctr.
Colleen Young

Springfield, MO
TC for ME!

Springfield, MO
TC/QG for ME!
Dr. Dean Cuebas

St. Louis, MO
Chinese Internal Arts
TC/QG/KF
Justin Meehan

St. Louis, MO
Feng Zhiqiang TC USA
Sifu Herb Parran

St. Louis, MO
Healing Qi/Tom Pasley

St. Louis, MO
Learn TC with Anna Lum

St. Louis, MO
Olivette Chai Chi/QG

St. Louis, MO
St. Louis Cheng Hsin TC

St. Louis, MO
STL TC Assn.
Michael David

St. Louis, MO
TC with Cis Hager

St. Louis, MO
Wu Hsing Chuan 5-Animal

St. Louis/Affton, MO
Shaolin Black Dragon
Joseph Kohl

Montana

Billings, MT
Billings TC Assc.

Clancy, MT
MountainSpirit QG

Eureka, MT
Dancing Dreamers Ctr.
QG/TC

Helena, MT
Sacred Mountain School
TC

Missoula, MT
Shen Yi School of TC

Red Lodge, MT
Access Holistic Health
TCC/QG

Nebraska

Hastings, NE
South Central Taekwondo

Lincoln, NE
TC Fitness

Omaha, NE
Omaha TC Assn.

Nevada

Las Vegas, NV
Lohan School of Shaolin

Las Vegas, NV
Vast Awakenings/Int'l. Arts

New Hampshire

Barrington, NH
Quest MA Acdmy.

Dover, NH
TC and QG Health with
Maya

Durham/Concord, NH
Red Lotus TC QG

Manchester, NH
Yang Chengfu TC
Michael Coulon

Nashua, NH
MA Ctr. for Personal Dev.

Newmarket, NH
Aryaloka Buddhist Rtrt. Ctr.

Sugar Hill, NH
Path of Harmony TC QG

New Jersey

Brick, NJ
China Hand KF Acdmy.

Cedar Grove, NJ
TC Chih

Clifton, NJ
TC Chih
Marion Mascone

Dunellen, NJ
Coiling Root Chen TC

Dunellen, NJ
Shaolin Circle TC

East Brunswick, NJ
Andy Lee Yang Chengfu
TC

Eastampton, NJ
QiSsage Body Systems,
LLC

Hamilton, NJ
Phoenix Acdmy. of MA

Hamilton, NJ
RWJ Ctr. for Health and
Fitness

Hamilton, NJ
TC Lee

Howell, NJ
TC Combat and Health

Keyport, NJ
Eagle TC Quan

Medford, NJ
Harmony TC

Metuchen, NJ
Black Belt Institute

Middletown, NJ
Kum Sung TC MA

Montclair, NJ
TC/QG with Joanne
Kornoelje

Morganville, NJ
QG with Maria Choy, M.D.

Mt. Laurel, NJ
Silver Tiger TC
William Ting

Mt. Laurel, NJ
QG Research Society

New Egypt, NJ
TC Chih/Siobhan
Hutchinson

North Plainfield, NJ
TC Chih

North Plainfield, NJ
TC Chih/Patricia Weber
Wilcomb

Ocean Grove, NJ
TC Chih/Daniel Pienciak

Oceanview, NJ
American Eagle TC/QG

Oceanview, NJ
Teacher Training TC/QG
Systems

Piscataway, NJ
Brian O'Connor's TC
Group

Piscataway, NJ
World Inst.—Self-Hlg.

Tinton Falls, NJ
Red Bank Acupnctr./Wellns.

Wantage, NJ
American Soc. of Internal
Arts

Wantage, NJ
Internal Gardens School of
Classical TC

Warren, NJ
Fran Maher/Brian Coffey
TC/QG

West Orange, NJ
Marcia Schoppik TC

Woodbridge, NJ
Wellness Through TC

New Mexico

Las Vegas, NM
QG/Peter Stege, D.O.M.

Santa Fe, NM
Heaven and Earth TC
Keith Cini

Santa Fe, NM
Spirit Warriors MAs
Acdmy./TC QG

New York

Albany, NY
Capital Dist. of NY TC and
KF Assn.

Amherst, NY
White's MAs Acdmy.

Batavia, NY
Watson Wlns. Ctr. TC/QG
Ray Watson

Bronxville, NY
TC School of Westchester

Brooklyn, NY
Full Aliveness QG
M. McComiskey

Brooklyn, NY
Patience TC Association

Brooklyn, NY
Xaverian TC/Joe Rubino

East Hampton, NY
TC/QG
Rachel Rudansky, Crtfd.
Rolfer

Elma, NY
Bill Adams's MA and Fitness

Endicott, NY
Sue Heavenrich

Garrison, NY
Hudson Valley TC Ch'uan

Glens Falls, NY
TC/QG with Mark Tolstrup

Hampton Bays, NY
TC Ctr. with Tina Curran

Huntington, NY
Inner Way with Roger
Sencer

Long Beach, NY
Toburan Wholistic Health

Long Island/Sound Beach,
NY
L.I. School of TC-Chuan

Medford, NY
Shaolin KF Studios

Monticello, NY
Cheng Man-Ching TC,
HTM

Morrisville, NY
Wu Style TC w/David
Dolbear

Mount Vernon, NY
Sadhana-Qi Wellness Ctr.

New York, NY
Adam Wallace

New York, NY
Ahn TC Studios

New York, NY
BlueSky TC
Carolyn Hearn

New York, NY (Queens)
Forest Hills TC
Michael Ferstendig

New York, NY
Gilda's Club
Ken Gray

New York, NY
H. Won T'ai-Chi Inst.

New York, NY
Int'l Yang Style TC Assn.
Bill Walsh

New York, NY
Lawrence Galante's TC

New York, NY
Lily Cohen's TC/QG

New York, NY
Mark Sabin TC Quan

New York, NY
Master Sam F. S. Chin's
I-Liq Chuan

New York, NY
Mind, Body, Shen
Derrick Trent

New York, NY
NY School of TC Chuan,
Inc.

New York, NY
Rama Krishnananda
Yoga/TC

New York, NY
Sai Guan Dao TC/Hlg. Arts
John Salgado

New York, NY
The Seed, Ctr. QG Dept.

New York, NY
Taoist Arts Ctr.

New York, NY
Taoist Yoga
Sharon Smith

New York, NY
TC Chih TC
Carolyn Perkins

New York, NY
The Universal Tao

New York, NY
William CC Chen TC, Inc.

New York, NY
Yang Chenfu TC Ctr.
Bill Walsh

New York, NY
Yang TC
Richard Jesaitis

Nyack, NY
Romain's KF/TC Acdmy.

Patchogue, NY
Water Tiger TC
Laurince D. McElroy

Pleasant Valley, NY
Master Sam F. S. Chin's
I-Liq Chuan

Queens, NY
Emei Acuptr./QG/TC/
Dachengquan

Queens, NY
Forest Hills TCC
Ann Harvey

Queens, NY
Laura Samuels TC/QG
Flushing YMCA

Rochester, NY
Kuan Yin TC
Diane Macchiavelli, L.Ac.

Rochester, NY
Northeastern MA

Rochester, NY
Rochester TC Ch'uan Ctr.

Rochester, NY
Wu Xing Institute

Saratoga Springs, NY
The TC Ctr.

Sound Beach, NY
LI School of TC

South Fallsburg, NY
Yang Style TC

Syracuse, NY
Central NY TC and QG
Ctr.

Syracuse, NY
Sun Style TCquan
Michael Walter

Tarrytown/Manhattan, NY
Everspring Acupuncture
Ctr.

Warwick, NY
Hudson Valley TC

Woodstock, NY
TC/QG/Qi Healing
Cassia Berman

Yonkers, NY
Taijiws with Sifu Wendy
Cali

Yorktown Heights, NY
Nat Costanzo's KF/TC Ctr.

North Carolina

Asheville, NC
Ctr. for Personal Mastery

Asheville, NC
Heaven and Earth TC

Asheville, NC
Lung Shan Hsing
I/Bagua/TC/KF

Chapel Hill, NC
Magic Tortoise TC School

Charlotte, NC
Peaceful Dragon Cultural
Ctr.

Charlotte, NC
TC Total Fitness/Mind and Body

Charlotte Norman, NC
Inner Power Fitness

Gibsonville, NC
Silk Tiger School of TC

Greensboro, NC
EarthStar TC

Greensboro, NC
East Gate Healing Arts Ctr.

Huntersville, NC
Peaceful Garden

Merritt, NC
Dragon Gate TC

Raleigh, NC
Inner Mtn. Jrny. TC Chih

Raleigh, NC
Qigong Wellness

Southern Pines, NC
Sandhills Combative Arts TC

Winston-Salem, NC
Golden Flower TC Assn.

North Dakota

Fargo, ND
The Spirit Room TC/QG

Ohio

Akron, OH
Wu Tang Ctr.
Tony Yang

Ashtabula, OH
Wellness/Total Lrng. Ctr.

Athens, OH
Three Treasures

Bayview, OH
TC Wu Style/Horn's MA

Bowling Green, OH
Chi Path

Brilliant, OH
Tai Chi Classes

Chagrin Falls, OH
QG Acdmy.

Cincinnati, OH
Creative Health Integrations/TCA

Cincinnati, OH
Have Qi Will Travel QG/TC

Cincinnati, OH
Mighty Vine Wellness Club

Cincinnati, OH
White Willow School of TC

Cleveland, OH
Healthy Hm., Healthy Body

Cleveland, OH
Hu's School-Chinese Int'l. MAs

Cleveland, OH
Immortal Palm Internal Arts

Cleveland, OH
Lucid Warrior Arts
Danny Kelly

Cleveland, OH
QG Acdmy.

Cleveland, OH
Susana Weingarten QG

Cuyahoga County, OH
QG Acdmy.

Dayton, OH
Stone River TC

Elyria, OH
OH Moo Duk Kwan MAs Ctr.

Georgetown, OH
TC for Health

Homerville, OH
TC Wu Style with Mary Cuchna

Kirtland/Lake County, OH
Prisma Ctr. QG/Wholstc.

Lakewood, OH
Tao's Healing Art

Lorain, OH
Lorain County Family YMCA

Mansfield, OH
Northern Shaolin Long Fist Style

Mansfield, OH
Richland Karate/Purple Bamboo Inst.

Maple Heights, OH
Golden Pyramid MA Ctr.

Marietta, OH
P.R.I.D.E. Dojo/Trng. Ctr.

Medina, OH
QG Acdmy.

Mentor, OH
Karate Kajukenpo Assn.

Middletown, OH
Miami University Club
Dr. Michael Steward Sr.

Monroe, OH
Quisno Wellness Ctr. Club
Dr. Michael Steward Sr.

North Canton, OH
Tai Ji 4 Health
Dave Parks

Norwalk, OH
Jasmine Dragon TC

Oxford, OH
Oxford Club, Univ. Campus
Dr. Michael Steward Sr.

Pomeroy, OH
HeartSong Ctr.

Stow, OH
White Birch Trad. MA

Strongsville, OH
Jeff Ellis' Int'l. Karate Ctrs.

Strongsville, OH
TC Wu Style with Jeff Ellis

Toledo, OH
Toledo TC
Talli Harman and T. R. Statum

Toledo/Pointe Place, OH
Asian MAs Acdmy.

Wapakoneta, OH
Greater Northwest TC

West Chester, OH
School TC/QG
Susan Evans

Wooster, OH
Acdmy. of Immortal Palm

Youngstown, OH
TC Step One

Oklahoma

Oklahoma City, OK
Mickey Sherman MAs

Tulsa, OK
Tulsa TC

Tulsa, OK
Yangs MAs Assn.

Oregon

Ashland, OR
Chi Healing Ctr.

Ashland, OR
TC with Gene Burnett

Ashland, OR
Wisdom Healing QG

Bend, OR
CenterPoint Health Inst.

Bend, OR
TC with Charla Quinn

Corvallis, OR
QG Assn. of America

Eugene, OR
Abode of the Eternal Tao

Eugene, OR
Better Balance TC

Eugene, OR
Natural Arts Ctr.

Eugene, OR
Strawberry Gatts School

Eugene, OR
Tranquility Thru Movement

Forest Grove, OR
Yang Cheng Fu TC Chuan Ctr.

Medford/Ashland, OR
Pond House TC-QG

Portland, OR
Acdmy. of Qi Dao

Portland, OR
Bob Lau's School of TCQuan

Portland, OR
Chinese Shamanic QG/TC

Portland, OR
Northwest QG Society

Portland, OR
Portland Qigong Clinic

Portland, OR
QG Educational Services

Portland, OR
School of TC Chuan

Portland, OR
Wu Dao Jing She Int'l QG Assn.

Pennsylvania

Abington, PA
Goldenlight:
Body/Mind/Spirit

Allentown, PA
Little Tiger TC and
Therapy

Allentown, PA
Manawa Universal Arts

Belle Vernon, PA
Chon's Korean Karate TC

Bethlehem, PA
Thomas Ardizzone TC/QG

Bristol, PA
Dragon Moon MA Assn.

Brodheadsville, PA
Gentle Strength QG Group

Doylestown, PA
Rolly Brown's TC

Douglassville, PA
The Open Door

Erie, PA
Body Awareness TC Quan

Fleetwood, PA
Manawa Universal Arts

Glenville, PA
TC Chih Joy Thru Mvmnt.
Pat Flynn

Hanover, PA
TC Chih
Margery Erickson

Harrisburg, PA
Jose Johnson's
MAs/Wellness Ctr.

Kingston, PA
Sakura MA Ctr./TC

Lancaster, PA
Unique Healing Solutions

Lebanon, PA
Bow Sim Mark's TC Arts

Leechburg, PA
Inner Strength, Inc.

Lehigh Valley, PA
Manawa Universal Arts

Lewisburg, PA
QG with Arlyne

Lock Haven, PA
TC/QG/Shiatsu/Reiki
Gerald Cierpilowski

Meadville/Franklin, PA
Cootie Harris School TC

New Holland, PA
QG Rainbow

North Wales, PA
I.E.F. MAs Acdmy.

Palmyra, PA
Judy Bayliss's Chi Lel QG

Philadelphia, PA
Ba Z TC/KF (Wu Tang
Sys.)

Philadelphia, PA
Holistic Hands

Philadelphia, PA
Martial Posture

Philadelphia, PA
PN Chen TC Quan Assn.

Philadelphia, PA
QG Class at PA Hospital

Philadelphia, PA
QG Research Society

Philadelphia, PA
Siu Lum MA Acdmy.

Philadelphia, PA
Tiger Mountain TC

Philadelphia, PA
TCquan Club

Pittsburgh, PA
Yin Cheng Gong Fa Assn.

Scranton, PA
Shen Lung Yi MAs

Uniontown, PA
White Dragon TC/Wlns.
Ctr.

Wayne, PA
TC with Carolee Parker

West Chester, PA
Peter Herman's TC

Westtown, PA
TC at the Concept School

Wilkes-Barre, PA
Chinese Health Institute

York, PA
TC Chih with Cathy
Lehman

Puerto Rico

Bayamón, PR
TC and QG Institute of PR

Bayamón, PR
Ancient Fitness

Dorado, PR
Pakua Health Studio

San Juan, PR
Blue Mountain TC Inst.

San Juan, PR
Hunyuan/Chen/Sun
Emma L. Mangual

San Juan, PR
Hunyuantaiji/Chen Style

San Juan, PR
School of TC/QG LI. Dinc.

San Juan, PR
Wutang Int'l TC/IIlg. Arts
of PR

San Juan, PR
Yang Style with Jorge
Melendez

Rhode Island

East Providence, RI
Way of the Dragon—
Hlth./Hlg./MAs

Harrisville, RI
Dalant Studio—Yang and
Soon TC/QG

Harrisville, RI
One Way Taijiquan
Leslie Mundy

North Kingstown, RI
N. K. Adult Education

Westerly, RI
Westerly TC

South Carolina

Beaufort, SC
Lowcountry TC

Bluffton, SC
Lowcountry TC

Charleston, SC
TC for Health
Chaz Walter

Columbia, SC
Lam Tang Shaolin KF
Acdmy.

Greenville, SC
Greenville TC

Greenville, SC
Qi Mountain

Hilton Head, SC
Lowcountry TC

Neeses, SC
Independent TC Inst.

South Dakota

Brookings, SD
Dakota TC

Rapid City, SD
QG for Health

Tennessee

Antioch, TN
One 80 Turn/LLC
Coach Bradley

Columbia, TN
BriLee Enterprises

Knoxville, TN
Flying Dragon Chinese MA

Knoxville, TN
Chen Style TC

Memphis, TN
TC with Shelia Rae

Memphis, TN
UT HELP Ctr.
Dr. Veronica Engle

Memphis, TN
YMAA TC of Memphis

Nashville, TN
TCC Assn., Nashville

Nashville, TN
TN Int'l. Inst. Medical QG
J. Michael Wood

Nashville, TN
YMCA with Tom Williams

Texas

Arlington, TX
John P. Painter, Ph.D., N.D.

Austin, TX
Dave Pickens Central Texas
MAs

Austin, TX
Global Wholeness
Sarah and Cobi Bentley

Austin, TX
Ip Sun TC (Korean)

Austin, TX
North Austin TC

Austin, TX
TC/QG with Heloise Gold

Austin, TX
TC Ohana with Stan Rossi

Austin, TX
Tom Gohring's TC

Austin, TX
Tukong MA

Austin, TX
USA KF Acdmy.

Cedar Park, TX
Dave Pickens Central TX
MAs

Corpus Christi, TX
QG Health Solutions

Dallas, TX
Lee's White Leopard
KF/TC

Dallas, TX
SimplyAware TC/KF
Chris Bouguyon

Deer Park, TX
Hassan Z. Saijyid
Judy Covin and Tandy
Robinson

El Paso, TX
Ctr. for Internal Arts

El Paso, TX
Texas TC with Sifu Ray
Abeyta

Fort Worth, TX
Ft. Worth TC with Justin
Harris

Georgetown, TX
TC Chih/TC with Jo
Trautmann

Grapevine/Ft. Worth, TX
Chi-Works

Houston, TX
EastWest Wellness Ctr.

Houston, TX
Medical QG/TC
Michael Powers

Houston, TX
Wu Shu KF Fed., Inc.

Laredo, TX
San Miguel TC/QG

Lake Jackson, TX
Nei Wai Chia MAs KF/TC
Sibok Dan Suchon

Lake Jackson/Houston, TX
Balance in Motion/TC for
Arthritis

League City (Houston), TX
Al Garza's MA America

League City, TX
A Taste of TC with Rick

Lubbock, TX
HealthPoint TC/QG/TCC
Larry Sava

Round Rock, TX
Dave Pickens Central Texas
MAs

San Angelo, TX
TC Concho

San Antonio, TX
Chen TC w/Salvador
DeLaRosa

San Antonio, TX
Yang Chengfu TC Ctrs.
Horacio Lopez

Sealy, TX
Far West Houston
TC/QG/RK/S/M

Waco, TX
Baylor University
Ruby Olar

Wichita Falls, TX
TC/KF Club—Wichita
Falls

Utah

Saint George, UT
Tai Chi Flow, Inc.

Salt Lake City, UT
Dao-Yin TC Study Grp.

Salt Lake City, UT
Dragon Studios TC
Quan/Hatha Yoga

Salt Lake City, UT
TaiChiME4Health/ZUKI
MAs

Salt Lake City, UT
WestWind T'ai Chi

Woods Cross, UT
Blue Dragon Dojo
Esther Van der Meide

Vermont

Burlington, VT
US/JMM and Assc. for
Waving Clouds

Virginia

Arlington, VA
White Birch School KF/TC

Arlington, VA
Skyvalley Tai Ji

Arlington/McLean, VA
Tai Chi
CenterArlington/Northern
VA
Peaceable Dragon

Arlington/Northern VA
Sheng Zhen QG

Charlottesville, VA
Hiromi TC

Chesapeake, VA
Peggy Tabor

Fairfax, VA
Cheng Ming MAs Assn.

Fredericksburg, VA
Highlander Hlth./Fitness
Ctr.

Herndon, VA
Qi Elements School TC/KF

Norfolk, VA
TC/QG Classes

Norfolk/Virginia Beach, VA
Tidewater TC Ctr.

Reston, VA
Walking Your Talk

Richmond, VA
Oriental Medicine
Specialists

Richmond, VA
Pa Kua KF School

Richmond/Southeastern VA
Jack Fuller

Virginia Beach/Newport
News, VA
Jow Ga KF and TC

Virginia Beach/Norfolk, VA
Bending Tree TC Kung

Winchester, VA
A Taste of China
Pat Rice

Winchester, VA
Yang Chengfu TC
Pat Rice

Washington

Anderson Island, WA
TC Chih with Rita Jacobsen

Bellingham, WA
Robert B. Bates

Edmonds, WA
Edmonds TC and QG

Freeland, WA
Island Athletic Club

Oak Harbor, WA
Tai Chi for Health TC/QG

Olympia, WA
PNW School

Port Orchard, WA
Holistic Healing and
Health, Inc.

Port Townsend, WA
Gilman Studio of TC
Chuan

Redmond, WA
Yang Chengfu TC Chuan
Ctr.

Seattle, WA
Chinese Wushu and TC
Acdmy.
Master Yijiao Hong

Seattle, WA
Embrace the Moon TC/QG

Seattle, WA
Ling Gui Int'l. Healing QG

Seattle, WA
QG Longevity Assn.

Seattle, WA
Tiantian School of QG

Seattle, WA
Tse QG Ctr.

Seattle Area, WA
Wu Dang Internal Arts

Seattle, WA
Yang Chengfu TC Chuan
Ctr

Seattle, WA
Yin Yang Arts Ctr.

Seattle, WA
ZY Qigong w/Grandmaster
Xu Mingtang

Spokane, WA
Northwest TC Assn.

Spokane, WA
Northwest TC/QG

Spokane, WA
NW TC Chuan Assn.

Spokane, WA
School of TC Chuan

Vancouver, WA
Mark Moy's KF/TC Acdmy.

Walla Walla, WA
Harmony and Health

Walla Walla, WA
Tien Shan QG with Steve
Smith

Walla Walla, WA
Wen Wu School of TC

Washington, D.C.

Washington, DC
Cloud Hands TC

Washington, DC
Skyvalley Tai Ji

Greater Wash. Area
David Chen Tai Chi

Wash. DC Metro Area
Dancing Mtn.
TCQuan/Taoist Arts

Wash. DC Metro Area
Tai Chi Center

West Virginia

Charles Town, WV
Blue Heron Martial/Healing
Arts

Huntington, WV
Eight-Treasures TC and
QG

Wisconsin

Appleton, WI
QG Life Enhancement Ctr.

Beloit, WI
Great Turtle TC/QG

Brookfield, WI
TC/QG
Master Jia-Jia Xiang,
O.M.D.

Butler, WI
Quest Int'l., Self-Defense

Eau Claire, WI
Healing Choices Massage
TC/QG

Franklin, WI
Innovative Health/Fitness

Franklin, WI
World TC Integrative Arts

Green Bay, WI
Balance from Within

Hudson, WI
Wind and Water QG

Madison, WI
Silver Dragon TC/QG

Madison, WI
TC Ctr.
Tricia Yu

Madison, WI
Yen-nien Daoguan
Don Coleman

Menomonie, WI
YamaMizu Ryui WI School
MA

Milwaukee, WI
Chen Zhonghua TC
Acdmy.—Milwaukee

Milwaukee, WI
Int'l. Inst. Holistic Med.-
TC/QG

Milwaukee, WI
Quest Int'l. Self-Defense

Milwaukee, WI
Shaolin Boxing, KF Inst.

Milwaukee, WI
TC Studies

Milwaukee, WI
White Crane

Milwaukee, WI
YMAA TC Quan of WI

New Berlin, WI
World TC Integrative Arts

Waukesha, WI
Shao Lin Boxing, KF Inst.

Waukesha and Milwaukee,
WI
Enhancing Balance
Patricia Culotti

Wausau, WI
WI Wen Wu School of TC

International Organizations and Schools

Australia

New South Wales

Ballina, NSW
Australian Acdmy. of
TC/QG

Blue Mountains/Bondi,
NSW
Nam Wah Pai QG/TC
Alex Galvan

Bossley Park, NSW
TC Healing Studio
Vera Bartolo

Central Coast, NSW
Australian Acdmy. of
TC/QG

Coffs Harbour, NSW
Sadhana School of Yoga/TC

Fairfield/Liverpool, NSW
Lima Eid

Gosford, NSW
Ray Martin and Heidi Cook

Jannali/Sydney, NSW
St. George College—TC
Arthritis/Diabetes

Lismore, NSW
CHEGS, Inc. TC

Liverpool, NSW
Liverpool TC
John Mills

Miranda, NSW
Australian Clg. of TC/QG
Sam Li and Rachel Addison

Newcastle, NSW
Australian Acdmy. of
TC/QG

Oatley/Sydney, NSW
Oatley RSL TC Arthritis
Jeni Afonso

Sydney, NSW
1 Better Health TC Chuan
2 TC Assn. of Australia

Sydney, NSW
Australian Acdmy. of
TC/QG

Sydney, NSW
Green Dragon TC/QG
Anthony Shing

Sydney, NSW
Sydney TC and QG Ctr.

Sydney, NSW
TC Assn. of Australia

Sydney Wide, NSW
TC Society

Sydney (Central/Southern),
NSW
SHARE—Southern Metro
Region, Inc.

Wollongong, NSW
Australian Acdmy. of
TC/QG

Queensland

Airlie Beach, Queensland
Soul Control

Biggenden, Queensland
TC Biggenden
Anne Buzaglo

Booyal, Queensland
TC with Margaret Smith

Brisbane, Queensland
Australian Acdmy. of
TC/QG

Brisbane, Queensland
Gentle Arts of Self-Defence

Buderim, Queensland
Rolling Waves QG w/Ian
Newton

Gold Coast, Queensland
Australian Acdmy. of
TC/QG

Gold Coast, Queensland
Gold Coast TC Acdmy.

Mackay, Queensland
Suzanne McLauchlan

Qld Ntrl. Therapies Clgs.
Mstr. Linage E. Montaigue

Redlands/Brisbane,
Queensland
Sun TC and Community
Fitness

Visit www.worldtaichiday.org for updated telephone, e-mail, and website information for all the teachers and schools listed in this appendix.

Rockhampton, Queensland
Australian Acdmy. of
TC/QG

Rockhampton, Queensland
TCquan QG Assn.
Lindsay Smith

Toowoomba, Queensland
Australian Acdmy. of
TC/QG

South Australia

Adelaide, SA
Australian Acdmy. of
TC/QG

Adelaide, SA
Moving Meditation/QG

Adelaide, SA
Seacliff TC/QG/Mulan
Quan

Moana, SA
Yueh Fei School of KF/TC

Port Lincoln, SA
TC/QG/TC for Arthritis
Corey Slade

Port Pirie, SA
YMCA, TC for Arthritis
and Diabetes

Tasmania

Hobart, Tasmania
Univ. of Tas. TC Club

Melbourne, Tasmania
TC Australia

Victoria

Bairnsdale/Gippsland/South
Coast, Victoria
TC and QG Acdmy.

Berwick, Victoria
Golden Lion Acdmy.

Melbourne, Victoria
Bayside TC with Jackie Watt

Melbourne, Victoria
Middle Park TC

Melbourne, Victoria
U3A Glen Eira, Inc.

Melbourne/Box Hill,
Victoria
Melbourne Push Hands
Club

Montrose, Victoria
TC for Health with Elaine D.

Moreland, Victoria
Moreland Cmty. Health Svc.

Morwell, Victoria
The TC Ctr. with Julie
Lucas

Morwell, Victoria
TC for Advanced Students
Stephen Lucas

Wattle Glen, Victoria
Cheng Ming-Miriam and
Neil Rosewarne

Western Australia

Perth, Western Australia
Australian Acdmy. of
TC/QG

Canada

Alberta

Calgary, Alberta
Paul Gandy

Edmonton, Alberta
Abundant Peace Aikido/TC

Fort McMurray, Alberta
Fort McMurray Study Grp.
TC/QG

British Columbia

Delta, BC
Riverbank TC

Fort St. John, BC
Rising TC Club

Kelowna, BC
Dancing Dragon School
TC/QG

Kelowna, BC
Crouching Tiger Yang
TC/QG

Kelowna, BC
Yang TC Chuan Club

Nelson, BC
Kootenay TC Ctr.

Parksville, BC
Easy TC

Salt Spring Island, BC
IQ-Balance

Salt Spring Island, BC
Seven Stars TC Club

Terrace, BC
Terrace TC Chuan

Vancouver, BC
Anthony Lee-Hem

Vancouver, BC
Wu's TC Chuan Acdmy.—
Van.

Manitoba

Winnipeg, Manitoba
The Arthritis Society

New Brunswick

Fredericton, NB
Wu's TC Chuan Acdmy.—
Fredericton

Miramichi City, NB
Miramichi TC and Aikido

Nova Scotia

Dartmouth, NS
TaiChiForArthritis (HRM)

Ontario

Barrie, Ontario
Flowing Rivers TC

Blenheim, Ontario
Harmony TC

Blyth, Ontario
Blyth TC Club

Brantford, Ontario
Yellow River TC School

Conestoga, Ontario
Eby Studio

Dundas, Ontario
TC Inst.
Reginald Duff Doel

Guelph, Ontario
Green Dragon QG/TC

Hamilton, Ontario
Innergy (TC)

Kitchener, Ontario
Atado TC School

Kitchener, Ontario
Cold Mtn. Internal Arts

London, Ontario
Phoenix TC Ctr.
Gloria Jenner

London, Ontario
Stephanie Hill

Madoc, Ontario
Greg Magwood TC

Mississauga, Ontario
TC and QG/TC Alumni

Muskoka, Ontario
Temple Knights Holistic
MA

Oakville, Ontario
TC/QG with Jill Heath

Ottawa, Ontario
World Institute for Self-
Hlg., Inc.

Peterborough, Ontario
Class Connections
Greg Magwood

Peterborough, Ontario
Peterborough TC Assn.

Toronto, Ontario
Chow QG Scarborough
East

Toronto, Ontario
Chow QG Etobicoke

Toronto, Ontario
Chow QG Toronto

Toronto, Ontario
Golden Pheasant TC and
Wellness

Toronto, Ontario
High Park MA Acdmy.

Toronto, Ontario
Int'l. Inst. with Zhi Neng

Toronto, Ontario
Mo's Society of TC

Toronto, Ontario
Nine Dragon Arts—
Baguazhang QG

Toronto, Ontario
North Star TC
Gordon Ainsley

Toronto, Ontario
Rising Sun School of TC

Toronto, Ontario
Sha Kin Practical Arts

Toronto, Ontario
Softworks TC

Toronto, Ontario
Temple Knights Holistic
MA

Toronto, Ontario
TC and Meditation Ctr.

Toronto, Ontario
TC Ch'uan Study Group

Toronto, Ontario
Wu's TC Chuan Acdmy.—
Toronto

Quebec

Montreal, Quebec
Dorothy Ramien

Montreal, Quebec
TCquan, École Gilles
Thibault

Salaberry de Valleyfield,
Quebec
La Voie du TC Chuan and
QG
Gilles D'Anjou

Sherbrooke, Quebec
Univ. of Sherbrooke
Raymond C. Benoit

Yukon Territory

Whitehorse, Yukon
Territory
TC Yukon

New Zealand

Auckland, NZ
Chen Style TaiChicise

Auckland, NZ
Sing Ong TC

Auckland, NZ
Wu Jao Acdmy.

Auckland, NZ
Wushu Culture Assn.

Auckland, NZ
Yang Style TC Chuan

Christchurch, NZ
Chen Style TaiChicise

Christchurch, NZ
Phoenix TC

Christchurch, NZ
Red Dragon TC

Christchurch, NZ
Shyng-Jian Tradt'l. Yang
TC

Greymouth, NZ
Internal KF

Hawke's Bay, NZ
QG Jleaf

Kapiti Coast, NZ
Belinda Hadfield

Takaka, NZ
TCA with Ann Marshall

Tauranga, NZ
TC with Rob McDonald

Wellington, NZ
Neale Svenson

Wellington, NZ
Wellington School of TC
Chuan

Wellington, NZ
Wu Tao Acdmy.
TC/QG/KF

Wellington, NZ
Yuan Tze Human Life
Science

South Africa

World TC Boxing Assn., SA
Morné Swanepoel

Cape Town, SA
European Assn. for Trad'l.
Wu TC
Robert Rudniak

Cape Town, SA
Shaolin with Leslie James
Reed

Cape Town (HQ), SA
U.S./U.K. Int'l. TC/Shaolin
Wushu

Durban, SA
TC Institute of Health

Johannesburg, SA
Int'l. Arts Resrch. Ctr. of SA

Johannesburg, SA
Living Tao S.A.

Johannesburg, SA
Shaolin MA Ctr.

United Kingdom

Note: All U.K. listings are
alphabetical by city, regard-
less of region. Therefore,
Scotland, Northern Ireland,
Wales, and similar listings
are found by city.

TC Quan and QG Fed. for
Europe—UK Hdqrtrs.
secretary@taichiunion.com

UK
Dr. Paul Lam TC for
Health

Practical TC Chuan

Altrincham, Cheshire
Zhong Ding Assn.
Colin Hoddes

Anglesey
Health Through TC/QG
Philip Mansfield

Ashburton/Newton Abbot,
Devon
Rainbow TC/QG School

Ashford, Kent
Wu Gong Academy
Barry Phelan

Barry/Cardiff/Cowbridge
Rising Phoenix TC and QG

Bedford Area, Bedfordshire
Greenfield TC

Bedford, Bedfordshire
Bicama TC/QG

Belfast, Northern Ireland
Making Moves TC
Petesy Burns

Belfast, Northern Ireland
Zhi-Ruo School of TC
Chuan

Belfast, Northern Ireland
Zhu Chang Hai Int'l.
Wushu Assn.

Belmont, Durham
Mei Shan TCQuan

Berkshire
Berkshire TC

Birmingham
Kai Ming Assn.
Mark Peters

Birmingham
Zhong Ding Assn.
Robert Wesley

Birmingham/Solihull, West
Midlands
Tai Chi for Health

Blackpool, Lancs
Everyday TC
Rosie Harrison

Bradford, Yorkshire
Lamas QG Assn.—Sf.
Wharton.

Bridgend
Swimming Dragon-Sun TC
Quan

Brighton, East Sussex
Brighton Yang
Richard Vahrman

Brighton, East Sussex
Tao Arts Tai Chi

Brighton
Wutan Int'l.
Eddie Turner

Brighton, East Sussex
Wuxing Wushu Xie Hui.

Bristol, Avon
The Bristol School of TC

Bristol
Bristol TC

Bristol, No County
QG Southwest

Broadstairs, Kent
TC QG 4 Healthy Lifestyle

Broomsgrove
Infinite TC with Jason
Chan

Bury, Manchester
British Chen Style TC
College

Cambridge
Cambridge Univ. TC
Chuan Soc.

Cambridge, Cambs
Grey Heron Internal Arts

Canterbury, Kent
Wu Gong Academy
Barry Phelan

Cheam, Surrey
The Chi Clinic

Chelmsford, Essex
Art of Energetics

Chesterfield, Derbyshire
Lamas QG Assn./Sifu Box

Cleckheaton, Yorkshire
Lee Family Arts (LFA)

Cleveleys, Lancashire
Zhong Ding Assn.
Joan Carlsson

Colchester, Essex
Art of Energetics

Colchester
Taoist TC Society—GB
Hdqtrs.

Cork
Infinite TC with Jason
Chan

Cornwall
St. Ives TC

Covent Garden, London
Rose Li School

Crouch End, London N8
European Assn. for Trad'l.
Wu Tai

Croydon, Surrey
Heaven Mountain
Paul Brewer

Deal, Kent
Red Dragon Retreats

Derby, Derbyshire
TC and Relaxation

Derby, Derbyshire
TC for Health/Carroll

Doncaster, South Yorkshire
LAMAS QG with Sifu
Jacquie Sham

Dublin
Infinite TC with Jason
Chan

Easingwold, North
Yorkshire
Vale of York—Sikung Box

Edinburch
Infinite TC with Jason
Chan

Edinburgh, Scotland
Wu Tao Kwoon
KF/Gennaro Ripa

Edinburgh, Scotland
Wutan TC Chuan
James Connachan

Epping, Essex
Art of Energetics

Epsom, Surrey
Heaven Mountain
Paul Brewer

Falkirk/Callander, Central
Scotland
Rising Moon TC

Farnborough, Hampshire
Five Elements

Fife, Scotland
Golden Gate TC

Folkestone, Kent
Art of Energetics

Forest of Dean,
Gloucestershire
Crystal TC

Forres/Moray, Scotland
White Crane TC Quan

Glossop, Derbyshire
Highpeak TC

Great Yarmouth, Norfolk
TC-QG Health Ctr.
Colin and Mitzi Orr

Harlow, Essex
Art of Energetics

Harrow, Middlesex
Zhong Ding Assn.
Adam Lammiman

Hebden Bridge, West
Yorkshire
Zhong Ding Assn.
Anne Whitehead

Hemel Hempstead, Essex
Art of Energetics

Hitchin, Hertfordshire
North Herts Internal Arts

Huddersfield, West
Yorkshire
Zhong Ding Assn.
Craig Jackson

Hull, Beverley, Bridlington
East-West Taoist Assn.
Howard and Gisela Gibbon

Hyde, Cheshire
School of TC Quan

Ipswich, Suffolk
Art of Energetics

Ivybridge, Devon
Zhong Ding Assn.
Richard Hopper

Jersey CI
East-West Taoist Assn.

Jersey, English Channel
Islands
Four Winds TC/QG
Master Freda Ruderham

Kingsteignton/Exeter,
Devon
Zhong Ding Assn.
Mike Bearne

Kingston, Surrey
Heaven Mountain
Paul Brewer

Kingston Upon Hull, KUH
Hull KF

Knebworth, Hertfordshire
North Herts Internal Arts

Leeds and York, North
Yorkshire
UKTC Five Winds School
of TC Chuan

Letchworth, Hertfordshire
Art of Energetics

Letchworth, Hertfordshire
North Herts Internal Arts

Leven, Leven
Leven TC

Lg. Eaton, Nottinghmshr.
White Cloud TC

London
Chi Moves

London
Chinese Heritage Inst.

London
Chiworks

London
GreenTC/Oriental Healing
Arts

London
Infinite TC with Jason
Chan

London
London School of
TC/Trad'l. Health

London
Lydia Wong

London
Nothing Special TC
Michael Metelits

London
Psi TC

London
Practical TC Int'l.

London
Sifu Lobo

London
TC UK

London
Templeton House Studio

London
Wu's TC Acdmy.
Don Spargo

London
Zhong Ding Assn.
Anthony Ulatowski

London
Zhong Ding Assn.
Brian Woodruff

London, Central
TC Kung

London, Croydon
Dynamic TC Assn.

London, London
Tse QG Ctr.

London, London
Tai Chi UK

London, London
School of Internal Arts

London, Surrey
The Chi Clinic

London/Bath
Yongquan TC Chuan

London/Brighton, East
Sussex
Gentle River TC

London/SW England
The Chin Woo Assn.

London/SW England
Three Treasures Trdt'l. MA
Assn.

London/SW England
Wu Style Hao Family TC
Assn.

London and Other
Locations
Tung Ying Jie TC Legacy
Gordon Joly

Long Ditton
Jean Anderson, TC Teacher

Loughborough,
Leicestershire
Jade Moon TCC
Stefan Esposito

Luton, Bedfordshire
Art of Energetics

Maidstone, Kent
Wu Gong Academy
Barry Phelan

Maldon, Essex
Art of Energetics

Manchester
Infinite TC
Jason Chan

Manchester
Tse QG Ctr.

Manchester, Lancashire
Zhong Ding Assn.
John Higginson

Mansfield, Nottinghamshire
LAMAS QG with Master
Edwards

Mansfield, Nottinghamshire
Zhong Ding Assn.
Darren Roberts

Margate, Kent
Wu Gong Academy
Barry Phelan

Midhurst, West Sussex
Five Elements

Milton Keynes
The Open University TC
Club

Newcastle, England
School of Internal Arts

Newcastle, Tyne and Wear
Dynamic Balancing TC

Newcastle Upon Tyne
School of Internal Arts

Newport/Penarth
Rising Phoenix TC and QG

No City, Devon
QG Southwest

North Dorset
COREhealth TC and QG

North Warwickshire
Midlands TC
Sifu G. Higham

Norwich
Norwich Tse TC and QG
Club

Norwich, Norfolk
Eastern Wave School/TC
Chuan

Norwich, Norfolk
Martyn Guest TC

Norwich, Norfolk
Taoist TC and KF

Norwich, UK and Int'l
Wellspring TC Ch'uan

Nottingham,
Nottinghamshire
Zhong Ding Assn.
Mike Roberts

Paddock Wood, Kent
Wu Gong Academy
Barry Phelan

Penicuik, Milothian,
Scotland
Wutan TC with James
Connachan

Plymouth, Devon
Zhong Ding Assn.
Roy Lancey

Pwllheli/Tremadog/Asersoch
Zhong Ding Assn.
Terry Higgins

Rainworth,
Nottinghamshire
Zhong Ding Assn.
Don Harradine

Ranby, Nottinghamshire
Lamas QG Assn.
Sifu Bailey

Redbridge, London
Art of Energetics

Reigate, Surrey
Heaven Mountain
Paul Brewer

Retford, Nottinghamshire
Lamas Qigong of America,
Inc.

Richmond, Surrey
Gentle River TC
Chris Long

Ruislip, Middlesex
Zhong Ding Assn.
David Spencer

Rye and Hastings, East
Sussex
XinSheng TC and QG with
Stuart

St. Albans, Hertfordshire
Art of Energetics

St. Albans, Hertfordshire
The School of TC Chuan

Scarborough, North
Yorkshire
East-West Taoist Assn.
Howard and Gisela Gibbon

Shrewsbury and Area,
Shropshire
LifeStyle TC and QG

Skelton, Stokesley, Redcar
East-West Taoist Assn.
Howard and Gisela Gibbon

Sothend-on-Sea, Essex
Art of Energetics

South Down, Northern
Ireland
Making Moves TC
Petesy Burns

South Somerset
COREhealth TC and QG

Stevenage, Hertfordshire
Art of Energetics

Stockport, Cheshire/
Manchester
Age Conern Stockport TC
for Health

Stockport, Greater
Manchester
Zhong Ding Assn.
Ben Jones

Stratford, London
Art of Energetics

Sunderland
East-West Taoist Assn.
Howard and Gisela Gibbon

Sutton, Nottinghamshire
Zhong Ding Assn.
Junior Mead

Swaffham, Norfolk
Acdmy. of Oriental Arts

Swansea, W. Glamorgan
Chanquanshu TC Quan
with Mike

Swindon, Wilts
Graham Pritchard &
Catherine Downes

Torquay, Devon
Wu Style Hao Family TC
Quan

Torquay, Devon
Zhong Ding Assn.
June Cole

Torquay, Devon
Zhong Ding Assn.
Peter Chapman

Town Bedworth, NR
Nuneaton Warwickshire,
Exhall TC Class

Uckfield, East Sussex
Zhong Ding Assn.
Lynn Gordon

Ulverston, Cumbria
Wayfinders TC Quan

Upminster, London
Art of Energetics

Welwyn Garden City,
Hertfordshire
Art of Energetics

West London
The Acdmy. of Eastern Arts
TC/QG

West Lothian
Bo'ness TCA
Robert Breslin

West Midlands, Solihull
Esther Gaynor, TC Teacher

Witham, Essex
Art of Energetics

Witney, Oxfordshire
Witney Wing Chun
01993-209377 or 07905-
628399

Worksop, Nottinghamshire
Lamas QG Assn.
Sifu Walker

Worthing, West Sussex
Zhong Ding Assn.

Yealmpton/Aveton Gifford,
Devon
Zhong Ding Assn.
Derek Bates

sit *www.worldtaichiday.org* for updated telephone, e-mail, and website information for all the teachers and schools listed in this appendix.

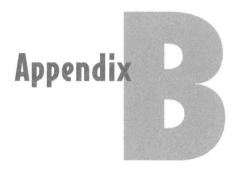

Suggested Readings

Bach, Richard. *Jonathan Livingston Seagull*. New York: The Macmillan Company, 1970.

Badgley, Laurence, M.D. *Healing AIDS Naturally*. Foster City, CA: Human Energy Press, 1987.

Batmanghelidj, F., M.D. *The Body's Many Cries for Water*. Falls Church, VA: Global Health Solutions, Inc., 1997.

Behr, Thomas E., Ph.D. *The Tao of Sales*. Rockport, MA: Element Books, Inc., 1997.

Benson, Herbert, M.D. *The Relaxation Response*. New York: Avon Books, 1975.

Booth, Jennifer. *Wind Blowing Lotus Leaf: The Way of Enlightened Action*. Huntington Beach, CA: Warrior of Light Publications, 1999.

Borysenko, Joan, Ph.D., and Miroslav Borysenko, Ph.D. *The Power of the Mind to Heal*. Carlsbad, CA: Hay House, Inc., 1994.

Capra, Fritjof (author of *The Tao of Physics*). *The Web of Life*. New York: Doubleday, 1996.

Chen Pan Ling. *Chen Pan Ling's Original Tai Chi Chuan Textbook*. New Orleans: Blitz! Design, 1998.

Chopra, Deepak. *Ageless Body, Timeless Mind*. New York: Harmony Books, 1993.

Cohen, Kenneth S. *The Way of Qigong: The Art and Science of Chinese Energy Healing*. New York: Ballantine Books, 1997.

Diller, Lawrence H., M.D. *Running on Ritalin: A Physician Reflects on Children, Society, and Performance in a Pill*. New York: Bantam Books, 1998.

Gerber, Richard, M.D. *Vibrational Medicine*. Santa Fe, NM: Bear and Company, 1988.

Greene, Brian. *The Elegant Universe: Superstrings, Hidden Dimensions, and the Quest for the Ultimate Theory.* New York, London: W.W. Norton and Company, 1999.

Lasorso, Vincent J. Jr. *Immortal's Gift: A Parable for the Soul.* Cincinnati, OH: White Willow School of Tai Chi, 2000.

Lee, Martin, Ph.D., with Melinda Emily and Joyce Lee. *The Healing Art of T'ai Chi.* New York: Sterling Publishing Co. Inc., 1996.

Leight, Michelle Dominique. *The New Beauty: East-West Teachings in the Beauty of Body and Soul.* New York: Kodansha America Inc., 1995.

Lipton, Bruce, Ph.D. *Biology of Belief.* Santa Rosa, CA: Mountain of Love/Elite Books, 2005.

Loupos, John. *Inside Tai Chi: Contemporary Views on an Ancient Art.* Roslindale, MA: YMAA Pub. Center, 2002.

Luk, Charles. *Taoist Yoga, Alchemy and Immortality.* York Beach, ME: Samuel Weisner, Inc., 1973.

Mann, Felix, M.B., L.M.C.C. *Acupuncture: The Ancient Chinese Art of Healing.* New York: Random House, 1978.

Mayer, Michael. *Secrets to Living Younger Longer: The Self Healing Path of Qigong, Standing Meditation and Tai Chi.* Orinda, CA: Bodymind Healing Pub., 2004.

McGaa, Ed (Eagle Man). *Mother Earth Spirituality—Native American Paths to Healing Ourselves and Our World.* San Francisco: Harper, 1990.

Moyers, Bill. *Healing and the Mind.* New York: Doubleday, 1993.

Rothstein, Larry, Ed.D., Lyle H. Miller, Ph.D., and Alma Dell Smith, Ph.D. *The Stress Solution.* New York: Pocket Books, 1993.

Sandifer, Jon. *Acupressure for Health, Vitality and First Aid.* Rockport, MA: Element Books Limited, 1997.

Sang, Larry. *The Principles of Feng Shui.* Monterey Park, CA: The American Feng Shui Institute, 1994.

Shanor, Karen Nesbitt, Ph.D. *The Emerging Mind: New Research into the Meaning of Consciousness, Based on the Smithsonian Institution Lecture Series.* Los Angeles: Renaissance Books, 1999.

Sheldrake, Rupert. *A New Science of Life: Morphic Resonance.* Rochester, VT: Park Street Press, 1995.

Star, Jonathan, trans. *Rumi: In the Arms of the Beloved.* New York: Jeremy P. Tarcher/Putnam, 1997.

Talbot, Michael. *The Holographic Universe.* New York: HarperCollins Publishers, Inc., 1991.

Watts, Alan. *The Way of Zen.* New York: Vintage Books, 1985.

Weil, Andrew, M.D. *Healthy Aging: A Lifelong Guide to Your Physical and Spiritual Well-Being.* New York: Rodale, Inc., 2005

———. *Spontaneous Healing.* New York: Ballantine Books, 1995.

Williams, Tom, Ph.D. *The Complete Illustrated Guide to Chinese Medicine.* Rockport, MA: Element Books, Inc., 1996.

Yang, Dr. Jwing-Ming. *Taijiquan, Classical Yang Style: The Complete Form and Qigong.* Roslindale, MA: YMAA Pub. Center 1999.

Yu-Cheng Huang. *Change the Picture.* Skokie, IL: Yu-Cheng Huang, 1998.

Yutang, Lin. *The Wisdom of Laotse.* New York: The Modern Library, 1948.

My Four-Hour Fully Instructional DVD Program, Plus ...

You've seen this book's valuable 1½-hour DVD, which contains many carefully selected useful excerpts from my world-acclaimed 4-hour *fully instructional* DVD (described later in this appendix) and from the nearly 80-minute *Mulan T'ai Chi* fully instructional video/DVD. However, because of time constraints, we couldn't fit all the great video on the book's DVD. The *full 4-hour program* and the *Mulan* DVD expand on the excerpts on the book's DVD with hours of instruction that's the closest thing to *private classes in the comfort of your own home.* As users have testified (see the following section), *my goal is to maximize your benefit from my acclaimed program.*

Sage Sifu Says

If questions arise as you view and enjoy my videos or DVDs, I accept and answer personal e-mail or phone queries from purchasers of the 4-hour DVD program.

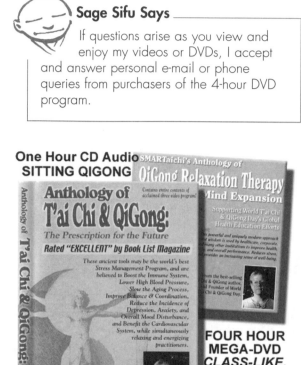

My entire 4-hour DVD program, *Anthology of T'ai Chi and QiGong: The Prescription for the Future*, gives a detailed breakdown of all 64 movements of the Long Form (see Chapter 15) through *lessons* accompanied by many *practice sessions* and *QiGong breathing instruction*. These richly explain how to perform each of the 64 movements shown on this book's DVD's *exhibition* of the forms (also described in Chapter 15). Therefore, the full 4-hour *real-time classlike instructional* provides details and tips to make the learning process not only fun and profoundly user-friendly, but also *a deeply relaxing experience, as the lessons are taught like relaxation therapies.*

Adding my 4-hour DVD to the resources you've already gained by using this book provides you with a profoundly high-level T'ai Chi and QiGong program, which brings my easygoing, personable instruction directly into the comfort of your own home. According to user reviews, this program has profoundly helped people worldwide with stress, anxiety, depression, pain reduction, mobility improvement, rehabilitation, creativity, and many other aspects of health improvement and life expansion.

The excerpts provided on this book's DVD insert greatly enhance its instructional value, but they also give you a feel for the high quality of *deeply detailed instruction* my full *4-hour* DVD program offers, which goes much further than this book's insert T'ai Chi forms exhibition. When you complete the 4-hour instructional, coupled with this book's resources, you will have a profound T'ai Chi and QiGong regimen that will last a lifetime and benefit you in *more ways than you can imagine.*

This appendix also provides details on instructional videos for the *Mulan Short Form* (see Chapter 16) and several Sitting QiGong audio therapies, in addition to the one described in Chapter 11. Excerpts from the *Mulan T'ai Chi* DVD/video are also included on this book's DVD. The *fully instructional 80 minute* Mulan T'ai Chi DVD/video offered here breaks down the *Mulan Form Exhibition* on this book's DVD into richly detailed instructional lessons and practice sessions.

To order this powerful program and other of my video, audio, and life-enhancement SMARTaichi products, see the end of the appendix.

Reviews of My T'ai Chi Instructional Program

"... I was skeptical to watch Bill's video ... since many of the videos I watched before were always 'over my head,' ... with no consideration for the simple needs of the student. ... *Bill Douglas's video was completely different!* ... I was able to grasp very easily what he was talking about. ... He goes through the practice in 'real time' so you get a full workout, not just the mini version, making it comfortable, effortless, and easy.

"I look forward to my practice and feeling like I'm doing it with a 'friend.' All in all, I get the feeling that Bill really wants people to get T'ai Chi and QiGong, rather than just *make a buck.* I highly recommend him and his instruction to everyone."

—*Linda Lyon, California*

"[I was] living with an extremely unhealthy lifestyle ... taking numerous medications for arthritis, depression, and pain. ... I ordered [Bill's videos]. ... [N]ow I am off most of my medications. People keep telling me I look 'different' [and] happy. Well, I am happy and I feel great! Thank you! Thank you! Thank you!"

—*Dave Long, Washington*

"[I was] suffering for years from chronic neck pain consequent to a whiplash injury ... and limited motion of the right shoulder. ... [Bill's T'ai Chi course] was initiated after unsuccessful sessions of various therapies. After two months of T'ai Chi, the pain in my cervical region disappeared while the range of motion of my right shoulder returned completely to normal."

—*Loredana Brizio-Molteni, M.D., F.A.C.S.*

DVD and Video Resources

Anthology of T'ai Chi and QiGong: The Prescription for the Future: My acclaimed 4-hour DVD (and VHS) program was rated "Excellent" by *Book List Magazine.* Having 4 hours *all on one DVD* is very convenient and allows you to go right to the lesson of the day. Brief excerpts of this video are contained on this book's DVD. You'll benefit from this complete instructional program for years and years.

Mulan Style Video: This VHS (soon to be DVD as well) video beautifully teaches in 17 detailed lessons the nuances of the *Mulan Basic Short Form* introduced in Chapter 16 and *exhibited* on this book's DVD. The *fully instructional* video is nearly 80 minutes long and breaks down the exhibition you see on this book's DVD into easy-to-follow lessons and a final practice session in a lovely park setting.

Audio Resources

Sitting QiGong is a powerful addition to any T'ai Chi or Moving QiGong practice. The resources here are a great place to start and have received rave reviews from users worldwide. Also, the *Children's QiGong* audio cassette is a fun filled way for young children (and their parents) to explore the inner world of health and relaxation.

CD

Anthology of QiGong Relaxation Therapy and Mind Expansion is a 72-minute, 4-track CD that offers three Sitting QiGong programs and an added introductory exercise at a great savings. It includes the exercises from *QiGong: Relaxation Therapy, QiGong: Expanding Awareness,* and *QiGong: An Earth Cleansing.*

Audio Cassettes

QiGong: Relaxation Therapy is a highly effective introduction to basic Sitting QiGong, or relaxation therapy, and this program has been used in major corporations and health network programs. (This exercise is included on the fully instructional DVD or VHS program *Anthology of T'ai Chi and QiGong*.)

QiGong: Expanding Awareness takes the basic relaxation therapy to an entirely different level, giving the user a way to cleanse and clear his or her entire field of awareness of the daily loads of stress and anxiety.

QiGong: An Earth Cleansing is what I call "The Meditation Tape for Those Who Can't Meditate!" It combines very tactile muscle tension and breath techniques to enable both mind and body to release their grip on the rat race and to find that calm center, *no matter how intense life is.*

QiGong: For Children's Health and Relaxation is a fanciful journey of awareness that teaches children (and teachers/parents) breathing techniques to manage stress while enjoying a fanciful flying adventure of the mind.

Instructors or retailers are offered wholesale discounts when ordering five or more of any product item. Call 913-648-2256.

Where to Find My Instructional Programs

You can order these instructional programs at Amazon.com; or find them in many Wild Oats health food markets; *or get them directly from me at my online store* where you'll find many life-enhancement, and lifestyle, products beyond T'ai Chi and QiGong resources at my website, www.smartaichi.com; or order by phone (Visa and MasterCard are accepted) or mail. The programs are also available in other select retail stores in the United States. (Ask your local DVD retailers if they carry them.)

In Australia/New Zealand, my DVDs are available from all leading online and retail DVD suppliers. In the United Kingdom/Europe, my DVDs are available from all leading online and retail DVD suppliers and from www.qleap.co.uk.

To order by phone, call 1-913-648-2256 or 1-877-482-4241 (toll-free in the United States). To order by mail, complete the following form and send it together with your check or money order to:

SMARTaichi
PO Box 7786
Shawnee Mission, KS 66207-0786

To order online, visit: www.SMARTaichi.com.

Allow 2 to 3 weeks for delivery, although orders usually arrive much more quickly.

Deliver to:

Name: _____

Address: _____

City/State/Zip: _____

Phone number (with area code): _____

E-mail: _____

Item	Quantity	Unit Price	Total
DVDs			
T'ai Chi and QiGong: The Prescription for the Future Series (4 hours)	_____	$69.88	_____
Mulan Style Video (approximately 80 minutes)	_____	$27.95	_____
Videos (VHS)			
T'ai Chi and QiGong: The Prescription for the Future Series (3-video set)	_____	$69.88	_____
Mulan Style Video (80 minutes)	_____	$27.95	_____
Audio Compact Disc			
Anthology of QiGong: Relaxation Therapy and Mind Expansion (contains all the exercises on the first three audio cassettes listed below)	_____	$19.88	_____
Audio Tapes			
QiGong: Relaxation Therapy	_____	$12.00	_____
QiGong: Expanding Awareness	_____	$12.00	_____
QiGong: An Earth Cleansing	_____	$12.00	_____
QiGong: For Children's Health and Relaxation	_____	$12.00	_____
Add $4.50 for the first item and $1.50 for each additional.		Shipping	_____
(Kansas residents add 7 percent sales tax.)		Tax	_____
		Total	_____

Send completed above form and make check payable to:

SMARTaichi
PO Box 7786
Shawnee Mission, KS 66207-0786

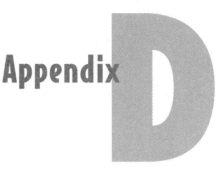

Glossary

abdominal breathing The QiGong breathing technique, whereby the abdominal area, or lower lungs, fills first and then the upper chest fills, fully inflating the lungs. On the exhale, the upper chest relaxes inward as the lungs deflate, followed by the abdominal muscles relaxing inward, allowing the lower lungs to deflate and fully expending the air from the lungs.

acupressure A massage technique of stimulating the acupuncture points without the use of acupuncture needles.

acupuncture A medical science that manipulates the flow of Qi, or life energy, through the body to maximize the body's health systems.

acupuncture maps Diagrams or models to help acupuncturists locate the acupuncture points on the body.

aura The sometimes visible aspect of life energy, whether seen with Kirlian photography or with the naked eye.

biofeedback A computer program often used to train people to relax under stress by showing their blood pressure, heart rate, and so on, while the participant uses relaxation techniques to normalize those indicators.

Bone Marrow Cleansing A Moving QiGong exercise designed to cleanse the bone marrow of stress that might inhibit the immune system.

Carry the Moon A Moving QiGong exercise designed to help the spine stay supple, support kidney function, and promote flexibility throughout the frame.

center The physical, mental, emotional, and spiritual clarity T'ai Chi and QiGong are designed to cultivate. Modern psychologists call this homeostasis.

Chen style   An ancient T'ai Chi style and the basis of the Yang style.

Chinese Drum, The   A QiGong warm-up for T'ai Chi preparation.

Chinese Medica   The bible of Traditional Chinese Medicine (TCM), encompassing all known knowledge on acupuncture, herbal medicine, and QiGong.

crisis   The Chinese character for *crisis* is made of two characters, the character for *danger* plus the one for *opportunity*.

dan tien   The physical energy center of the body, located approximately 1½ to 3 inches below the navel, near the center of the body.

DHEA (dehydroepiandrosterone) Adequate dehydroepiandrosterone levels are related to youthfulness and a more functional immune system. QiGong practice is believed to elevate DHEA levels.

Dong Gong   *See* Moving QiGong.

energy meridians   In Chinese, *jing luo*, or channel network. Modern acupuncturists may refer to these meridians as "bioenergetic circuits." These are the paths that Qi moves through to circulate within the body, although they are not physical vessels like veins or arteries. They are energy channels where energy appears to flow more easily through the body's tissue. There are 14 main meridians, and 12 of those are directly associated with bodily organs, such as the heart and liver.

External QiGong   A TCM practice whereby the provider allows his or her Qi, cultivated through internal QiGong practice, to flow, usually from the hands, out into the patient to help the healing process.

fan lao huan tong   In Chinese, this means "reverse old age and return to youthfulness." This is the goal of T'ai Chi and QiGong.

Feng Shui   The Chinese design art for creating flow and balance of energy within homes and other structures.

fight or flight response   The body's reflex response to stress that involves elevated blood pressure, increased heart rate, and feelings of subdued panic.

free radicals   Atoms with an extra electron, believed to contribute to the aging process. Regular T'ai Chi practice may reduce the cell damage these free radicals cause.

Grand Terminus   The yin-yang symbol, and also the final movement of the Kuang Ping Yang style of T'ai Chi.

holistic   Chinese philosophy that sees the entire universe within each individual part, in much the same way the body's building blocks of DNA coding are contained within each individual cell in the body.

homeostasis   Modern therapists use this term to describe a chemical, emotional, and mental sense of health and well-being. This is what T'ai Chi is designed to promote.

horary clock   TCM's understanding of the ebb and flow of life energy patterns within the body. This understanding is used to treat various conditions using acupuncture, herbal, or QiGong therapy for optimum results.

Horse Stance   The basic stance for T'ai Chi, QiGong, and most martial arts.

hypertension   High blood pressure caused most often by unmanaged stress. High blood pressure is the cause of most heart disease.

I Ching   Also known as *The Book of Changes*, the *I Ching* is an ancient Chinese book of divination. The book is used to tell fortunes or to inspire people to look more deeply into themselves and their lives before making life decisions.

Jing Gong   *See* Sitting QiGong.

Kirlian photography   A photography method that appears to capture images of Qi or life energy.

Kuang Ping Yang style   The 64-movement long form of T'ai Chi brought to the West by master Kuo Lien Ying.

Lao-Tzu The founder of Taoist philosophy.

master One who cultivates a clarity in life, enabling her to be a nurturing force to herself and the world.

Moving QiGong Moving exercises, such as T'ai Chi, that stimulate the flow of Qi through the body.

Mulan Quan Style A relatively modern form, rooted in a more ancient style. This may be the most elegant form of T'ai Chi, incorporating both dance and martial arts forms.

postbirth breathing Normal abdominal T'ai Chi breathing.

prebirth breathing A form of breathing that requires the abdominal muscles to draw in on an in-breath and relax out on an exhale.

psychoneuroimmunology The modern science of studying how the mind's attitudes and beliefs affect physical health.

Push Hands A sparring tool and/or a subtle tool for self-awareness, whereby two partners (or opponents) engage in a dancelike exchange, becoming aware of one another's posture and balance. This can be carried to an extreme of pushing the opponent down when he is vulnerable, or merely becoming gently conscious of when he is vulnerable without actually pushing him down.

Qi Life energy. The Chinese character for *Qi* is also the character for air, as in breath.

QiGong "Breath work" or "energy exercise." There are about 7,000 QiGong exercises in the Chinese Medica (the bible of Chinese medicine).

Sensei A teacher; a term of respect often used in martial arts circles.

Sifu Chinese for "one who has mastered an art." This term applies not only to martial arts: a master chef or artist might be a Sifu as well.

sinking Qi Settling the weight of the body into the leg you are shifting onto.

Sitting QiGong Meditative exercises to promote the flow of Qi throughout the body.

Soong Yi-Dien "Loosen up"; also a T'ai Chi instruction to loosen the body, mind, and heart, encouraging the student to be more flexible and adaptable to all changes.

spirit The Latin root of *spirit* is *spir*, "to breathe," similar to the Chinese Qi, or life energy, expressed by the same word as *air*.

stress In TCM, the result of unmanaged stress is blocked energy and is the source of most physical, mental, emotional, and social problems.

T'ai Chi A moving form of QiGong. Most Moving QiGong forms have only a few simple movements and lack the continuous flow of the many multiple movements that T'ai Chi forms weave together.

T'ai Chi Ch'uan "Supreme ultimate fist" or highest martial art.

Taoism An ancient Chinese philosophy of life that holds that the Tao, the way of life, or the invisible force of nature's laws, can be accessed in states of alert calm. Regular immersion in the effortless power of life energy (through QiGong meditation) is believed to access the Tao for our lives, leading us to the most effortless and meaningful way to live.

Taoist Canon An ancient book that held all the early writing on QiGong, although at that time QiGong was called Tao-yin.

Taoist philosophy Often thought of as T'ai Chi philosophy because the subtle awareness of self and life energy is so directly applicable to Taoism's goal of getting in touch with the Tao's natural laws and quiet power.

Tao-yin "Leading or guiding the energy"; another ancient name for QiGong.

T-cells Cells that are believed to support the immune system by consuming viruses, bacteria, and even tumor cells. T'ai Chi practice is believed to boost the body's production of T-cells.

To gu na xin "Expelling the old energy, absorbing the new"; which was another name for QiGong used in the past.

Traditional Chinese Medicine (TCM) The Chinese health sciences that see the body and mind as a holistic entity united by the flow of life energy, or Qi. The three main branches of TCM are acupuncture, herbal medicine, and exercises such as T'ai Chi and QiGong, often used in combination.

vertical axis The postural alignment for T'ai Chi.

Wan Yang-Ming Philosopher who fused the physical motions of T'ai Chi Ch'uan with the philosophy of Taoism.

Wu style A formidable martial art form of T'ai Chi popular in many countries.

Yang Lu-Chan The great grand master of Kuang Ping Yang style, who created it after studying the Chen family style.

Yang style A form of T'ai Chi very popular in the United States and China.

Yellow Emperor's Classic of Chinese Medicine, The The bible of Chinese Medicine in 200 B.C.E. It stressed that "true medicine" is curing disease before it develops.

yin and yang The Chinese concepts of universal forces. All things are an eternally flowing interaction of two opposites; the ideal is healthful balance in all things. Yin is internal, dark, feminine, and receptive. Yang is external, light, masculine, and dynamic.

Zang Fu In Chinese, "solid-hollow." A system that indicates how Qi, or life energy, flows throughout and between organs. It is the model of how the entire body is interlinked by that flow, and shows how treating associated organs or energy meridians can improve others.

zazen The Zen art of meditation. Directly translated, it means "just sitting."

Zen An oriental art of being here and now, allowing the mind and heart to let go of past and future attachments so one can be fully immersed in the moment.

Index

K

kicks, 87
Kidney Channel, 28
kidneys, 31
kids. See children
Kirlian photography, 110-111
knee to chest exercise, 126
Kuang Ping Yang style, 66, 145-146
Kuang Ping Yang style movements, 149, 153
    Apparent Closing, 160
    Block Up/Fist Down, 180
    Brush Knee Twist Step, 158
    Chop Opponent with Fist, 185
    Cross Wave of Water Lily, 206
    Cross Wave of Water Lily Kick, 202
    Fair Lady Works at Shuttles, 191
    Fan Through the Arms, 170
    Fan Through the Arms (Backhand Slap), 198
    Fist Under Elbow, 163
    Golden Cock Stands on One Leg, 195
    Grand Terminus, 209
    Grasp the Bird's Tail, 154, 193, 207
    Green Dragon Rising from the Water, 170
    High Pat on Horse, 201
    High Pat on Horse/Guarding the Temples, 174
    Lower Block/Upper Block, Separation of Left Foot, 175
    Lower Block/Upper Block, Separation of Right Foot, 175, 184
    Parry and Punch, 182, 185
    Parry Up, Downward Strike, 202
    Partition of Wild Horse's Mane, 189
    Push Turn and Carry Tiger to Mountain, 160
    Raise Right Hand and Left, Turn and Repeat, 166
    Repulse the Monkey, 163, 197
    Retreat to Ride the Tiger, 204
    Single Whip, 155, 171, 174
    Single Whip Down, Return to the Earth, 194
    Sink to the Earth/Backward Elbow Strike, 188
    Slanting Body/Turn the Moon, 204
    Slow Palm Slant Flying, 165
    Spiraling Hands to Focus Mind Toward the Temple to Parry and Punch, 161
    Step Back/Lower Block/Upper Block, Kick Front, 182
    Step Push/Box Opponent's Ears/Cannon Through Sky, 198
    Step Up to Form Seven Stars, 203
    Stork Covers Its Wing/Sword in Sheath, 165
    Stretch Bow to Shoot Tiger, 206
    Strike Palm to Ask Blessings, 154
    Turn and Double kick, 180
    Turn and Kick with Sole, 177
    Wave Hand Over Light/Fly Pulling Back, 169
    Wave Hands Like Clouds, 172, 194, 200
    White Crane Cools Its Wings, 156
    Wing Blowing Lotus Leaves, 178
kung fu, 7
Kuo Lien-ying (Kuang Ping Yang style creator), 66

L

lactic acids, 18
Lao Tzu, 17
large classes, 73
Large Intestine Channel, 28
law enforcement, 272
learning movements, 84
lengthening muscles, 134-135
leukemia, 254
Level Sword, Turn Body, and Lift Knee movement, 230
Level Sword to Lift Leg Movement, 230

N-O

P

T

U

V

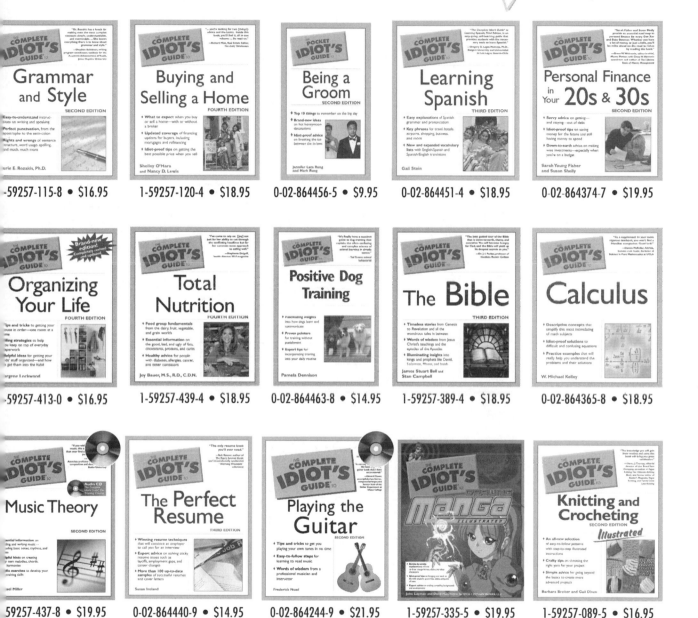

On the DVD

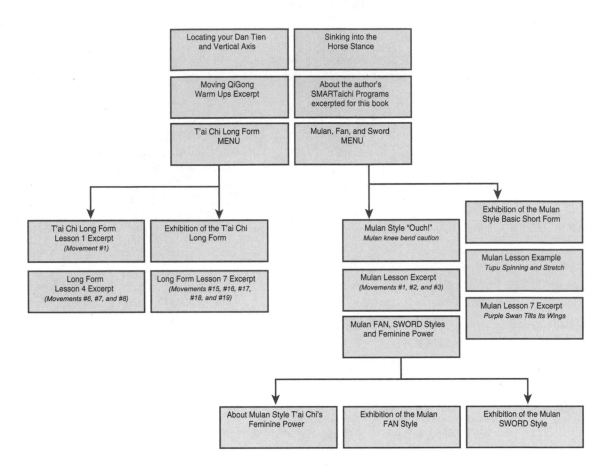

WARRANTY LIMITS

READ THIS ENCLOSED AGREEMENT BEFORE OPENING MEDIA PACKAGE.

BY OPENING THIS SEALED VIDEO PACKAGE, YOU ACCEPT AND AGREE TO THE TERMS AND CONDITIONS PRINTED BELOW. IF YOU DO NOT AGREE, **DO NOT OPEN THE PACKAGE.** SIMPLY RETURN THE SEALED PACKAGE.

This DVD is distributed on an "AS IS" basis, without warranty. Neither the authors, the publisher, and/or Penguin Group (USA) Inc./Alpha Books make any representation or warranty, either express or implied, with respect to the DVD, its quality, accuracy, or fitness for a specific purpose. Therefore, neither the author, the publisher, and/or Penguin Group (USA) Inc./Alpha Books shall have any liability to you or any other person or entity with respect to any liability, loss, or damage caused directly or indirectly by the content contained on the DVD or by the DVD itself. If the DVD is defective, you may return it for replacement.